T0264067

Diagnosis, Evaluation, and Treatment of Non-Muscle Invasive Bladder Cancer

Editor

SAM S. CHANG

UROLOGIC CLINICS OF NORTH AMERICA

www.urologic.theclinics.com

Consulting Editor
SAMIR S. TANEJA

MAY 2013 • Volume 40 • Number 2

ELSEVIER

1600 John F. Kennedy Boulevard • Suite 1800 • Philadelphia, Pennsylvania, 19103-2899

http://www.theclinics.com

UROLOGIC CLINICS OF NORTH AMERICA Volume 40, Number 2
May 2013 ISSN 0094-0143, ISBN-13: 978-1-4557-7345-9

Editor: Stephanie Donley

Urologic Clinics of North America (ISSN 0094-0143) is published quarterly by Elsevier Inc., 360 Park Avenue South, New York, NY 10010-1710. Months of issue are February, May, August, and November. Business and Editorial Offices: 1600 John F. Kennedy Blvd., Suite 1800, Philadelphia, PA 19103-2899. Periodicals postage paid at New York, NY and additional mailing offices. Subscription prices are $339.00 per year (US individuals), $583.00 per year (US institutions), $396.00 per year (Canadian individuals), $713.00 per year (Canadian institutions), $492.00 per year (foreign individuals), and $713.00 per year (foreign institutions). Foreign air speed delivery is included in all *Clinics* subscription prices. All prices are subject to change without notice. **POSTMASTER:** Send address changes to *Urologic Clinics of North America*, Elsevier Health Sciences Division, Subscription Customer Service, 3251 Riverport Lane, Maryland Heights, MO 63043. Customer Service: 1-800-654-2452 (US). From outside the United States, call 1-314-447-8871. Fax: 1-314-447-8029. E-mail: JournalsCustomerServiceusa@elsevier.com (for print support) and JournalsOnlineSupport-usa@elsevier.com (for online support).

Reprints. For copies of 100 or more, of articles in this publication, please contact the Commercial Reprints Department, Elsevier Inc., 360 Park Avenue South, New York, New York 10010-1710. Tel.: 212-633-3813; Fax: 212-462-1935; E-mail: reprints@elsevier.com.

Urologic Clinics of North America is covered in MEDLINE/PubMed (*Index Medicus*), *Excerpta Medica, Current Contents/Clinical Medicine, Science Citation Index,* and *ISI/BIOMED*.

Printed and bound by CPI Group (UK) Ltd, Croydon, CR0 4YY

Transferred to digital print 2012

Contributors

CONSULTING EDITOR

SAMIR S. TANEJA, MD
The James M. Neissa and Janet Riha Neissa Professor of Urologic Oncology, Professor of Urology and Radiology, Director, Division of Urologic Oncology, Co-Director, Smilow Comprehensive Prostate Cancer Center, Department of Urology, NYU Langone Medical Center, New York, New York

EDITOR

SAM S. CHANG, MD, FACS
Professor, Department of Urologic Surgery, Vanderbilt University Medical Center, Nashville, Tennessee

AUTHORS

JENNIFER J. AHN, MD
Postgraduate Residency Fellow, Department of Urology, Columbia University Medical Center, New York, New York

PETER E. CLARK, MD
Department of Urologic Surgery, Vanderbilt University Medical Center, Nashville, Tennessee

JOSHUA A. COHN, MD
Resident, Section of Urology, The University of Chicago Medical Center, Chicago, Illinois

SIAMAK DANESHMAND, MD
Associate Professor of Urology (Clinical Scholar), Director of Urologic Oncology, USC Institute of Urology, Norris Comprehensive Cancer Center, Los Angeles, California

JOSEPH A. GILLESPIE, MD
Resident (PGY3), Department of Urology, University of Iowa, Iowa City, Iowa

JOHN L. GORE, MD, MS
Assistant Professor, Department of Urology, University of Washington; Adjunct Assistant Professor, Department of Surgery, Affiliate Investigator, Fred Hutchinson Cancer Research Center, University of Washington, Seattle, Washington

JOSHUA G. GRIFFIN, MD
Assistant Professor, Department of Urology, University of Kansas Medical Center, Kansas City, Kansas

DONNA E. HANSEL, MD, PhD
Pathology and Laboratory Medicine Institute; Glickman Urological and Kidney Institute; Taussig Cancer Institute; Genomic Medicine Institute, The Cleveland Clinic, Cleveland, Ohio

JEFF HOLZBEIERLEIN, MD
Associate Professor, Department of Urology, University of Kansas Medical Center, Kansas City, Kansas

JOHANN P. INGIMARSSON, MD
Urology Resident, Section of Urology, Department of Surgery, Dartmouth Hitchcock Medical Center, Norris Cotton Cancer Center, Geisel School of Medicine, Lebanon, New Hampshire

ANDREW C. JAMES, MD
Clinical Instructor, Department of Urology, University of Washington, Seattle, Washington

DAVID C. JOHNSON, MD
Resident in Urology, Department of Urology, University of North Carolina, Chapel Hill, North Carolina

J. STEPHEN JONES, MD
Glickman Urological and Kidney Institute, The Cleveland Clinic, Cleveland, Ohio

ASHISH M. KAMAT, MD
Associate Professor and Fellowship Director, Department of Urology, MD Anderson Cancer Center, Houston, Texas

BADRINATH R. KONETY, MD, MBA
Department of Urology, University of Minnesota, Minneapolis, Minnesota

RIANNE J.M. LAMMERS, MD
PhD-candidate, Department of Urology, Radboud University Medical Centre, Nijmegen, The Netherlands

MICHAEL C. LARGE, MD
Fellow, Section of Urology, The University of Chicago Medical Center, Chicago, Illinois

CHERYL T. LEE, MD
Associate Professor, Department of Urology, University of Michigan, Ann Arbor, Michigan

WILLIAM T. LOWRANCE, MD, MPH
Division of Urology, Huntsman Cancer Institute, University of Utah, Salt Lake City, Utah

JAMES M. MCKIERNAN, MD
George F. Cahill Professor of Urology, Department of Urology, Columbia University Medical Center, New York, New York

TODD M. MORGAN, MD
Assistant Professor, Department of Urology, University of Michigan, Ann Arbor, Michigan

MICHAEL A. O'DONNELL, MD
Professor and Director of Urologic Oncology, Department of Urology, University of Iowa, Iowa City, Iowa

BROCK B. O'NEIL, MD
Division of Urology, University of Utah, Salt Lake City, Utah

RAJ S. PRUTHI, MD, FACS
Professor and Chair, Department of Urology, University of North Carolina, Chapel Hill, North Carolina

CHAD R. RITCH, MD
Department of Urologic Surgery, Vanderbilt University Medical Center, Nashville, Tennessee

JOSEPH SANFRANCESCO, MD
Pathology and Laboratory Medicine Institute, The Cleveland Clinic, Cleveland, Ohio

JOHN D. SEIGNE, MB, FACS
Associate Professor of Surgery, Section of Urology, Department of Surgery, Dartmouth Hitchcock Medical Center, Norris Cotton Cancer Center, Geisel School of Medicine, Lebanon, New Hampshire

JAY B. SHAH, MD
Assistant Professor, Department of Urology, MD Anderson Cancer Center, Houston, Texas

GARY D. STEINBERG, MD, FACS
The Bruce and Beth White Family Professor of Surgery, Vice Chairman and Director of Urologic Oncology, Section of Urology, The University of Chicago Medical Center, Chicago, Illinois

RICHARD J. SYLVESTER, ScD
Professor, Department of Biostatistics, EORTC Headquarters, Brussels, Belgium

JEFFREY M. TOMASINI, MD
Department of Urology, University of Minnesota, Minneapolis, Minnesota

J. ALFRED WITJES, MD, PhD
Professor, Department of Urology, Radboud University Medical Centre, Nijmegen, The Netherlands

MICHAEL E. WOODS, MD, FACS
Associate Professor, Department of Urology, University of North Carolina, Chapel Hill, North Carolina

Contents

PROGRAM OBJECTIVE:

The goal of *Urologic Clinics of North America* is to keep practicing urologists and urology residents up to date with current clinical practice in urology by providing timely articles reviewing the state of the art in patient care.

TARGET AUDIENCE

Practicing urologists, urology residents and other health care professionals practicing in the discipline of urology.

LEARNING OBJECTIVES

Upon completion of this activity, participants will be able to:

- Describe when to use perioperative chemotherapy.
- Recognize the role of cystectomy for high grade T1 urothelial carcinoma.
- Review side effects of perioperative intravesical treatment.

ACCREDITATION

The Elsevier Office of Continuing Medical Education (EOCME) is accredited by the Accreditation Council for Continuing Medical Education (ACCME) to provide continuing medical education for physicians.

The EOCME designates this journal-based CME activity for a maximum of 14*AMA PRA Category 1 Credit*(s)™. Physicians should claim only the credit commensurate with the extent of their participation in the activity.

All other health care professionals completing continuing education credit for this activity will be issued a certificate of participation.

DISCLOSURE OF CONFLICTS OF INTEREST

The EOCME assesses conflict of interest with its instructors, faculty, planners, and other individuals who are in a position to control the content of CME activities. All relevant conflicts of interest that are identified are thoroughly vetted by EOCME for fair balance, scientific objectivity, and patient care recommendations. EOCME is committed to providing its learners with CME activities that promote improvements or quality in healthcare and not a specific proprietary business or a commercial interest.

The planning committee, staff, authors and editors listed below have identified no financial relationships or relationships to products or devices they or their spouse/life partner have with commercial interest related to the content of this CME activity:

Jennifer J. Ahn, MD; Sam S. Chang, MD; Peter E. Clark, MD; Joshua A. Cohn, MD; Stephanie Donley; Joseph A. Gillespie, MD; John L. Gore, MD, MS; Joshua G. Griffin, MD; Donna E. Hansel, MD, PhD; Johann P. Ingimarsson, MD; Andrew C. James, MD; David C. Johnson, MD; Indu Kumari; Rianne J.M. Lammers, MD; Michael C. Large, MD; Sandy Lavery; Cheryl T. Lee, MD; William T. Lowrance, MD, MPH; Jill McNair; Brock B. O'Neil, MD; Raj S. Pruthi, MD; Chad R. Ritch, MD; Joseph Sanfrancesco, MD; Jay B. Shah, MD; Richard J. Sylvester, MD; Jeffrey M. Tomasini, MD; Yvette Williams; and J. Alfred Witjes, MD, PhD.

The planning committee, staff, authors and editors listed below have identified financial relationships or relationships to products or devices they or their spouse/life partner have with commercial interest related to the content of this CME activity:

- Siamak Daneshmand, MD is a consultant/advisor for ENDO and is on speakers bureau for ENDO and Cubist.
- Jeffrey Holzbeierlein, MD is on speakers bureau for Janssen and Amgen.
- J. Stephen Jones, MD is a consultant/advisor for Photocure.
- Ashish M. Kamat, MD has a research grant from Alere, Inc. and is a consultant/advisor for Archimedes, Photocure, Endo Pharmaceuticals, sanofi-aventis, Taris, and Cubist & Allergan.
- Badrinath R. Konety, MD, MBA is a consultant/advisor for Amgen, Inc., Spectrum Pharmaceuticals, Allergan, Inc. and Dendreon, Inc.; is on speakers bureau for Amgen, Inc., and has royalties/patents with McGraw Hill, Inc.
- James M. McKiernan, MD has research grants from Celgene and the Prostrate Cancer Foundation.
- Todd M. Morgan is a consultant/advisor for Endo Health.
- Michael A. O'Donnell is a consultant/advisor for Viventia, Spectrum, Allergan, Endo Pharmaceuticals, Merck and Medical Enterprises.
- John D. Seigne, MD has stock ownership in Johnson & Johnson and Novartis.
- Gary D. Steinberg, MD is a consultant/advisor for Photocure, Abbott Molecular, Endo Pharmaceuticals, Tengion, Predictive Biosciences and Taris Biomedical; is on speakers bureau for Photocure, Abbott Molecular and Endo Pharmaceuticals; and has a research grant from Abbott Molecular.
- Samir S. Taneja, MD is on Speakers Bureau for Janssen, and is a consultant/advisor for Elgen, GTX, Bayer and Healthtronics
- Michael E. Woods, MD is a consultant/advisor for Beacon LBS.

UNAPPROVED/OFF-LABEL USE DISCLOSURE

The EOCME requires CME faculty to disclose to the participants:

1. When products or procedures being discussed are off-label, unlabelled, experimental, and/or investigational (not US Food and Drug Administration (FDA) approved); and
2. Any limitations on the information presented, such as data that are preliminary or that represent ongoing research, interim analyses, and/or unsupported opinions. Faculty may discuss information about pharmaceutical agents that is outside of FDA-approved labelling. This information is intended solely for CME and is not intended to promote off-label use of these medications. If you have any questions, contact the medical affairs department of the manufacturer for the most recent prescribing information.

TO ENROLL

To enroll in the *Urologic Clinics of North America* Continuing Medical Education program, call customer service at 1-800-654-2452 or sign up online at http://www.theclinics.com/home/cme. The CME program is available to subscribers for an additional annual fee of $243 USD.

METHOD OF PARTICIPATION

In order to claim credit, participants must complete the following:

1. Complete enrolment as indicated above.
2. Read the activity.
3. Complete the CME Test and Evaluation. Participants must achieve a score of 70% on the test. All CME Tests and Evaluations must be completed online.

CME INQUIRIES/SPECIAL NEEDS

For all CME inquiries or special needs, please contact elsevierCME@elsevier.com.

UROLOGIC CLINICS OF NORTH AMERICA

FORTHCOMING ISSUES

August 2013
Urologic Trauma and Reconstruction
Alan F. Morey, MD, and Steven J. Hudak, MD, *Editors*

November 2013
Office Based Procedures
J. Stephen Jones, MD, *Editor*

February 2014
Early Stage Prostate Cancer: Screening and Detection
Stacy Loeb, MD, and Matthew Cooperberg, MD, *Editors*

RECENT ISSUES

February 2013
The Multidisciplinary Management of Urinary Stone Disease
Ojas Shah, MD, *Editor*

November 2012
Castrate-Resistant Prostate Cancer
Adam S. Kibel, MD, *Editor*

August 2012
Controversies in Female Pelvic Reconstruction
Roger Dmochowski, MD, and Mickey Karram, MD, *Editors*

Foreword

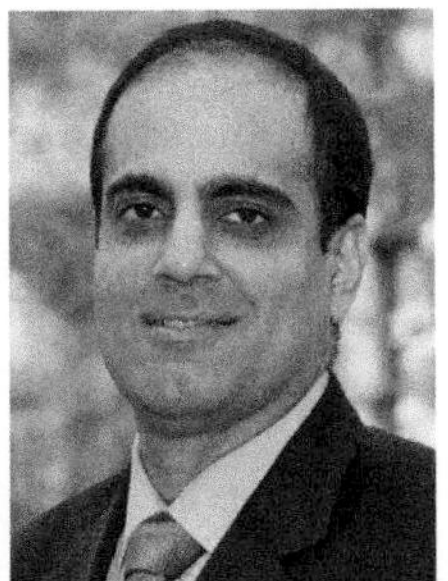

Samir S. Taneja, MD
Consulting Editor

Non-muscle invasive bladder cancer (NMIBC) represents, in effect, a constellation of diseases. Among cancers labeled as "non-muscle invasive" are those with virtually benign behavior and those with a highly lethal phenotype. As such, the management has evolved greatly in the past 30 years, and the current "state of the art" reflects one of the most well-developed risk-stratification schemes in urologic cancers. Identification of high-risk disease leads to a completely different treatment paradigm than that carried out in the remaining patients.

The prevalence of the NMIBC, along with the high rate of recurrence, makes it a disease with tremendous financial implications in the upcoming era of health care reform. Proper, evidence-based management has the potential to not only improve patient outcome but also reduce overall costs associated with the care of these patients. This will secondarily influence the allocation of dollars to urologic disease overall.

Although there are now a number of national and international guidelines published regarding the management of NMIBC, the entire story of how to manage these patients is far from written. Ongoing controversies in risk stratification, timing of therapy, and sequence of therapy continue to fuel controversy. I am deeply indebted to Dr Sam Chang for his willingness to serve as guest editor for this issue of the *Urologic Clinics* and to put much of the ongoing controversy into a cohesive framework. He has solicited articles from the brightest and best in formulating this fantastic issue. In keeping with our ongoing effort to provide a multidisciplinary perspective on urologic disease, the articles in this issue cover a range of topics including both the management of NMIBC and the impact of the disease itself on Urology. I am confident that this issue will both educate you regarding the management of your patients and challenge you to explore the ongoing controversies.

Samir S. Taneja, MD
Division of Urologic Oncology
Smilow Comprehensive Prostate Cancer Center
Department of Urology
NYU Langone Medical Center
150 East 32nd Street, Suite 200
New York, NY 10016, USA

E-mail address:
samir.taneja@nyumc.org

Urol Clin N Am 40 (2013) xi
http://dx.doi.org/10.1016/j.ucl.2013.01.016
0094-0143/13/$ – see front matter

Preface
Non-Muscle Invasive Bladder Cancer

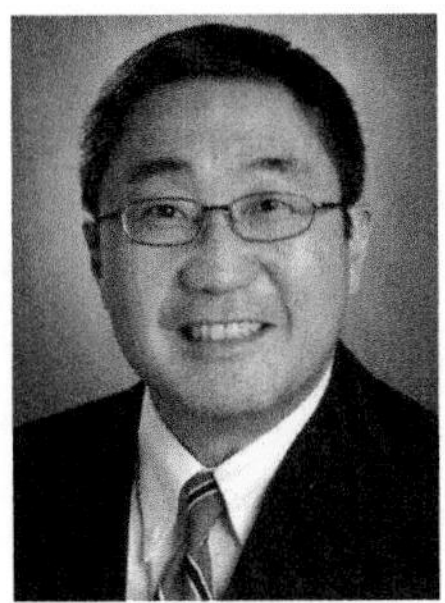

Sam S. Chang, MD, FACS
Editor

As the second most frequent genitourinary malignancy, non-muscle invasive bladder represents a significant, heterogeneous disease that urologists commonly diagnose, evaluate, and treat. The range of this disease process from an innocuous single, small papillary tumor to multiple T1 bladder tumors is impressive. Overtreatment and undertreatment are considerations for each of us as we attempt to individualize and optimize our care. Ever present as well are patient quality-of-life concerns and the economic health cost burden.

Over the past decade new discoveries have improved diagnosis and management of this disease, but despite these, we still follow certain practice patterns based only on historical precedent. There is much we need to learn and much we need to research. Herein, leaders in this field contribute articles focusing on specific areas of controversy and need. The reader will find up-to-date information on cancer diagnosis, evaluation, and treatment that includes practical solutions to difficult clinical situations.

I hope you learn as much as I have from this volume.

Sam S. Chang, MD, FACS
Professor, Department of Urologic Surgery
Vanderbilt University Medical Center
MCN A1302
Nashville, TN 37232, USA

E-mail address:
sam.chang@vanderbilt.edu

Urol Clin N Am 40 (2013) xiii
http://dx.doi.org/10.1016/j.ucl.2013.01.011

NMIBC Risk Calculators

How Useful Are They for the Practicing Urologist and How Can Their Clinical Utility Be Improved?

Rianne J.M. Lammers, MD[a], Richard J. Sylvester, ScD[b], Cheryl T. Lee, MD[c], J. Alfred Witjes, MD, PhD[a,*]

KEYWORDS

• Non-muscle invasive bladder cancer • EORTC • Risk table • Prognostic model

KEY POINTS

- The natural history of non-muscle invasive bladder cancer in individual patients can be unpredictable.
- Although there are known clinical and molecular factors associated with tumor recurrence and progression, it is challenging to reconcile these data during a typical patient encounter within a busy clinic.
- Prognostic models, such as risk tables and nomograms, aim to facilitate risk stratification, patient counseling, and treatment decision making.
- There are many prognostic models available for non-muscle invasive bladder cancer, but they are not commonly used in daily practice because of their complexity and limited usefulness in treatment decision making.
- To make prognostic models more useful, the focus should be on the clinical implications of the model for the patient, such as by focusing on negative and positive predictive value, rather than *P* values, sensitivity, and specificity. The net benefit of the model should be compared with the standard model by means of classification tables and decision analytic techniques to test its additional clinical value.
- Biomarkers do not have sufficient additional value, and markers undergoing investigation should first stand the test of time.
- Ultimately, even good models will not be translated into clinical practice unless they can be integrated into the standard clinical workflow.

BACKGROUND

Overall, bladder cancer (BC) is the seventh most common malignancy in men and the 17th in women.[1] The incidence increases with age and is highest at 50 to 70 years of age. Eighty percent of patients with BC are men.[2] Important risk factors are chemical and environmental exposures, such as smoking and aromatic amines, and chronic irritation.[3,4] In the Western world,

Funding Sources: None for all authors.
Conflict of Interest: None for all authors.

[a] Department of Urology, Radboud University Medical Centre, Geert Grooteplein Zuid 10 (659), P.O. Box 9101, Nijmegen 6500 HB, The Netherlands; [b] Department of Biostatistics, EORTC Headquarters, 83 Avenue E. Mounier, Brussels 1200, Belgium; [c] Department of Urology, University of Michigan, 7303 CCGC, 1500 East Medical Center Drive, Ann Arbor, MI 48109-0946, USA
* Corresponding author.
E-mail address: f.witjes@uro.umcn.nl

Urol Clin N Am 40 (2013) 155–164
http://dx.doi.org/10.1016/j.ucl.2013.01.002
0094-0143/13/$ – see front matter

more than 90% of BC are urothelial carcinomas or transitional cell carcinoma.[5]

On average, 70% of patients with BC present with non-muscle invasive BC (NMIBC) and the remainder with muscle-invasive disease (MIBC). In the non-muscle invasive group, approximately 70% present as Ta lesions (noninvasive papillary carcinoma), 20% as T1 lesions (invasion into subepithelial connective tissue), and 10% as carcinoma in situ (CIS or Tis lesions; high-grade noninvasive flat tumor).[6] For grading, both the World Health Organization's (WHO) 1973 and the WHO's 2004 classifications are advised. The WHO's 1973 grading system recognizes 3 groups: grade 1 to 3. The WHO's 2004 classification defines 4 groups of papillary lesions: urothelial papilloma (benign), papillary urothelial neoplasm of low malignant potential, low-grade papillary urothelial carcinoma, and high-grade papillary urothelial carcinoma.[7] For staging, the TNM classification is used.[8]

Another way to stratify patients is by prognostic factors and, thus, outcome. The European Organization for Research and Treatment of Cancer (EORTC) developed a prognostic model for recurrence and progression for patients with NMIBC,[9] which the authors discuss in this article. Other prognostic models with applications in urological practice have been created recently using other techniques: nomograms, neuro-fuzzy models, and artificial neural networks (ANN).

The most well-known prognostic model is the risk table, which divides patients into risk groups based on their score. It gives the probability of an event (recurrence, progression) for patients within a given risk group. It assumes that all patients within a given risk group have a similar prognosis; however, the choice of cutoff values when stratifying patients into groups is somewhat artificial. It is unlikely that all patients within a given group will have the same prognosis, and patients with similar scores who fall into different risk groups might not have different prognoses. Furthermore, when one variable is missing, it is not possible to calculate the probabilities. Nevertheless, risk tables can easily identify the very low- and very high-risk patients.

A nomogram is a graphical device that is used to calculate an individual patient's probability of an event based on a multivariable model with their specific prognostic factors and, hence, gives a more individualized risk calculation. Nomograms are based on a (continuous) score, whereas risk tables subdivide patients into different categories based on their score. They provide a more individualized probability of the event of interest, and software is usually developed to make them easy to use. Because the nomogram probabilities come directly from the multivariable model, it is important that the model is well calibrated, that is, it has an excellent goodness of fit. Otherwise, the probabilities provided by the model will be incorrect. However, when one of the variables is missing for a patient, the nomogram cannot be used for that patient. As mentioned by Hernandez and colleagues,[10] nomograms are usually developed with very large series, and it has to be determined if they are applicable to lower-volume centers.

More advanced prognostic models are neuro-fuzzy models and ANN. The latter is a mathematical model based on a biologic neural network. It can handle complex relationships between input and output and can find patterns in the data. ANN are adaptive systems that can change their structure during the learning phase. A neuro-fuzzy model is a combination of an ANN and fuzzy logistics, which is a form of logistics that can handle reasoning. Because there is little experience in NMIBC with these models, they are not discussed further.

In the next paragraphs, the advantages and disadvantages of the most well-known prognostic model, the EORTC risk tables, are discussed. Then, several other NMIBC prognostic models are described; the authors discuss the lack of use of prognostic models in the daily urological practice. Finally, the authors provide a future perspective on prognostic models: how should we develop and use prognostic models for patients with NMIBC?

EORTC RISK TABLES

Development of the EORTC Risk Tables

In 2006, Sylvester and colleagues[9] published the EORTC scoring system for NMIBC. They combined individual patient data of 2596 patients from 7 EORTC trials (inclusion period: January 1979–September 1989). The aim was to provide simple tables that would allow urologists to easily calculate the probability of recurrence and progression after transurethral resection of the bladder tumor (TURBT) for patients with NMIBC. The most appropriate adjuvant treatment after TURBT and the frequency of follow-up can then be determined in an individual patient based on their prognosis. Data on patient and tumor characteristics and the endpoints of time to first recurrence and time to progression to MIBC were merged. The most important variables were then determined by regression models. Patients were divided into 4 risk groups for both recurrence and progression according to their total score. Probabilities of recurrence and progression at 1 year and 5 years were calculated. Also, software was provided to calculate these probabilities at 1, 2, 3, 4, and 5 years. The model accuracy using Harrell's bias corrected concordance index (c index) was calculated. The c index is the probability that for 2 patients chosen at random, the patient who had the actual event first had a higher probability of having the event according to the model; an uninformative model will have a c index of 0.5 or 50% (flipping a coin), and a perfect model will have a c index of 1 or 100%. Area under the curve (AUC) can also provide this information but only for binary outcomes (recurrence yes/no). To adjust for bias (overfitting, overoptimism), models were refit 200 times using the bootstrap technique (internal validation). Bootstrapping is a resampling method in which analyses are repeated many times but with different random samples of subjects each: in each analysis some subjects might not be included, others are included once, twice, and so forth. The 2596 eligible patients had mainly favorable characteristics. A total of 22% received no adjuvant intravesical treatment before recurrence; 78% of the patients received intravesical therapy, mostly chemotherapy. The median follow-up was 3.9 years. In total, 47.8% of patients experienced a recurrence with a median time to recurrence of 2.7 years. The most important factors that influenced the time to first recurrence were prior recurrence rate, number of tumors, and tumor size. Only 10.7% of patients experienced progression to muscle-invasive disease. The median time to progression was not observed, with progression rates at 5 years varying from 0.8% to 45%. The most important factors influencing time to progression were T category, CIS, and grade. Scores were calculated for each patient, varying from 0 to 17 for recurrence and 0 to 23 for progression. **Table 1** gives an overview of the probabilities of recurrence and progression. Furthermore, Sylvester and colleagues[9] found that concomitant CIS is the most important prognostic factor in patients with pT1G3-tumors, and that recurrence at first follow-up cystoscopy at three months is associated with a higher chance of progression.

As mentioned in an editorial comment by Karakiewicz, the internal validation yielded a c index of 0.66 for recurrence at both 1 and 5 years, which means that 66% of recurrences were accurately predicted at 1 and 5 years. The c index for progression was 0.74 at 1 year and 0.75 at 5 years.[9]

In 2013, the EORTC will start updating these risk tables for patients treated with maintenance bacillus Calmette-Guerin (BCG).

The NMIBC guidelines panel of the European Association of Urology (EAU) classified patients into subgroups of low, intermediate, and high risk based on these tables (**Table 1**, last column) and provided treatment and follow-up recommendations depending on a patient's risk group.[11]The American Urological Association (AUA) also specified therapy based on clinical risk. However, the panel of the AUA defined only 2 risk groups: low-risk patients (pTa, low grade) and high-risk patients (pT1, high grade, and/or CIS).[12]

Table 1
Probability of recurrence and progression according to total score[9] and classification system by the NMIBC guidelines panel of the European Association of Urology[11]

	Probability of Recurrence at 1 y		Probability of Recurrence at 5 y		
Recurrence Score	**(%)**	**(95% CI)**	**(%)**	**(95% CI)**	**Recurrence Risk Group**
0	15	(10–19)	31	(24–37)	Low risk
1–4	24	(21–26)	46	(42–49)	Intermediate risk
5–9	38	(35–41)	62	(58–65)	Intermediate risk
10–17	61	(55–67)	78	(73–84)	High risk
	Probability of Progression at 1 y		**Probability of Progression at 5 y**		
Progression Score	**(%)**	**(95% CI)**	**(%)**	**(95% CI)**	**Progression Risk Group**
0	0.2	(0–0.7)	0.8	(0–1.7)	Low risk
2–6	1	(0.4–1.6)	6	(5–8)	Intermediate risk
7–13	5	(4–7)	17	(14–20)	High risk
14–23	17	(10–24)	45	(35–55)	High risk

Abbreviation: CI, confidence interval.

Disadvantages

As mentioned earlier, patient and tumor characteristics influence the probability of recurrence and progression. However, it should be taken into account that 22% of patients received no intravesical treatment at all, and the treatment that was given consisted mostly of intravesical chemotherapy. Only 171 of the patients (7%) received BCG and none received BCG maintenance. Also, less than 10% of patients received a single immediate postoperative instillation with chemotherapy, and a re-TURBT was not performed in high-risk patients. As mentioned in the discussion by Sylvester and colleagues,[9] data for other factors that might be of prognostic importance were not available: depth of lamina propria invasion, location of the tumor on the bladder wall, lymphovascular invasion, and micropapillary tumors. Also, recent developments, such as molecular markers, fluorescence cystoscopy and re-TURBT, that are likely to further reduce the risks of recurrence and progression were not taken into account.[13] Unfortunately, long-term follow-up is not available in most large series of patients where these new treatment developments and more recently identified prognostic factors have been assessed.

Many of the patients included in the EORTC series, particularly those in the high-risk category, would be undertreated according to today's standards. As such, the recurrence rates and especially the progression rates are likely to be somewhat higher than those found in contemporary practice. Thus, the progression rates and to a lesser extent the recurrence rates published in the EORTC series should be similar to the untreated natural history of the disease, enabling one to determine the most important prognostic factors without having to take into account treatment as a confounding factor. One can, however, ask what the real value of these risk tables is in the treatment decision process because the positive predictive value (PPV) of the EORTC risk table for progression in high-risk patients is low, only 21%. This subject is discussed in more detail later in this article.

External Validation

Several groups have independently validated the EORTC risk tables.[10,14–18] Fernandez-Gomez and colleagues[18] performed an external validation in 1062 patients with NMIBC treated with maintenance BCG. For recurrence, Fernandez-Gomez and colleagues found a lower risk in each group of patients than Sylvester and colleagues,[9] but the c index was comparable. For progression, lower risks were found in the cohort from Fernandez-Gomez and colleagues,[18] especially in the highest-risk group at 5 years. The limitations as discussed by the investigators are the lack of re-TURBT and a short maintenance regimen. The investigators also mention the difference in the distribution of patients: there are more patients with aggressive tumor characteristics in this cohort than in the EORTC cohort. As mentioned in an editorial comment by Sylvester,[13] application of the EORTC scoring system in the BCG series to predict progression yields a sensitivity of 88% and a negative predictive value (NPV) of 95%, but the PPV is only 17%. PPV is the proportion of positive test results that are true positive; thus, it reflects the probability that a positive test reflects the underlying condition being tested for. NPV is the proportion of subjects with a negative test result who are correctly diagnosed and, thus, without the investigated disease. Overall, this is a well-performed external validation, which shows that although the EORTC risk tables provided an adequate discrimination between patients with a different prognosis, their calibration was poor in patients treated with BCG.

Van Rhijn and colleagues[16] validated the EORTC risk scores in 230 Dutch patients with primary NMIBC. Additionally, they proposed an alternative to pathologic grade with molecular grade (mG) based on fibroblast growth factor receptor 3 (FGFR3) gene mutation and MIB-1 expression. The median follow-up was 8.6 years. In general, 5-year recurrence-free survival (RFS) and progression-free survival (PFS) rates were lower in the cohort of Van Rhijn and colleagues than in the EORTC-cohort. According to the authors, the differences in PFS may be explained by the lower number of patients, by the selection of only primary patients, by the longer median follow-up, or because 32% of patients died of other causes. Furthermore, they found that mG was related to progression and disease-specific survival, and adding mG increased the predictive accuracy for progression from 74.9% to 81.7%. These data suggest a potential advantage to incorporating molecular markers into the EORTC risk score.

Sakano and colleagues[14] validated the EORTC risk group stratification in 529 Japanese patients with NMIBC. The investigators concluded that the risk stratification as mentioned in the EAU's guidelines is probably not applicable for Japanese patients but the subgroup classification on intermediate risk could be. Seo and colleagues[15] compared recurrence and progression rates between the EORTC risk tables and their own cohort of 251 Korean patients. All recurrence rates of the Korean patients were lower than in the

EORTC cohort, except for the 1-year recurrence rate in the intermediate-risk group, which was comparable with that of the EORTC cohort. In general, rates for progression in the Korean cohort were quite comparable with the rates in the EORTC risk tables despite the more aggressive patient and tumor characteristics of the Korean cohort. Hernandez and colleagues[10] performed an external validation in 417 patients with primary NMIBC. In general, probabilities for both recurrence and progression in this cohort were higher than in the EORTC cohort. Their results validate the EORTC risk tables in terms of recurrence but not in terms of progression because of the low number of patients that progressed. Pillai and colleagues[17] validated the EORTC risk model in 109 patients with primary and recurrent NMIBC. They found significantly higher 1- and 5-year probabilities of recurrence for all 4 groups compared with the EORTC model. However, it was not possible to draw firm conclusions about the validity because of the low number of patients in the individual groups.

In all, it is likely that the recurrence and especially progression rates reported by the EORTC risk tables are higher than those found in current clinical practice. As mentioned earlier, the progression probabilities and to a lesser extent the recurrence probabilities mentioned in the EORTC study are likely to be similar to the untreated natural history of the disease.

OTHER BC PROGNOSTIC MODELS

There are many prognostic models for NMIBC[19–26] as well as for muscle-invasive disease.[27–33] In this section, the authors discuss some of the other prognostic models for NMIBC. The prognostic models on MIBC are not discussed.

Club Urologico Español de Tratamiento Oncologico Scoring Model

The scoring model from the Spanish Urological Club for Oncological Treatment (Club Urologico Español de Tratamiento Oncologico [CUETO]) is the most commonly known prognostic model for NMIBC besides the EORTC risk tables. Fernandez-Gomez and colleagues[26] used the data of 1062 patients treated with BCG in 4 studies between 1990 and 1999. All patients received BCG maintenance treatment regimens (12 instillations within 5–6 months after TURBT) and had identical follow-up schedules, but the BCG dose did differ (13.5–81.0 mg). Only 4.2% received less than 6 BCG instillations, and less than 30% of patients discontinued therapy. The median follow-up was 69 months. In total, 346 patients (32.6%) had recurrences, and 142 patients (13.4%) had progression to muscle-invasive disease. Prognostic factors for time to recurrence were gender, age, tumor status, number of tumors, associated CIS, and grade. For time to progression, age, tumor status, T category, and grade were of significant influence. A scoring system from 0 to 16 was developed for recurrence and from 0 to 14 for progression. Then recurrence and progression probabilities at 1, 2, and 5 years were calculated. Finally, these probabilities were compared with the EORTC recurrence probabilities. All recurrence probabilities were lower in the CUETO model than in the EORTC model. The progression probabilities were lower for high-risk patients; but in most intermediate-risk patients, the 2 scoring systems gave similar progression probabilities. As mentioned in the discussion by Fernandez-Gomez and colleagues,[13] limitations of this study are the retrospective analyses and the use of the old TNM classification. Furthermore, no re-TURBT or immediate postoperative instillations were done, and the parameters of possible influence that were missing in the EORTC risk tables, such as tumor location, are also missing in the CUETO scoring model. Also, an internal validation to test accuracy is lacking and, as mentioned in the editorial comment, the lower significance of CIS is likely to be caused by the small number of patients with CIS. The sensitivity of this scoring model is 60%, the NPV is 92%, but the PPV is only 24%.

Rosevaer and colleagues[34] conducted an external validation of the CUETO model in 718 patients treated with BCG plus interferon-alpha. The 3-year RFS was much lower in this study than in the CUETO study. However, comparing RFS between the 4 groups categorized according to the CUETO score showed a significant difference between the groups ($P<.001$). Therefore, the discrimination when using this scoring model is good. Nevertheless, currently accepted practices, such as immediate postoperative instillations, re-TURBT, and long-term maintenance BCG instillations, were not taken into account for both this group and the CUETO model, which is of influence on the clinical outcome of these patients.

Other Prognostic Models for NMIBC

Besides the most well-known EORTC risk tables and the CUETO scoring model, several other models have been developed[19–24]; but because these models are not commonly used in daily practice, they are beyond the scope of this review. However, in general, the most frequently cited prognostic factors for the time to first recurrence are the number of tumors, whether the tumor is primary or recurrent, and if recurrent, the prior recurrence rate and the tumor size. For the time to progression to MIBC, the most important prognostic factors are grade, stage, and the presence of CIS. The most frequently cited prognostic factors for the course of the disease in patients with CIS are age, response to BCG, type of CIS (primary, secondary, concurrent), extent of CIS (unifocal, multifocal, or diffuse), the presence of irritative bladder symptoms, hematuria, and extravesical extension.[35]

USE OF PROGNOSTIC MODELS IN UROLOGICAL PRACTICES

In general, a good prognostic model discriminates between disease and illness, gives an accurate prognosis, has a good calibration, is generalizable, and is easy to use. Good sensitivity and specificity are required for proper discrimination. But, depending on how the model will be used, the NPV and PPV might be more important than sensitivity and specificity. The accuracy of a model can be assessed by internal validation (apparent validation, split-sample validation, cross-validation, or bootstrapping) or, even better, by external validation with a new cohort. The latter also tests the generalizability of the model. A model with a good calibration has a good agreement between the observed/true outcome and the predicted outcome.[36] Unfortunately, none of the existing prognostic models for NMIBC have all of these requirements. Common problems are overfitting of the model because validation is done on the data used to derive it from, leading to a poor generalizability, a low c index, or a poor calibration when applied to external datasets, resulting in either overtreatment or undertreatment of patients, which is not in concordance with the current treatment guidelines. And if the c index or calibration is high, the next question is whether it is high enough to justify the use of the model in clinical practice.

For use in daily practice, other variables, such as patient comorbidity and risk of major surgery, are also important in making a final decision on which treatment best suits a given patient. Another current problem is the lack of validation. Prognostic models that have not had an external validation are less reliable and clinicians may be less eager to incorporate them into their clinic workflow. Practice patterns are also very difficult to change. The very practical nature of a busy clinic may undermine the provider's use of any prognostic models unless it is readily incorporated into an electronic health record that will automate the calculation of risk category or disease outcome. It is likely that urologic trainees exposed to these models during their residency and fellowship will use them, or subsequent versions, later in practice. All these factors are responsible for the fact that few urologists currently use prognostic models in their daily practice.

Some risk models, such as the EORTC risk tables, are incorporated into guidelines. But guidelines are not commonly followed, as shown by Chamie and colleagues.[37] They investigated practice patterns concerning treatment in 4545 American patients with high-grade NMIBC. The American guideline, the European guideline, and the National Comprehensive Cancer Network's (NCCN) guideline were all investigated for their use in daily practice. An extremely low number of patients received all the diagnostic and therapeutic steps in concordance with the guidelines, namely, only one patient. However, 25.8% of patients did receive 6 or more instillations with BCG. Upper tract imaging and a single postoperative instillation with intravesical chemotherapy were especially lacking.

Despite the disadvantages of the prognostic models, clinical reasoning is not flawless; omission bias (bias against action) and outcome bias (it is easier to evaluate outcome than it is to evaluate a decision process) can influence treatment decisions,[38] and medical doctors tend to recommend the treatment they deliver themselves.[39] Several studies have shown that predicting clinical outcome by medical doctors is less accurate than when using prognostic models.[40,41]

The International Bladder Cancer Group (IBCG) recognized these flaws and provided uniform terminology and recommendations for the risk classification and management of patients with NMIBC.[42] Based on the 4 existing guideline recommendations (EAU, AUA, NCCN, and First International Consultation on Bladder Tumors guidelines), they developed a simple algorithm for the treatment and management of patients with primary NMIBC based on 3 easily definable risk groups: low risk was defined as a solitary, primary low-grade pTa tumor, whereas high risk was any pT1 and/or high-grade tumor and/or CIS. This model is a fine example of a useful model for day-to-day urological practice. However, the algorithm is only for primary patients, and recommendations for the management of treatment failure and recurrence are less clearly defined because of the major differences between the 4 guidelines.

Should we then decide to stop developing and using prognostic models? The authors of this article do not advise to stop, but statistical concepts, such as discrimination (c index, AUC), calibration, *P* values, hazard ratios, odds ratios, and even sensitivity and specificity, do not really help clinicians when it comes to making clinical decisions in a given patient. It remains very important to give an adequate treatment as soon as possible because delay and inadequate therapy are associated with a worse outcome.[43–45] The authors discuss their view on improving the use of prognostic models in the next paragraph.

FUTURE PERSPECTIVES ON BC PROGNOSTIC MODELS

Before developing new models, one should carefully think about the clinical purpose of the model: what is the goal of the prognostic model and how will it be used in clinical practice? For BC, one could consider to try to identify high-risk patients for immediate cystectomy or to identify low-risk patients who do not need further treatment or would be candidates for low-intensity surveillance. When developing a model, clinically meaningful statistics should be used, such as PPV and NPV. For example, the PPV of the EORTC risk tables for progression in high-risk patients is only 21%, which means that if a patient is classified as high-risk and would go for cystectomy, this would be overtreatment in 79% of the cases. Thus, the EORTC risk tables are not useful for determining what the best treatment is for high-risk patients.

One option is to update the existing models with data that were not previously available. Data on recent advances that are currently recommended by the guidelines should be included in the current models, such as data on re-TURBT, fluorescence cystoscopy, and postoperative instillations. External validation should always be performed when a prognostic model is to assess its generalizability.

As mentioned by Shariat and colleagues,[46] larger data sets, better data collection methods, and more sophisticated modeling procedures are needed to improve predictive accuracy. In addition, better accuracy might be accomplished by modeling physician- or hospital-specific data for patients being treated by that physician or at that hospital. Finally, prognostic models that predict the likelihood of metastatic progression, cancer-specific mortality, and the long-term quality of life are likely to have great utility for patients and physicians when exploring treatment alternatives.

Should we update models by combining patient and tumor characteristics with biomarkers? Ideally, biomarkers should help to identify patients at high risk of recurrence and could, therefore, increase the accuracy of prognostic models. Several groups have already attempted to combine biomarkers to improve the outcome of NMIBC.[16,21,47–49] Shariat and colleagues[21] combined their nomogram with nuclear matrix protein 22 (NMP22). This combination had a good accuracy (AUC >80%), but the investigators did not compare models with and without NMP22, so the additional value of adding NMP22 was not investigated. Another example of combining a biomarker with clinical data is the previously mentioned article of Van Rhijn and colleagues[16] in which they combined molecular grading (FGFR3 gene mutation status and MIB-1 expression) with the EORTC risk scores. They found an additional value of this combination: the predictive accuracy of the EORTC risk scores increased from 74.9% to 81.7%. Members of this group also combined 4 molecular markers (FGFR3 gene mutation status, Ki67, P53, and P27 expression) with T1 substaging (2 types: T1e vs T1m and T1a vs T1b vs T1c) and EORTC risk scores.[49] P53 was not of any value, and the additional value of the other 3 markers was only 1.3% ($P>.05$). However, the T1e/T1m substaging was one of the most important variables for progression.

Before adding biomarkers to prognostic models, we should take into account which (statistical) steps are necessary to make a model of additional value. According to Sylvester, 4 steps are needed: first the identification of interesting biomarkers, then the defining of a function used to combine the biomarkers together into a classification rule, next a validation to show its reproducibility, and finally investigating whether the biomarkers improves the predictive accuracy of the model.[50] Also, we should investigate whether we need one biomarker or a panel of markers. We have to improve the scientific rigor related to biomarker evaluation and testing and the feasibility of their use in day-to-day clinical practice as compared with the currently available biomarkers.

Another, and perhaps the best, possibility would be to simplify the current prognostic models to make them more useable in daily practice. We should improve their PPV and/or NPV and pay more attention to calibration, as suggested by Sylvester.[50] Classification tables including NPV and PPV express the results of prognostic models in clinical terms and can be used to compare them. Once there is a model that is clinically useful (ie, with high NPV and PPV) the model should be evaluated. As mentioned earlier, *P* values, hazard ratios, c index, and so forth have little or no direct consequences for day-to-day practice. A more relevant method has been suggested by Vickers and Cronin[51] to calculate the net benefit of a new model compared with the standard model as part of a decision curve analysis. This analysis is based on 2 principles: models may influence medical decisions and decisions have consequences that can be directly incorporated into analyses by using weights. Decision analytic techniques may be used to determine whether a model is worth using at all, which of the 2 (or more) models is preferable, and whether an additional predictor is worth measuring.

If we know what the important prognostic factors in a certain group of patients are, we can personalize their treatment based on their level of risk. As mentioned earlier, the IBCG has already published a simple algorithm for the treatment and management of patients with primary NMIBC.[42] The EAU NMIBC Guidelines Panel is working to simplify the risk group definitions for their day-to-day use in the clinic. The EORTC will be updating their risk tables in patients treated with maintenance BCG, and several authors of this article are working on outcome probabilities after intravesical chemotherapy. All of these are practical examples of work that is being done to make it easier for clinicians to classify patients according to their level of risk and, thus, to provide the most appropriate treatment in individual patients.

SUMMARY

Currently, there are many prognostic models available for NMIBC but they are not commonly used in daily practice because of their complexity and limited usefulness in treatment decision making. To make prognostic models more useful, the focus should be on the clinical implications of the model for the patient, such as by focusing on NPV and PPV rather than *P* values, sensitivity, and specificity. The net benefit of a model should be compared with the standard model by means of classification tables and decision analytic techniques to test its additional clinical value. Currently, biomarkers do not have sufficient additional value, and markers under investigation should first stand the test of time.

Ultimately, even good models will not be translated into clinical practice unless they can be integrated into the standard clinical workflow and prove their importance in improved therapeutic results. Despite the efforts of many, these predictive models have not replaced a practicing clinician's treatment experience.

REFERENCES

1. Wu X, Ros MM, Gu J, et al. Epidemiology and genetic susceptibility to bladder cancer. BJU Int 2008;102(9 Pt B):1207–15.
2. Jemal A, Bray F, Center MM, et al. Global cancer statistics. CA Cancer J Clin 2011;61(2):69–90.
3. Zeegers MP, Tan FE, Dorant E, et al. The impact of characteristics of cigarette smoking on urinary tract cancer risk: a meta-analysis of epidemiologic studies. Cancer 2000;89(3):630–9.
4. Pelucchi C, Bosetti C, Negri E, et al. Mechanisms of disease: the epidemiology of bladder cancer. Nat Clin Pract Urol 2006;3(6):327–40.
5. Messing EM. Urothelial tumors of the bladder. In: Wein AJ, Kavoussi LR, Novick AC, et al, editors. Campbell-walsh urology, vol. 9, 9th edition. Philadelphia: Saunders Elsevier; 2007. p. 2419–31.
6. Kirkali Z, Chan T, Manoharan M, et al. Bladder cancer: epidemiology, staging and grading, and diagnosis. Urology 2005;66(6 Suppl 1):4–34.
7. Sauter G, Algaba F, Amin MB, et al. Tumours of the urinary system: non-invasive urothelial neoplasias. In: Eble JN, Sauter G, Epstein JI, et al, editors. WHO classification of classification of tumors of the urinary system and male genital organs. Lyon (France): IARC Press; 2004. p. 29–34.
8. Sobin LH, Gospodariwicz M, Wittekind C. Urinary bladder. In: Sobin LH, Gospodariwicz M, Wittekind C, editors. TNM classification of malignant tumors. UICC Union International Contre le Cancer, vol. 7. Hoboken (NJ): Wiley-Blackwell; 2009. p. 262–5.
9. Sylvester RJ, van der Meijden AP, Oosterlinck W, et al. Predicting recurrence and progression in individual patients with stage Ta T1 bladder cancer using EORTC risk tables: a combined analysis of 2596 patients from seven EORTC trials. Eur Urol 2006;49(3):465–77.
10. Hernandez V, De La Pena E, Martin MD, et al. External validation and applicability of the EORTC risk tables for non-muscle-invasive bladder cancer. World J Urol 2011;29(4):409–14.
11. Babjuk M, Oosterlinck W, Sylvester R, et al. EAU guidelines on non-muscle-invasive urothelial carcinoma of the bladder, the 2011 update. Eur Urol 2011;59(6):997–1008.
12. Hall MC, Chang SS, Dalbagni G, et al. Guideline for the management of non muscle invasive bladder cancer (stages Ta, T1, and Tis): 2007 update. J Urol 2007;178(6):2314–30.
13. Sylvester RJ. How well can you actually predict which non-muscle-invasive bladder cancer patients will progress? Eur Urol 2011;60(3):431–3 [discussion: 433–4].
14. Sakano S, Matsuyama H, Takai K, et al. Risk group stratification to predict recurrence after transurethral resection in Japanese patients with stage Ta and T1 bladder tumours: validation study on the European Association of Urology guidelines. BJU Int 2011;107(10):1598–604.
15. Seo KW, Kim BH, Park CH, et al. The efficacy of the EORTC scoring system and risk tables for the

prediction of recurrence and progression of non-muscle-invasive bladder cancer after intravesical bacillus Calmette-Guerin instillation. Korean J Urol 2010;51(3):165–70.
16. van Rhijn BW, Zuiverloon TC, Vis AN, et al. Molecular grade (FGFR3/MIB-1) and EORTC risk scores are predictive in primary non-muscle-invasive bladder cancer. Eur Urol 2010;58(3):433–41.
17. Pillai R, Wang D, Mayer EK, et al. Do standardised prognostic algorithms reflect local practice? Application of EORTC risk tables for non-muscle invasive (pTa/pT1) bladder cancer recurrence and progression in a local cohort. ScientificWorldJournal 2011; 11:751–9.
18. Fernandez-Gomez J, Madero R, Solsona E, et al. The EORTC tables overestimate the risk of recurrence and progression in patients with non-muscle-invasive bladder cancer treated with bacillus Calmette-Guerin: external validation of the EORTC risk tables. Eur Urol 2011;60:423–30.
19. Kiemeney LA, Witjes JA, Heijbroek RP, et al. Predictability of recurrent and progressive disease in individual patients with primary superficial bladder cancer. J Urol 1993;150(1):60–4.
20. Millan-Rodriguez F, Chechile-Toniolo G, Salvador-Bayarri J, et al. Primary superficial bladder cancer risk groups according to progression, mortality and recurrence. J Urol 2000;164(3 Pt 1):680–4.
21. Shariat SF, Zippe C, Ludecke G, et al. Nomograms including nuclear matrix protein 22 for prediction of disease recurrence and progression in patients with Ta, T1 or CIS transitional cell carcinoma of the bladder. J Urol 2005;173(5):1518–25.
22. Hong SJ, Cho KS, Han M, et al. Nomograms for prediction of disease recurrence in patients with primary Ta, T1 transitional cell carcinoma of the bladder. J Korean Med Sci 2008;23(3):428–33.
23. Yamada T, Tsuchiya K, Kato S, et al. A pretreatment nomogram predicting recurrence- and progression-free survival for nonmuscle invasive bladder cancer in Japanese patients. Int J Clin Oncol 2010;15(3): 271–9.
24. Pan CC, Chang YH, Chen KK, et al. Constructing prognostic model incorporating the 2004 WHO/ISUP classification for patients with non-muscle-invasive urothelial tumours of the urinary bladder. J Clin Pathol 2010;63(10):910–5.
25. Shapur N, Pode D, Katz R, et al. Predicting the risk of high-grade bladder cancer using noninvasive data. Urol Int 2011;87(3):319–24.
26. Fernandez-Gomez J, Madero R, Solsona E, et al. Predicting nonmuscle invasive bladder cancer recurrence and progression in patients treated with bacillus Calmette-Guerin: the CUETO scoring model. J Urol 2009;182(5):2195–203.
27. Catto JW, Abbod MF, Linkens DA, et al. Neurofuzzy modeling to determine recurrence risk following radical cystectomy for nonmetastatic urothelial carcinoma of the bladder. Clin Cancer Res 2009; 15(9):3150–5.
28. Gakis G, Todenhofer T, Renninger M, et al. Development of a new outcome prediction model in carcinoma invading the bladder based on preoperative serum C-reactive protein and standard pathological risk factors: the TNR-C score. BJU Int 2011;108(11): 1800–5.
29. Morgan TM, Keegan KA, Barocas DA, et al. Predicting the probability of 90-day survival of elderly patients with bladder cancer treated with radical cystectomy. J Urol 2011;186(3):829–34.
30. Shariat SF, Chromecki TF, Cha EK, et al. Risk stratification of organ confined bladder cancer after radical cystectomy using cell cycle related biomarkers. J Urol 2012;187(2):457–62.
31. Sonpavde G, Khan MM, Svatek RS, et al. Prognostic risk stratification of pathological stage T2N0 bladder cancer after radical cystectomy. BJU Int 2011; 108(5):687–92.
32. Sonpavde G, Khan MM, Svatek RS, et al. Prognostic risk stratification of pathological stage T3N0 bladder cancer after radical cystectomy. J Urol 2011;185(4): 1216–21.
33. Taylor JM, Feifer A, Savage CJ, et al. Evaluating the utility of a preoperative nomogram for predicting 90-day mortality following radical cystectomy for bladder cancer. BJU Int 2012;109(6):855–9.
34. Rosevear HM, Lightfoot AJ, Nepple KG, et al. Usefulness of the Spanish Urological Club for Oncological Treatment scoring model to predict nonmuscle invasive bladder cancer recurrence in patients treated with intravesical bacillus Calmette-Guerin plus interferon-alpha. J Urol 2011;185(1):67–71.
35. Sylvester RJ. Natural history, recurrence, and progression in superficial bladder cancer. ScientificWorldJournal 2006;6:2617–25.
36. Steyerberg EW. Clinical prediction models. A practical approach to development, validation, and updating, vol. 1. New York: Springer Science; 2009.
37. Chamie K, Saigal CS, Lai J, et al. Compliance with guidelines for patients with bladder cancer: variation in the delivery of care. Cancer 2011;117(23): 5392–401.
38. Elstein AS. Heuristics and biases: selected errors in clinical reasoning. Acad Med 1999;74(7):791–4.
39. Fowler FJ Jr, McNaughton Collins M, Albertsen PC, et al. Comparison of recommendations by urologists and radiation oncologists for treatment of clinically localized prostate cancer. JAMA 2000;283(24): 3217–22.
40. Ross PL, Gerigk C, Gonen M, et al. Comparisons of nomograms and urologists' predictions in prostate cancer. Semin Urol Oncol 2002;20(2):82–8.
41. Specht MC, Kattan MW, Gonen M, et al. Predicting nonsentinel node status after positive sentinel lymph

biopsy for breast cancer: clinicians versus nomogram. Ann Surg Oncol 2005;12(8):654–9.
42. Brausi M, Witjes JA, Lamm D, et al. A review of current guidelines and best practice recommendations for the management of nonmuscle invasive bladder cancer by the International Bladder Cancer Group. J Urol 2011;186(6):2158–67.
43. Schrier BP, Hollander MP, van Rhijn BW, et al. Prognosis of muscle-invasive bladder cancer: difference between primary and progressive tumours and implications for therapy. Eur Urol 2004;45(3):292–6.
44. Hollenbeck BK, Dunn RL, Ye Z, et al. Delays in diagnosis and bladder cancer mortality. Cancer 2010; 116(22):5235–42.
45. Skolarus TA, Ye Z, Montgomery JS, et al. Use of restaging bladder tumor resection for bladder cancer among Medicare beneficiaries. Urology 2011;78(6):1345–9.
46. Shariat SF, Margulis V, Lotan Y, et al. Nomograms for bladder cancer. Eur Urol 2008;54(1):41–53.
47. Shariat SF, Karakiewicz PI, Ashfaq R, et al. Multiple biomarkers improve prediction of bladder cancer recurrence and mortality in patients undergoing cystectomy. Cancer 2008;112(2):315–25.
48. Riester M, Taylor JM, Feifer A, et al. Combination of a novel gene expression signature with a clinical nomogram improves the prediction of survival in high-risk bladder cancer. Clin Cancer Res 2012; 18(5):1323–33.
49. van Rhijn BW, Liu L, Vis AN, et al. Prognostic value of molecular markers, sub-stage and European Organisation for the Research and Treatment of Cancer risk scores in primary T1 bladder cancer. BJU Int 2012;110:1169–76.
50. Sylvester RJ. Combining a molecular profile with a clinical and pathological profile: biostatistical considerations. Scand J Urol Nephrol Suppl 2008;(218):185–90.
51. Vickers AJ, Cronin AM. Traditional statistical methods for evaluating prediction models are uninformative as to clinical value: towards a decision analytic framework. Semin Oncol 2010;37(1): 31–8.

Urinary Markers/Cytology
What and When Should a Urologist Use

Jeffrey M. Tomasini, MD, Badrinath R. Konety, MD, MBA*

KEYWORDS

• Non-muscle invasive bladder cancer • Cytology • UroVysion FISH • NMP22 • BTA • ImmunoCyt

KEY POINTS

- 80% of urothelial carcinoma is non-muscle invasive at diagnosis, and up to 70% will have recurrence within 5 years.
- Urine-based tumor markers are an important adjunct in both screening and surveillance of urothelial carcinoma.
- Cystoscopy remains the most cost-effective method for identifying bladder cancer recurrence.
- Urine cytology is highly specific but lacks sensitivity in detection of non-muscle invasive bladder cancer.
- Use of urine tumor markers may best be served when cytology is indeterminate or likely to be inaccurate.

INTRODUCTION

It is estimated that there are 585,390 people in the United States living with bladder cancer, and an additional 73,510 cases will be newly diagnosed in 2012. As of 2012, bladder cancer is the fourth most common cancer afflicting men and ninth most common cancer in women.[1] Nearly 80% of all bladder cancer diagnoses are non-muscle invasive at presentation.[2] Of patients with non-muscle invasive urothelial carcinoma, 50% to 70% will have at least one recurrence in 5 years, and up to 20% will progress to a more advanced stage during that time.[3] Identifying a test to both screen and facilitate surveillance for bladder cancer is of paramount importance. At present, diagnosis and surveillance of urothelial cancer includes imaging of the upper urinary tracts with computed tomography (CT) urography, urinary cytologic evaluation, and cystoscopy.

A test that is inexpensive, noninvasive, and reproducible and that provides excellent sensitivity and specificity is an ideal candidate for a screening marker. Currently, there are 4 Food and Drug Administration (FDA)–approved bladder cancer tumor markers available for use in the United States. These have been used with varying success. However, the data regarding the consistency and reliability of these markers have been mixed, and the precise role for these new markers other than cytology is yet to be clearly defined. Some of these markers are also more expensive than urine cytology and even cystoscopy. Thus, it is imperative to clearly define a strategy for using these tests in the diagnosis and follow-up of both non-muscle invasive bladder cancer (NMIBC) and muscle invasive bladder cancer.

CYTOLOGY

Urinary cytology, first described for use in evaluating urothelial cancer in 1945 by Papanicolaou,[4] has been a standard test in the evaluation of bladder cancer. A urine sample is collected, centrifuged, and the sediment resuspended, stained, and evaluated with light microscopy (**Fig. 1**). The sample is then read by a pathologist who classifies the sample as normal, atypical, or indeterminate; suspicious; or malignant.[5] A malignant sample was previously assigned a grade of 1, 2, or 3. The new standard is to designate a malignant sample as either low-grade or high-grade based on architectural and cytologic criteria to reduce ambiguity and improve interobserver reproducibility.[6]

Department of Urology, University of Minnesota, MMC 394, 420 Delaware Street, Minneapolis, MN 55455, USA
* Corresponding author.
E-mail address: brkonety@umn.edu

Urol Clin N Am 40 (2013) 165–173
http://dx.doi.org/10.1016/j.ucl.2013.01.015

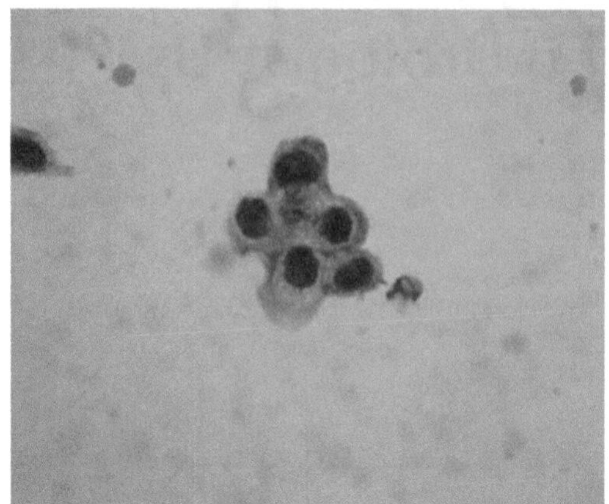

Fig. 1. A voided urine sample revealing low-grade urothelial carcinoma.

Several factors affect the utility of urinary cytology. Cancer cells must be sloughed into the urine to be collected. High-grade cancers are more apt to slough into urine than low-grade cancers because of weaker intercellular attachments.[2] The sample is subjectively diagnosed and graded by a cytopathologist, and as such there is both interobserver and intraobserver variability. Inflammatory conditions of the bladder including cystitis and bladder calculi can affect the results.[7] Given these factors, sensitivity of urinary cytology for non-muscle invasive disease is quite variable. Pooled data reveal overall sensitivity for non-muscle invasive disease ranging from 29% to 77%. Overall specificity of cytology ranges from 71% to 100%, with most studies reporting more than 90% specificity for both low-grade and high-grade urothelial cancer.[8–13]

One of the problems with interpreting urine cytology is that the result is sometimes ambiguous. A result of atypical, atypical suspicious, or suspicious is hard to judge and use in management decisions.[14] Individuals who have undergone recent instrumentation or have evidence of inflammation or stone disease may demonstrate an atypical cytology. However, if these individuals also have a history of urothelial carcinoma, the interpretation of the urine cytology reading is difficult. This could lead to unnecessary work up and related morbidity and cost. The use of some of the alternative urine-based markers could potentially serve to improve the accuracy of urine cytology or arbitrate indeterminate results.

UROVYSION (FLUORESCENCE IN-SITU HYBRIDIZATION)

The UroVysion (Abbott Molecular Inc, Des Plaines, IL, USA) test uses fluorescence in-situ hybridization (FISH) to detect increased copy numbers, or aneuploidy, of chromosomes 3, 7, and 17, as well as homozygous deletions of loci at chromosome 9p21.[15] A positive test is determined by presence of either (1) 5 or more cells with 2 or more chromosomal gains (chromosomes 3, 7, 17), or (2) 12 or more cells with gain of a single chromosome, or (3) 12 or more cells with homozygous detection of 9p21 locus (**Fig. 2**).[16,17] False-positive results can occur when a barbotage sample is used because of probe uptake in multinucleated umbrella cells, which are dislodged and can be falsely elevated in barbotage specimens. These cells typically constitute only 2% of the cells in a urine sample,[18] but up to 11% in a barbotage sample.[19] Other explanations for a false-positive FISH include the presence of an inclusion body such as a polyoma virus and seminal vesicle cells. False-negative FISH is seen in the presence of degenerated cells, hyphae, excess lubricant, squamous cells, and autofluorescent bacteria. Positivity with aneuploidy of chromosomes 7 and 17 is more commonly associated with the presence of tumor compared with

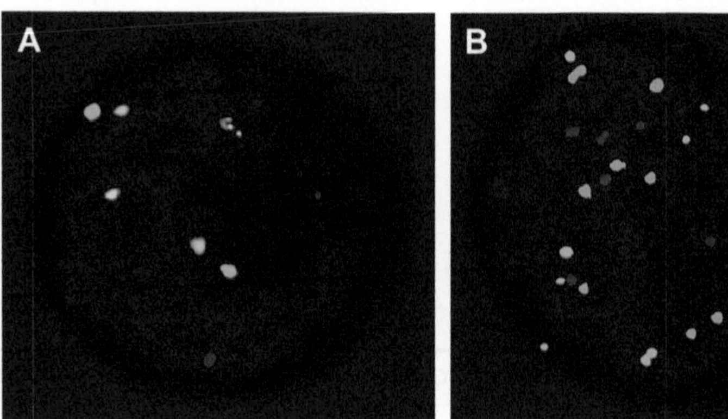

Fig. 2. UroVysion FISH test of voided urine. (*A*) A negative test with 2 copies of each probe present. (*B*) A positive test with multiple copies of each probe visible.

positivity with aneuploidy of chromosome 3 or loss of 9p21. The loss of 9p21 is also more commonly associated with the presence of low-grade, non-muscle invasive tumors. Additionally, the result of an UroVysion FISH test may be positive in the absence of a positive cystoscopic or cytologic evaluation; this occurs in 35% to 63% of patients up to 6 to 20 months before development of a macroscopically visible urothelial malignancy and has been deemed an "anticipatory positive" FISH test.[13,20–22]

UroVysion FISH is more sensitive for high-grade and invasive urothelial malignancies, with reported sensitivity ranging between 83% and 100%. It is also fairly sensitive at detecting non-muscle invasive tumors, with sensitivity ranging from 64% to 76%. UroVysion FISH is nearly as specific as urinary cytology with reported specificity ranging from 89% to 96%.[8,13,23,24] FISH has also been shown to have utility in surveillance for urothelial carcinoma recurrence after intravesical bacillus Calmette-Guerin (BCG) therapy. Both cystoscopy and cytology are often inconclusive following BCG therapy because of the confounding effect of BCG-induced inflammation. Patients with a positive FISH following BCG therapy have demonstrated nearly 10-fold higher likelihood of muscle invasive disease as compared with patients with a negative FISH after BCG.[22] A positive FISH test after intravesical BCG therapy is also associated with a higher likelihood of nonresponse to BCG and recurrent tumor (**Table 1**).

More recently, UroVysion FISH has also been used to adjudicate the results of urine cytology, which are read as "atypical." Given that FISH examines the chromosomal abnormalities in a cell that are less susceptible to conditions that may affect cell morphology such as inflammation or BCG therapy, it may serve as an attractive second level test in patients with hard to interpret urine cytology results. Schlomer and colleagues[25] examined the utility of reflex FISH testing in 120 patients with atypical urine cytology. They found that in patients with a positive cystoscopy, additional FISH testing was of little value. In those with an equivocal cystoscopy or with a negative cystoscopy, the negative predictive value (NPV) of FISH was 100%. They concluded that reflex FISH testing could eliminate the need for further workup and biopsy in patients with an atypical cytology, negative FISH and equivocal or negative cystoscopy. They found no patients with an atypical cytology and a false-positive FISH test.

FISH testing has also been able to detect patients with bladder cancer of nonurothelial histology as well as cancers in adjacent organs such as colon and prostate.[26] Sensitivity for detection of adenocarcinoma is as high as 79%. FISH testing of other body fluids such as pleural effusion fluid can help detect tumor cells.[27]

NUCLEAR MATRIX PROTEIN 22

Nuclear matrix proteins (NMPs) are structural components of the cell nucleus, and also function in regulation of gene expression and DNA replication. NMP22 is a protein specific to mitosis and is involved in the distribution of chromatids to daughter cells. The concentration of NMP22 has been shown to be up to 25 times greater in bladder cancer cell lines than normal urothelium.[28] Inflammatory conditions including cystitis, pyuria, urolithiasis, and hematuria can result in elevated urinary NMP22 levels.[29] NMP22 is available as a point-of-care assay called BladderChek (Stellar Pharmaceutics, Inc, London, Ontario) (**Fig. 3**) that provides immediate results at half the cost of urine cytology.[30]

Several studies have evaluated patients with NMP22 and have examined cohorts that were further subdivided as superficial and invasive disease. Sensitivity of NMP22 in non-muscle invasive disease ranged from 54% to 63% and 70% to 100% sensitive for muscle invasive disease. Overall specificity of NMP22 in urothelial carcinoma ranged from 55% to 90%.[8,11,31–33] Grossman,

Table 1
Utility of urinary FISH testing in assessing response to intravesical BCG therapy

		Tumor Recurrence Post-BCG			
	No. Patients	(%)	Positive FISH with Recurrent Tumors	Negative FISH with Recurrent Tumors	% MIBC (≥T2)
Kipp et al,[22] 2005	37	67	100%	52%	58
Whitson et al,[58] 2009	42	43	89%	26%	5
Mengual et al,[59] 2007	65	36	52%	25%	10
Savic et al,[60] 2009	68	38	76%	26%	
Kamat et al,[61] 2012	126	31	50%	18%	28

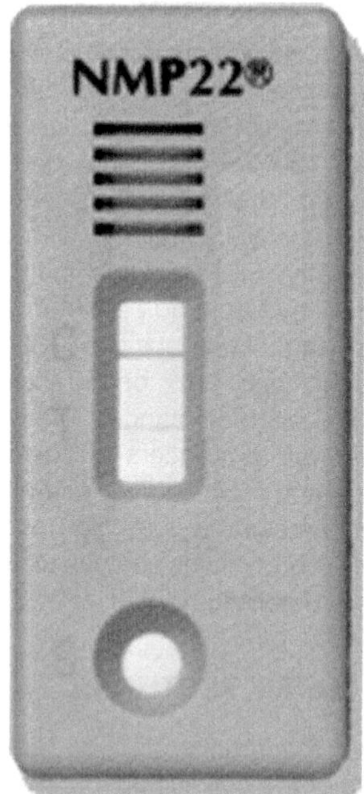

Fig. 3. The BladderChek NMP22 point of care test.

and colleagues[30] evaluated 1331 patients at high risk for urothelial carcinoma with NMP22, cytology, and cystoscopy. Seventy-nine cancers were biopsy proven, 62 of which were non-muscle invasive disease. The sensitivity of NMP22 in this group was 50% compared with 16% for cytology.

A Canadian group prospectively evaluated patients with high-risk superficial disease (tumors that are high-grade, carcinoma in-situ or T1, >3 cm, and recurrent disease at initial 3-month cystoscopy) with NMP22. Fifteen patients out of 94 tested had a positive NMP22 test result and 9 of the 15 patients developed a subsequent recurrence (60%), which is compared with 30 patients with recurrence and a negative NMP22 test (37%). The group concluded that NMP22 may be helpful to risk-stratify patients on surveillance, but NMP22 results in this population did not predict progression-free survival or overall survival.[34] The combination of cystoscopy and NMP22 has been shown to have a higher sensitivity than the combination of cytology and cystoscopy (99% vs 94%), which along with the immediate availability of results, makes it more attractive to use NMP22 BladderChek as an adjunct to cystoscopy.[35] However, the higher false-positive rate of NMP22 has hampered the wide adoption of this approach.

NMP22 along with other markers has also been used in several studies testing the concept of screening for bladder cancer. The ease of use and rapid availability of the results from the NMP22 BladderChek test render it attractive in this context. However, results from the studies suggest that the BladderChek test does not significantly aid in identification of patients with bladder cancer.[36,37] The false negative rate of NMP22 was found to be too high. NMP22 can also yield false-positive tests in the presence of inflammation and hematuria, which raises concerns regarding its use in the setting of screening.

BLADDER TUMOR ANTIGEN

The bladder tumor antigen (BTA) test is available in 2 formats: BTA stat and BTA TRAK (Polymedco, Inc, Cortlandt Manor, NY, USA). Both assays detect complement factor H-related protein in urine, which is responsible for preventing activation of the complement cascade. This test is based on a presumed selectivity of bladder cancer cells to avoid immunologic detection, and complement factor-H related protein is not found in normal bladder cancer cells.[38,39] BTA stat is FDA approved for surveillance, but not initial diagnosis of bladder cancer, and is provided as a point-of-care qualitative assay similar to that of NMP22 (**Fig. 4**). Results are provided in less than 30 minutes. BTA TRAK is a quantitative standard enzyme-linked immunosorbent assay.[2] False-positive results may occur in presence of hematuria, urolithiasis, inflammation, and recent urologic instrumentation.[17,40] Intravesical BCG therapy has also been associated with false-positive BTA tests.[41,42]

In a meta-analysis that included numerous studies evaluating BTA stat, the sensitivity of this rapid point-of-care test for non-muscle invasive urothelial carcinoma ranged from 45% to 75%.[8] The BTA stat test was significantly more sensitive for muscle invasive disease, sensitivity ranging from 67% to 100%. Overall specificity of this test was 64% to 89%.[8,9,11,23,24,31,33,43–45]

IMMUNOCYT

ImmunoCyt/uCyt+ (Scimedex, Corp., Denville, NJ, USA) is an assay using fluorescent-labeled antibodies to 3 glycoprotein antigens commonly

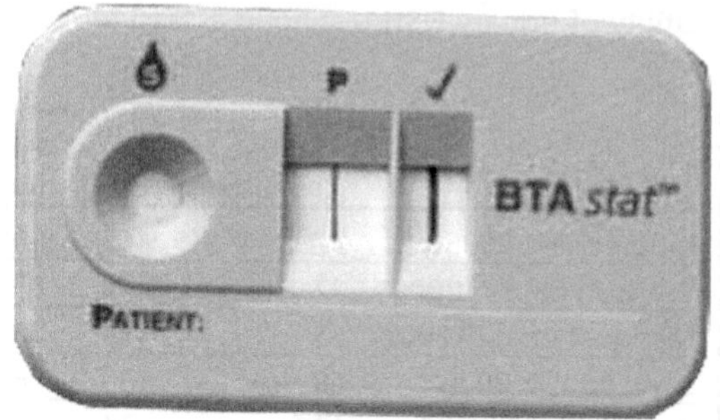

Fig. 4. The BTA stat point of care test.

found on urothelial carcinoma cells. Texas red stain (red) is used to identify 19A211, a high molecular weight form of carcinoembryonic antigen (**Fig. 5**). Fluorescein-tagged antibodies (green) are directed at mucins LDQ10 and M344, both of which are specific to cancer cells.[46] A test is considered positive if at least one cell has a green or red fluorescence and negative if no fluorescently labeled cells are identified after counting 500 cells.[47] Limitations of ImmunoCyt include necessity to evaluate at least 500 cells per slide to ensure a complete evaluation, difficult detection of green fluorescence when present in low concentration, and requirement of adequate training to perform and read the test.[41]

The antigens detected by ImmunoCyt are commonly present even on low-grade and non-muscle invasive tumor cells. M344 is expressed in 71% of Ta and T1 tumor cells, and 19A211 is detectable in 90% of the same tumor cells.[48] Sensitivity of ImmunoCyt in non-muscle invasive urothelial cancers is 60% and increased to 80% for muscle invasive cancers. Overall specificity is 78%.[10] Sensitivity for low-grade tumors increased to 79% when ImmunoCyt is performed in addition to urinary cytology and to 99% for high-grade tumors.[49]

ImmunoCyt has been combined with urine cytology to enhance the sensitivity and specificity of urine cytology. The combination of the 2 tests has been used particularly effectively in reducing the frequency of surveillance cystoscopy in patients with low-grade non-muscle invasive disease.[49,50] ImmunoCyt has also been used as a second level test to arbitrate atypical cytology.[51] A reflex ImmunoCyt test appears to be able to predict the findings on cystoscopy in patients with atypical cytology. A reflex ImmunoCyt test had an NPV of 90% in those with a prior history of urothelial carcinoma, whereas in those without such a history, reflex ImmunoCyt had an NPV of 94%.

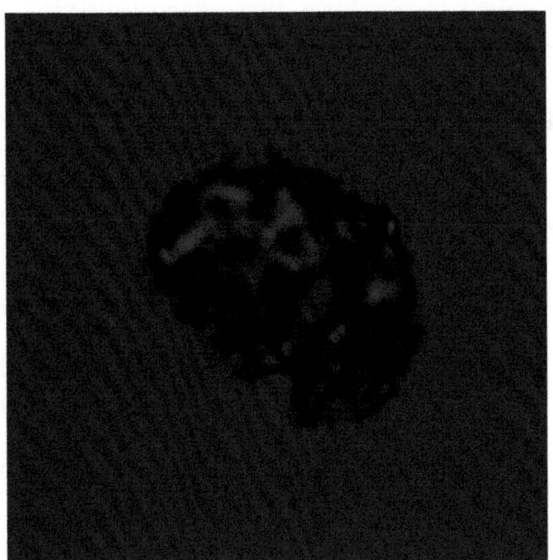

Fig. 5. Positive Immunocyt test of a voided urine specimen.

DISCUSSION

Bladder cancer has a very high recurrence rate, up to 70% within 5 years of initial diagnosis.[3] As such, patients with bladder cancer require close surveillance for a prolonged period of time. Cystoscopy is the gold-standard modality for detection of recurrence of bladder cancer. Although it is generally well tolerated, cystoscopy is an invasive procedure. The high rate of tumor recurrence in bladder cancer mandates a frequent surveillance interval, thus many patients undergo cystoscopy several times per year. This has resulted in bladder cancer being the most expensive malignancy to treat per patient from diagnosis to death.[52]

Most bladder cancers are detected on evaluation for gross hematuria. Three quarters of these tumors are non-muscle invasive at diagnosis. Institution of a screening program, particularly in high-risk populations such as heavy smokers or those with occupational exposure, would ideally identify tumors earlier than if presenting with gross hematuria, thus decreasing the rate of invasive disease at diagnosis. Using mathematical modeling, Lotan and colleagues[53] determined that screening is cost-effective for bladder cancer. Several studies have prospectively evaluated the efficacy of screening for bladder cancer. Steiner and colleagues[36] screened 183 patients deemed high-risk based on smoking history greater than 40 pack-years. Urine dipstick for microscopic hematuria, cytology, NMP22, and UroVysion were used for screening, and a positive result in any test led to cystoscopy and CT urography for diagnosis. This resulted in diagnosis of 6 malignancies, half of which were of the upper tracts. One false-negative result was identified. Use of urine dipstick, cytology, and UroVysion was recommended for screening in high-risk patients.

Cancer screening programs should be cost-effective, and the prevalence of disease must be sufficient within a population to justify testing. Lotan found a significant improvement in overall survival, downstaging of disease, and cost reduction when incidence of bladder cancer was more than 1.6%.[53] However, these studies that have used marker-based screening have not proved very effective. One reason has been the relatively low prevalence of the disease in a general population. More effectively, identification of an "at risk" population and availability of better makers with higher specificity while retaining the ease of use of the currently available point of care tests such as NMP22 BladderChek may ultimately help facilitate these efforts.

BTA stat and BTA TRAK, NMP22 and NMP22 BladderChek, UroVysion, and ImmunoCyt tests are currently the only FDA-approved urine-based bladder tumor markers. These tests are all approved for use in surveillance of bladder cancer, and with the exception of ImmunoCyt, for the initial diagnosis of bladder cancer as well. To be effective in replacing cystoscopy for the surveillance of NMIBC, a urinary tumor marker should have high sensitivity and a low false-negative rate or a high NPV. The sensitivity (63%–76%) and NPV for markers such as FISH are high (>80%). However, this level may not be sufficient for most patients. Surveys of patients undergoing cystoscopic surveillance indicate that 75% of patients would require a test to have a sensitivity greater than 95%, and an additional 21% would accept a marker sensitivity of 90% to 95% before foregoing cystoscopic surveillance.[54] None of the currently available markers are able to achieve this level of sensitivity consistently. Hence at this time, eliminating cystoscopy from surveillance of NMIBC does not appear to be a viable option. Cystoscopic surveillance may also be the most cost-effective method of monitoring NMIBC at this time. In a prospective trial of 200 patients with prior diagnosis of non-muscle invasive bladder cancer, patients underwent surveillance cystoscopy as well as evaluation with urinary cytology, NMP22 BladderChek, and UroVysion FISH.[55] The investigators concluded that cystoscopy remains the most cost-effective method to identify bladder cancer recurrence. Detection was not improved with addition of these markers to cystoscopy and simply added to cost. The cost per tumor detected by cystoscopy alone was $7,692, compared with $11,143 for cystoscopy and NMP22, $19,111 for cystoscopy and UroVysion, and 10,267 for cystoscopy and cytology.[55] Hence the International Consultation on Urologic Diseases – European Association of Urology panel concluded that at this time white light cystoscopy remains the most cost-effective method of surveillance of the lower urinary tract for tumor recurrence.[56]

Future applications of urinary markers can be designed based on the type of marker, that is, protein-based or cytologic/molecular. Protein-based markers tend to lend themselves to point of care determination, which is most attractive for use in the context of screening and perhaps even patient self-testing. These tests are also more easily applied during episodes of surveillance as the results are more immediately available and clearly defined without a gradation between positive and negative as can be the case with urine cytology. At least one study suggests that availability of the results of urinary marker testing at the time of surveillance can lead to higher rates of biopsy/resection and recurrence detection.[57] This represents a diagnostic review bias that favors use of urinary markers at the time of cystoscopy. Cytologic or molecular markers on the other hand, may have more prognostic ability. They could optimally be applied for assessment of tumor response to intravesical therapy and to determine risk of progression. They could also be better used to arbitrate atypical or suspicious urine cytology readings. Reflex testing of all specimens with an atypical reading could lead to reduced diagnostic workup and therefore reduced morbidity and costs.

Over the past 2 decades, significant efforts have been made to identify and apply urinary tumor markers to enhance the diagnosis of bladder cancer and to overcome the shortcomings of urine cytology. Although several attractive markers have been identified, follow-up studies and phase IV post-FDA approval clinical experience have not consistently borne out the initial favorable results; this has led to confusion regarding optimal applicability of these markers. With continued careful study, it is very likely that we will define more precise indications for the use of these markers. At the current time, they seem most appropriate for use as an adjunct to cystoscopy, particularly in situations where cytology is likely to be inaccurate (eg, postintravesical therapy, inflammation) or if cytology is itself indeterminate. They could also be used if cytology is hard to obtain or unreliable.

REFERENCES

1. Siegel R, DeSantis C, Virgo K, et al. Cancer treatment and survivorship statistics, 2012. CA Cancer J Clin 2012;62(4):220–41.
2. Villicana P, Whiting B, Goodison S, et al. Urine-based assays for the detection of bladder cancer. Biomark Med 2009;3(3):265.
3. Donat SM. Evaluation and follow-up strategies for superficial bladder cancer. Urol Clin North Am 2003;30(4):765–76.
4. Papanicolaou GN, Marshall VF. Urine sediment smears as a diagnostic procedure in cancers of the urinary tract. Science 1945;101(2629): 519–20.
5. Wild PJ, Fuchs T, Stoehr R, et al. Detection of urothelial bladder cancer cells in voided urine can be

improved by a combination of cytology and standardized microsatellite analysis. Cancer Epidemiol Biomarkers Prev 2009;18(6):1798–806.

6. Miyamoto H, Miller JS, Fajardo DA, et al. Noninvasive papillary urothelial neoplasms: the 2004 WHO/ISUP classification system. Pathol Int 2010; 60(1):1–8.
7. Talwar R, Sinha T, Karan SC, et al. Voided urinary cytology in bladder cancer: is it time to review the indications? Urology 2007;70(2):267–71.
8. Lokeshwar VB, Habuchi T, Grossman HB, et al. Bladder tumor markers beyond cytology: international consensus panel on bladder tumor markers. Urology 2005;66(6 Suppl 1):35–63.
9. Schroeder GL, Lorenzo-Gomez MF, Hautmann SH, et al. A side by side comparison of cytology and biomarkers for bladder cancer detection. J Urol 2004;172(3):1123–6.
10. Hautmann S, Toma M, Lorenzo Gomez MF, et al. Immunocyt and the HA-HAase urine tests for the detection of bladder cancer: a side-by-side comparison. Eur Urol 2004;46(4):466–71.
11. Boman H, Hedelin H, Holmang S. Four bladder tumor markers have a disappointingly low sensitivity for small size and low grade recurrence. J Urol 2002; 167(1):80–3.
12. Babjuk M, Kostirova M, Mudra K, et al. Qualitative and quantitative detection of urinary human complement factor H-related protein (BTA stat and BTA TRAK) and fragments of cytokeratins 8, 18 (UBC rapid and UBC IRMA) as markers for transitional cell carcinoma of the bladder. Eur Urol 2002;41(1): 34–9.
13. Sarosdy MF, Schellhammer P, Bokinsky G, et al. Clinical evaluation of a multi-target fluorescent in situ hybridization assay for detection of bladder cancer. J Urol 2002;168(5):1950–4.
14. Layfield LJ, Elsheikh TM, Fili A, et al. Review of the state of the art and recommendations of the Papanicolaou Society of Cytopathology for urinary cytology procedures and reporting: the Papanicolaou Society of Cytopathology Practice Guidelines Task Force. Diagn Cytopathol 2004;30(1):24–30.
15. Cajulis RS, Haines GK 3rd, Frias-Hidvegi D, et al. Cytology, flow cytometry, image analysis, and interphase cytogenetics by fluorescence in situ hybridization in the diagnosis of transitional cell carcinoma in bladder washes: a comparative study. Diagn Cytopathol 1995;13(3):214–23 [discussion: 224].
16. Placer J, Espinet B, Salido M, et al. Clinical utility of a multiprobe FISH assay in voided urine specimens for the detection of bladder cancer and its recurrences, compared with urinary cytology. Eur Urol 2002;42(6):547–52.
17. Konety BR. Molecular markers in bladder cancer: a critical appraisal. Urol Oncol 2006;24(4): 326–37.
18. Schwarz S, Rechenmacher M, Filbeck T, et al. Value of multicolour fluorescence in situ hybridisation (UroVysion) in the differential diagnosis of flat urothelial lesions. J Clin Pathol 2008;61(3):272–7.
19. Bergman J, Reznichek RC, Rajfer J. Surveillance of patients with bladder carcinoma using fluorescent in-situ hybridization on bladder washings. BJU Int 2008;101(1):26–9.
20. Zellweger T, Benz G, Cathomas G, et al. Multi-target fluorescence in situ hybridization in bladder washings for prediction of recurrent bladder cancer. Int J Cancer 2006;119(7):1660–5.
21. Yoder BJ, Skacel M, Hedgepeth R, et al. Reflex UroVysion testing of bladder cancer surveillance patients with equivocal or negative urine cytology: a prospective study with focus on the natural history of anticipatory positive findings. Am J Clin Pathol 2007;127(2):295–301.
22. Kipp BR, Karnes RJ, Brankley SM, et al. Monitoring intravesical therapy for superficial bladder cancer using fluorescence in situ hybridization. J Urol 2005;173(2):401–4.
23. Friedrich MG, Toma MI, Hellstern A, et al. Comparison of multitarget fluorescence in situ hybridization in urine with other noninvasive tests for detecting bladder cancer. BJU Int 2003;92(9):911–4.
24. Halling KC, King W, Sokolova IA, et al. A comparison of BTA stat, hemoglobin dipstick, telomerase and Vysis UroVysion assays for the detection of urothelial carcinoma in urine. J Urol 2002;167(5):2001–6.
25. Schlomer BJ, Ho R, Sagalowsky A, et al. Prospective validation of the clinical usefulness of reflex fluorescence in situ hybridization assay in patients with atypical cytology for the detection of urothelial carcinoma of the bladder. J Urol 2010;183(1):62–7.
26. Reid-Nicholson MD, Ramalingam P, Adeagbo B, et al. The use of Urovysion fluorescence in situ hybridization in the diagnosis and surveillance of non-urothelial carcinoma of the bladder. Mod Pathol 2009;22(1):119–27.
27. Flores-Staino C, Darai-Ramqvist E, Dobra K, et al. Adaptation of a commercial fluorescent in situ hybridization test to the diagnosis of malignant cells in effusions. Lung Cancer 2010;68(1):39–43.
28. Carpinito GA, Stadler WM, Briggman JV, et al. Urinary nuclear matrix protein as a marker for transitional cell carcinoma of the urinary tract. J Urol 1996; 156(4):1280–5.
29. Ponsky LE, Sharma S, Pandrangi L, et al. Screening and monitoring for bladder cancer: refining the use of NMP22. J Urol 2001;166(1):75–8.
30. Grossman HB, Messing E, Soloway M, et al. Detection of bladder cancer using a point-of-care proteomic assay. JAMA 2005;293(7):810–6.
31. Giannopoulos A, Manousakas T, Gounari A, et al. Comparative evaluation of the diagnostic performance of the BTA stat test, NMP22 and urinary

bladder cancer antigen for primary and recurrent bladder tumors. J Urol 2001;166(2):470–5.

32. Mian C, Lodde M, Haitel A, et al. Comparison of the monoclonal UBC-ELISA test and the NMP22 ELISA test for the detection of urothelial cell carcinoma of the bladder. Urology 2000;55(2):223–6.
33. Serretta V, Pomara G, Rizzo I, et al. Urinary BTA-stat, BTA-trak and NMP22 in surveillance after TUR of recurrent superficial transitional cell carcinoma of the bladder. Eur Urol 2000;38(4):419–25.
34. Lau P, Chin JL, Pautler S, et al. NMP22 is predictive of recurrence in high-risk superficial bladder cancer patients. Can Urol Assoc J 2009;3(6):454–8.
35. Nguyen CT, Jones JS. Defining the role of NMP22 in bladder cancer surveillance. World J Urol 2008; 26(1):51–8.
36. Steiner H, Bergmeister M, Verdorfer I, et al. Early results of bladder-cancer screening in a high-risk population of heavy smokers. BJU Int 2008;102(3): 291–6.
37. Lotan Y, Elias K, Svatek RS, et al. Bladder cancer screening in a high risk asymptomatic population using a point of care urine based protein tumor marker. J Urol 2009;182(1):52–7 [discussion: 58].
38. Poulakis V, Witzsch U, De Vries R, et al. A comparison of urinary nuclear matrix protein-22 and bladder tumour antigen tests with voided urinary cytology in detecting and following bladder cancer: the prognostic value of false-positive results. BJU Int 2001; 88(7):692–701.
39. Parker J, Spiess PE. Current and emerging bladder cancer urinary biomarkers. ScientificWorldJournal 2011;11:1103–12.
40. Oge O, Atsu N, Sahin A, et al. Comparison of BTA stat and NMP22 tests in the detection of bladder cancer. Scand J Urol Nephrol 2000; 34(6):349–51.
41. Konety B, Lotan Y. Urothelial bladder cancer: biomarkers for detection and screening. BJU Int 2008;102(9 Pt B):1234–41.
42. Raitanen MP, Hellstrom P, Marttila T, et al. Effect of intravesical instillations on the human complement factor H related protein (BTA stat) test. Eur Urol 2001;40(4):422–6.
43. Mian C, Lodde M, Haitel A, et al. Comparison of two qualitative assays, the UBC rapid test and the BTA stat test, in the diagnosis of urothelial cell carcinoma of the bladder. Urology 2000;56(2):228–31.
44. Sarosdy MF, Hudson MA, Ellis WJ, et al. Improved detection of recurrent bladder cancer using the Bard BTA stat Test. Urology 1997; 50(3):349–53.
45. Toma MI, Friedrich MG, Hautmann SH, et al. Comparison of the ImmunoCyt test and urinary cytology with other urine tests in the detection and surveillance of bladder cancer. World J Urol 2004; 22(2):145–9.
46. Fradet Y, Lockhard C. Performance characteristics of a new monoclonal antibody test for bladder cancer: ImmunoCyt trade mark. Can J Urol 1997; 4(3):400–5.
47. Vriesema JL, Atsma F, Kiemeney LA, et al. Diagnostic efficacy of the ImmunoCyt test to detect superficial bladder cancer recurrence. Urology 2001;58(3):367–71.
48. Allard P, Fradet Y, Tetu B, et al. Tumor-associated antigens as prognostic factors for recurrence in 382 patients with primary transitional cell carcinoma of the bladder. Clin Cancer Res 1995;1(10): 1195–202.
49. Mian C, Maier K, Comploj E, et al. uCyt+/ImmunoCyt in the detection of recurrent urothelial carcinoma: an update on 1991 analyses. Cancer 2006; 108(1):60–5.
50. Mian C, Lodde M, Comploj E, et al. The value of the ImmunoCyt/uCyt+ test in the detection and follow-up of carcinoma in situ of the urinary bladder. Anticancer Res 2005;25(5):3641–4.
51. Odisho AY, Berry AB, Ahmad AE, et al. Reflex ImmunoCyt testing for the diagnosis of bladder cancer in patients with atypical urine cytology. Eur Urol 2012. [Epub ahead of print].
52. Botteman MF, Pashos CL, Redaelli A, et al. The health economics of bladder cancer: a comprehensive review of the published literature. Pharmacoeconomics 2003;21(18):1315–30.
53. Lotan Y, Svatek RS, Sagalowsky AI. Should we screen for bladder cancer in a high-risk population?: a cost per life-year saved analysis. Cancer 2006; 107(5):982–90.
54. Yossepowitch O, Herr HW, Donat SM. Use of urinary biomarkers for bladder cancer surveillance: patient perspectives. J Urol 2007;177(4):1277–82 [discussion: 1282].
55. Kamat AM, Karam JA, Grossman HB, et al. Prospective trial to identify optimal bladder cancer surveillance protocol: reducing costs while maximizing sensitivity. BJU Int 2011;108(7):1119–23.
56. Kamat AM, Hegarty PK, Gee JR, et al. ICUD-EAU international consultation on bladder cancer 2012: screening, diagnosis, and molecular markers. Eur Urol 2013;63(1):4–15.
57. van der Aa MN, Steyerberg EW, Bangma C, et al. Cystoscopy revisited as the gold standard for detecting bladder cancer recurrence: diagnostic review bias in the randomized, prospective CEFUB trial. J Urol 2010;183(1):76–80.
58. Whitson J, Berry A, Carroll P, et al. A multicolour fluorescence in situ hybridization test predicts recurrence in patients with high-risk superficial bladder tumours undergoing intravesical therapy. BJU Int 2009; 104(3):336–9.
59. Mengual L, Marin-Aguilera M, Ribal MJ, et al. Clinical utility of fluorescent in situ hybridization for the

surveillance of bladder cancer patients treated with bacillus Calmette-Guerin therapy. Eur Urol 2007; 52(3):752–9.

60. Savic S, Zlobec I, Thalmann GN, et al. The prognostic value of cytology and fluorescence in situ hybridization in the follow-up of nonmuscle-invasive bladder cancer after intravesical Bacillus Calmette-Guerin therapy. Int J Cancer 2009; 124(12):2899–904.
61. Kamat AM, Dickstein RJ, Messetti F, et al. Use of fluorescence in situ hybridization to predict response to bacillus Calmette-Guerin therapy for bladder cancer: results of a prospective trial. J Urol 2012;187(3):862–7.

Office-based Bladder Tumor Fulguration and Surveillance
Indications and Techniques

Brock B. O'Neil, MD[a], William T. Lowrance, MD, MPH[b,*]

KEYWORDS

• Bladder cancer • Fulguration • Electrocoagulation • Laser • Recurrence

KEY POINTS

- Low-grade (LG) noninvasive bladder cancer is a heterogeneous disease with variable recurrence and progression rates, and helpful tools are available to appropriately risk-stratify patients.
- Substantial cost is accrued from management of recurrent LG bladder cancer in operating rooms.
- Office-based management of LG noninvasive bladder cancer is a cost-effective, well-tolerated, and safe strategy when applied to suitable patients.

INTRODUCTION

Bladder cancer is the fourth most common malignancy among men in the United States, with 52,050 expected newly diagnosed cases in 2011 and 17,320 cases among women. Although 14,990 deaths were expected during the same time period, most cases of bladder cancers are noninvasive and LG.[1,2] Despite the low risk for lethality, non-muscle invasive bladder cancer (NMIBC) has a substantial risk for recurrence and progression occurs in some cases.[3]

Recurrent disease has long been managed with resection and fulguration.[4] This is often performed in an operating room, resulting in significant expense, possible morbidity, and repeated exposure to general anesthesia. Some investigators have proposed alternative strategies for managing LG NMIBC, including office-based interventions in attempts to control cost and improve quality of life without exposing patients to unnecessary risks. This article examines the rationale, efficacy, and logistics of managing NMIBC in the office setting, thereby avoiding the need for intraoperative management for all recurrent LG NMIBC.

LOW-GRADE NON-MUSCLE INVASIVE BLADDER CANCER

In efforts to clarify confusion surrounding papillary bladder tumors, the World Health Organization and the International Society of Urological Pathology created a more stringent pathology classification scheme for bladder cancer. This system classifies non-muscle invasive papillary tumors into papilloma, papillary urothelial neoplasm of low malignant potential, LG, and high grade.[5] There are significant differences in recurrence rates between tumors in this schema (**Fig. 1**).[6] The risk for the first 3 of these groups for progression to invasive disease is low, with 0% to 1.2% for papillomas, 0% to 8% for papillary urothelial neoplasms of low malignant potential, and 5% to 13% for LG papillary tumors in contrast to progression rates greater than 45% for high-grade tumors.[3,6–8] Although investigators report a variety of predictors for recurrence and progression, the strongest seem to include tumor stage, size, number, early previous recurrences, and presence of carcinoma in situ (CIS).[3]

The updated classification scheme provides additional information to better risk-stratify patients,

Disclosures: None.

[a] Division of Urology, University of Utah, 30 North 1900 East, Salt Lake City, UT 84132, USA; [b] Division of Urology, Huntsman Cancer Institute, University of Utah, 1950 Circle of Hope, Salt Lake City, UT 84112, USA
* Corresponding author.
E-mail address: will.lowrance@hci.utah.edu

Urol Clin N Am 40 (2013) 175–182
http://dx.doi.org/10.1016/j.ucl.2013.01.007

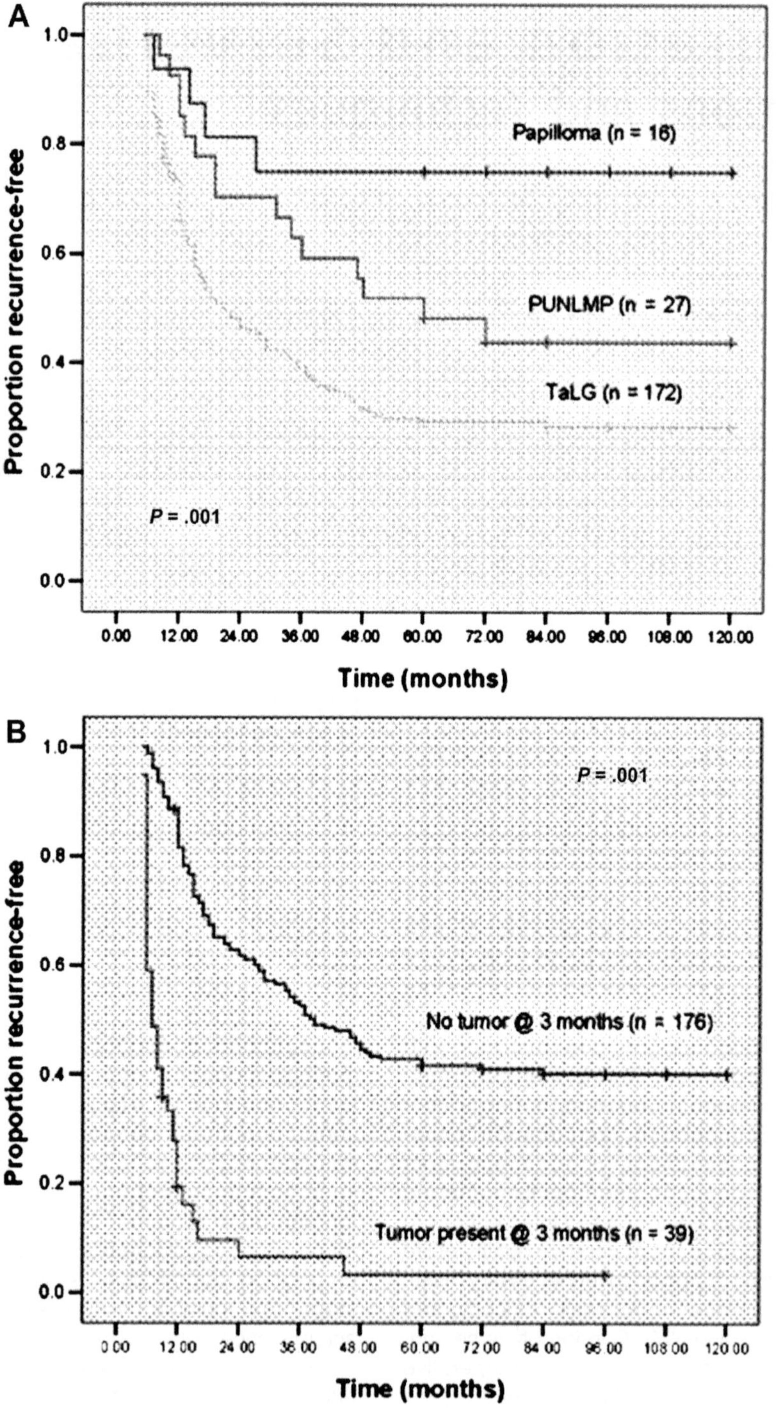

Fig. 1. (*A*) Recurrence-free survival by tumor type. (*B*) Recurrence-free survival by 3-month cystoscopy. (*From* Herr HW, Donat SM, Reuter VE. Management of low grade papillary bladder tumors. J Urol 2007;178(4 Pt 1):1201–5 [discussion: 1205]; with permission.)

distinguishing those who may need more-aggressive therapy from those who do not.[9] Yet many perform cystoscopy every 3 months for the first 2 or 3 years, every 6 months for the following 2 years, and yearly thereafter, regardless of the risk of recurrence and progression. However, this strategy has not been shown more effective than less-rigorous surveillance protocols and subjects patients to frequent interventions that may not be of benefit and increase the cost of care. As a result, most argue for an approach tailored to patients' risk of recurrence and progression.[10]

Not all investigators agree with this approach. Leblanc and colleagues[11] presented data for patients initially diagnosed with Ta grade 1 disease and with follow-up of more than 5 years. They reported an overall recurrence rate of 55%, with 14% having recurrences more than 5 years from initial diagnosis. Progression to higher grade or stage was identified in 37%, but only 3.3% developed muscle invasive disease. These investigators argue for frequent cystoscopic evaluation continuing beyond 5 years.

VISUAL GRADING

An additional key to appropriately offer less-invasive treatment without harming those who require more-aggressive care is the ability to reliably differentiate between low-risk and high-risk tumors based on visual appearance. Herr and colleagues[12] found that experienced urologists were able to correctly identify 93% of lesions that had recurred after initial diagnosis of NMIBC as Ta grade 1 tumors. When voided urine cytology was added, accuracy increased to 99% for Ta grade 1 tumors. The investigators did not outline specific cystoscopic criteria that the performing urologist used but rather this determination was made by an overall impression of the surgeon based on experience. Other investigators have attempted to more rigorously outline criteria for higher-risk tumors. Satoh and colleagues[13] found that tumors greater than 1 cm, those sessile in nature, and nonpapillary tumors were more likely to have muscle invasion.

COST

Management of bladder cancer has the highest cost of any malignancy per patient covered by Medicare, with lifetime costs per patient ranging from $96,000 to $187,000.[14] When modeling for patients of all ages, including those younger than 65 years, another group estimated the lifetime costs for patients presenting with bladder cancer between $99,270 and $120,684. They found that 60% of these cost were related to surveillance and treatment of recurrences, with patients averaging 2.9 cystoscopies per patient per year.[15]

Study of cost-effective treatment of bladder cancer is limited and has not been incorporated into treatment guidelines.[16] However, it is intuitive that substantial cost reductions may be achieved by shifting surveillance from frequent invasive procedures to less-frequent, risk-stratified protocols that use office-based management strategies in appropriately selected patients. Strategies that risk-stratify patients for surveillance cystoscopy and upper-tract imaging can reduce the frequency with which patients who have low-risk disease undergo costly and invasive procedures without exposing them to additional risk.[17]

Treatment and surveillance schedules for early-stage bladder cancer vary greatly by provider[18] and higher intensity does not seem to prevent later treatments or need for major medical interventions, such as cystectomy. Furthermore, those who used high-intensity treatment and surveillance were more likely to use major medical interventions later on, contributing to higher costs.[19]

Office-based fulguration instead of resection in operating rooms has the benefit of avoiding outpatient facility, anesthesia, and pathologist fees in addition to decreasing patient time commitment and convalescence. Recognizing the potential cost savings of in-office procedures for the management of NMIBC, the Centers for Medicare and Medicaid Services increased physician reimbursement for office-based endoscopic procedures by a factor of almost 10 for office fulguration and by 3 for biopsy. However, in one faculty practice, this change in reimbursement did not decrease the overall cost for treating patients but instead resulted in an almost doubling in charges.[20]

OFFICE-BASED MANAGEMENT

Several investigators have reported various approaches to office-based management of LG NMIBC with good outcomes. Outpatient fulguration with electrocautery of LG bladder tumors was described more than 30 years ago with substantial cost savings over inpatient management.[21] Herr[22] then described management of 185 patients with superficial bladder tumors using a flexible cystoscope, fulguration with a Bugbee electrode, and only local anesthethsia. No patient requested that the procedure be stopped and at 24 months, 63% remained tumor-free. Wedderburn and coworkers[23] reported on office-based treatment of 103 consecutive patients with recurrent LG Ta lesions using only nonanesthetizing lubricant gel, with 80% reporting negligible or mild discomfort and only

2 patients reporting that they would have preferred the procedure to be done under a general anesthetic. No recurrence was found in 50.5%, with a median follow-up of 21 months, but 25.5% of those that recurred did so at the original treatment site. An update of the experience at Memorial Sloan-Kettering Cancer Center reported outcomes of office-based fulguration alone in 123 patients with recurrent NMIBC. Median follow-up was 6.84 years, and 73% had no evidence of disease, 21.7% were alive with disease, and 2.2% died from disease.[24]

Variations on the use of traditional fulguration with electrocautery have been reported. Muraishi and colleagues[25] described using a biopsy forceps with electrocautery to simultaneously cauterize and obtain a specimen for pathologic evaluation. They subsequently updated this procedure by insufflating the bladder with CO_2, injecting the tumor with a mixture of 2% xylocaine and indigo carmine, and then resecting the tumor with hot biopsy cup forceps.[26]

Use of the holmium:YAG laser alone or in combination with intravesical agents has also been reported for management of NMIBC. Jonler and colleagues[27] described ablation with a holmium laser in an office setting, using urethral lidocaine alone in 52 patients. No pain was reported in 86% and all stated they preferred this method to traditional transurethral resection (TUR). Unfortunately, no follow-up data were provided to assess the adequacy of treatment. Other investigators have reported limited follow-up but with acceptable recurrence rates.[28,29]

In a nonrandomized study comparing holmium laser with traditional TUR, Zhu and colleagues[30] reported using the laser to resect rather than just ablate NMIBC under epidural anesthesia. They reported no difference in recurrence rate between the 2 therapies with mean follow-up of 34 months but with the advantage of fewer bladder perforations and bleeding complications. However, resection rather than ablation with laser may be too difficult or uncomfortable to do in the office and access to the laser generator in this setting may limit its use. For these and other logistical reasons, the authors favor office-based ablation with electrocautery rather than office-based holmium laser ablation.

PATIENT SELECTION

Proper risk stratification is critical for appropriate application of office-based management of NMIBC to those patients who are likely to benefit without exposing other patients to undue risk for recurrence or progression. Millan-Rodriguez and colleagues[31] risk-stratified patients with NMIBC into low-risk, intermediate-risk, and high-risk groups with good discriminative ability for recurrence, progression, and mortality using data from 1529 patients. The European Organisation for Research and Treatment of Cancer (EORTC) combined data from 7 randomized trials comparing treatments after initial diagnosis of Ta, T1, and CIS bladder cancer in more than 2500 patients to create tables that allow for calculation of short-term and long-term risks of recurrence and progression.[3] Number of tumors, tumor size, prior recurrence rate, stage, presence of CIS, and grade are used to place each patient into a 4-tier risk group both for recurrence and progression at 1 year and 5 years (**Tables 1** and **2**). A calculator based on these data is available at: http://www.eortc.be/tools/bladdercalculator/.

Combining these tables with an experienced eye at determining recurrent LG bladder lesions based on appearance,[12] appropriate patients can

Table 1
Weights for calculating EORTC recurrence and progression scores

Factor	Recurrence	Progression
Number of tumors		
Single	0	0
2 to 7	3	3
≥8	6	3
Tumor size		
<3 cm	0	0
≥3 cm	3	3
Prior recurrence rate		
Primary	0	0
≤1 Rec/y	2	2
>1 Rec/y	4	2
T category		
Ta	0	0
T1	1	4
CIS		
No	0	0
Yes	1	6
Grade		
G1	0	0
G2	1	0
G3	2	5
Total score	0–17	0–23

Abbreviation: Rec, recurrence.

From Sylvester RJ, van der Meijden AP, Oosterlinck W, et al. Predicting recurrence and progression in individual patients with stage Ta T1 bladder cancer using EORTC risk tables: a combined analysis of 2596 patients from seven EORTC trials. Eur Urol 2006;49(3):466–5 [discussion: 475–7]; with permission.

Table 2
Probability of recurrence and progression according to total EORTC score

	Probability Recurrence, 1 y (95% CI)	Probability Recurrence, 5 y (95% CI)
Recurrence score		
0	15% (10%, 19%)	31% (24%, 37%)
1–4	24% (21%, 26%)	46% (42%, 49%)
5–9	38% (35%, 41%)	62% (58%, 65%)
10–17	61% (55%, 67%)	78% (73%, 84%)
Progression score		
0	0.2% (0%, 0.7%)	0.8% (0%, 1.7%)
2–6	1.0% (0.4%, 1.6%)	6% (5%, 8%)
7–13	5% (4%, 7%)	17% (14%, 20%)
14–2	17% (10%, 24%)	45% (35%, 55%)

From Sylvester RJ, van der Meijden AP, Oosterlinck W, et al. Predicting recurrence and progression in individual patients with stage Ta T1 bladder cancer using EORTC risk tables: a combined analysis of 2596 patients from seven EORTC trials. Eur Urol 2006;49(3):466–5 [discussion: 475–7]; with permission.

be selected for office-based management. A hypothetical patient presenting with 4 small, LG, noninvasive-appearing recurrent tumors found more than 12 months from the primary resection is a reasonable patient for offering this approach. This patient would have 1-year and 5-year risks of recurrence of 38% and 62%, and progression rates of 1% and 6%, respectively.

Although no prospective work has provided a cutoff of risk stratification at which it is safe to offer office-based management, a suggested treatment algorithm has been proposed by Donat and colleagues[24] (**Fig. 2**). The authors typically offer this strategy to patients who have fewer than 5 recurrent tumors that are smaller than 1 cm, appear to be LG Ta, and have a progression score that puts them in the bottom 2 risk groups (EORTC progression score <7).

PATIENT PREPARATION AND PROCEDURE TECHNIQUE

After appropriately selecting patients based on the previously outlined criteria, the authors discuss the benefits of office-based management, including avoiding an intraoperative procedure and associated morbidity, decreased time commitment, convalescence, and cost. Then, what patients will experience during the procedure is outlined, including distinguishing the procedure from diagnostic cystoscopy, describing the sensation of the cautery device as a light pinprick, and that the procedure will be stopped at any time if requested. Informed consent is obtained before proceeding.

Prior to the procedure, patients provide a voided urine specimen that is checked with a dipstick urinalysis to ensure there is no sign of a urinary tract infection. Patients are given a single dose of oral antibiotics for urinary tract infection prophylaxis. The authors follow recommendations by Herr and colleagues[12] to obtain a cytology specimen at the time of fulguration to increase the discriminative power of visual inspection for correctly identifying LG NMIBC. If cytology is later found positive for high-grade disease, patients are taken to an operating room for formal TUR and pathologic evaluation. The authors do not routinely obtain tumor fragments for pathology during office-based fulguration because this increases the cost of the procedure and has not proved necessary beyond visual diagnosis and cytology. However, biopsy devices are available for obtaining specimens for those who desire that pathologic information.

Patients are positioned on a procedure table in the supine position for men or low lithotomy for women. The authors typically instill 2% lidocaine gel per urethra. Others administer a lidocaine solution into the bladder with a catheter and allow the solution to dwell in combination with or instead of the urethral lidocaine gel.

The authors use a 17-French flexible cystoscope with a 5-French working port and a camera displaying the image on a monitor at the bedside. Sterile water is used for irrigation and a flexible monopolar Bugbee electrode is passed through the scope to fulgurate tumors. Typically, the coagulation setting is turned to 25 W. The authors begin cauterizing the papillary fronds, move centrally, and finish at the base; the base tends to be more sensitive, and the authors find it better tolerated in this order. Some clinics do not have access to a cautery generator, limiting the ability to perform office-based fulguration. This generator, or even the more expensive holmium:YAG laser generators, may be borrowed from an operating room when needed instead of purchasing a dedicated device for a clinic.

Descriptions of holmium:YAG settings and technique vary and are flexible, depending on surgeon experience and preference. Published series report use of 200-μm to 550-μm laser fibers, power settings of 10 W to 40 W (1–2.2 J at 10–40 Hz), and vaporization with or without tumor resection.[27,29,30]

An indwelling catheter is not routinely left in place after the procedure. Patients are educated on expected findings of bladder spasms, mild hematuria, and irritative voiding symptoms and instructed to monitor for signs and symptoms of

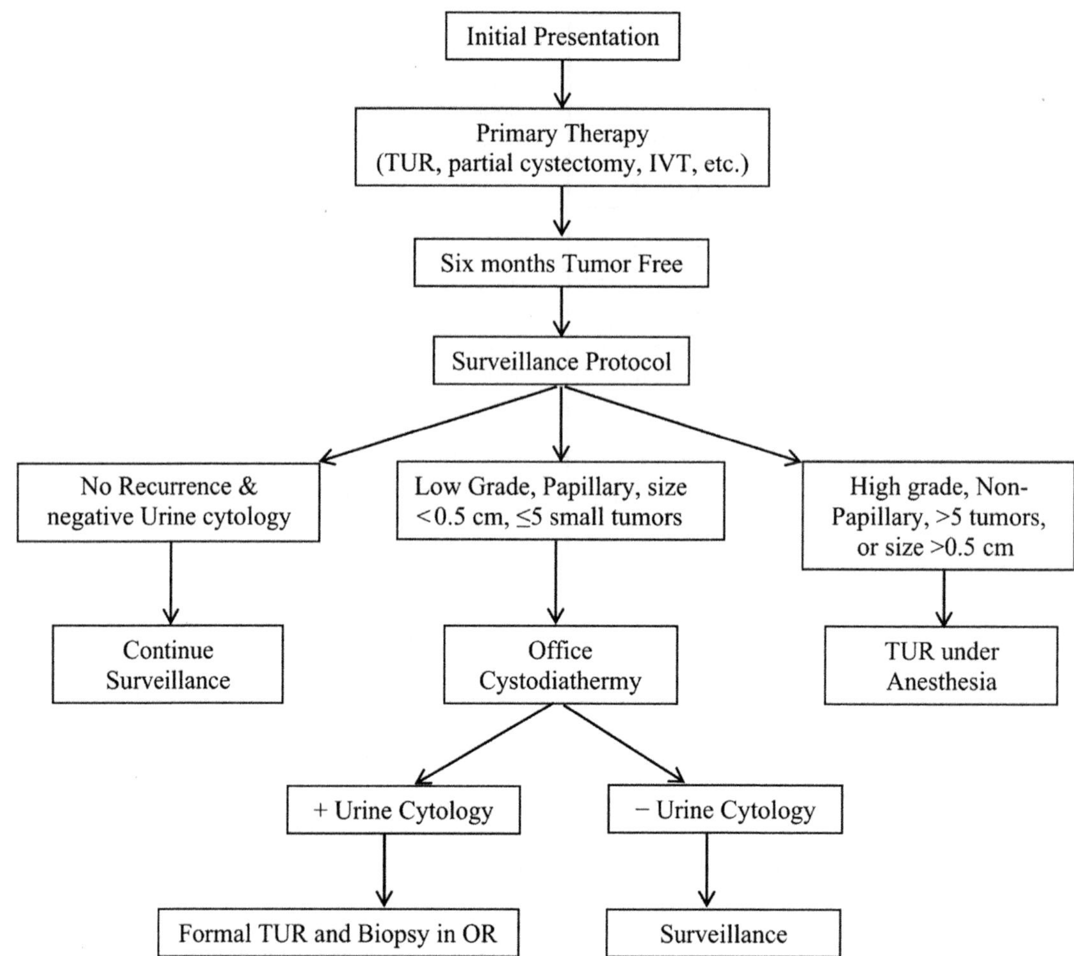

Fig. 2. Treatment algorithm for LG NMIBC. IVT, intravesical therapy; OR, operating room. (*From* Donat SM, North A, Dalbagni G, et al. Efficacy of office fulguration for recurrent low grade papillary bladder tumors less than 0.5 cm. J Urol 2004;171(2 Pt 1):636–9; with permission.)

urinary tract infections. The authors provide a prescription for a few doses of narcotic pain medication and an anticholinergic for bladder spasms but do not routinely continue antibiotics beyond a single preoperative dose. Patients are required to void before discharge from clinic to minimize the risk of urinary retention at home.

FOLLOW-UP

In the absence of guidance from level I medical evidence, the follow-up schedules for surveillance cystoscopy after treatment of NMIBC tend to be variable. Most agree that a risk-adapted strategy should be used to personalize patients' follow-up cystoscopies according to their individual risk of tumor recurrence or disease progression. The authors tend to follow patients with LG NMIBC who undergo office-based fulguration in the following manner: history and physical examination, urine cytology, and surveillance cystoscopy at 3 months; then, every 6 months through 2 years; and then, annually, unless there are tumor recurrences. The National Comprehensive Cancer Network and the European Association of Urology provide further guidelines on surveillance for NMIBC at the following Web addresses: https://subscriptions.nccn.org/login.aspx; http://www.uroweb.org/guidelines/online-guidelines/.

ALTERNATIVES

An initial expectant management approach has been proposed by other investigators who argue that resection or fulguration is not needed at the initial finding of recurrent lesions in patients with LG NMIBC. Soloway and colleagues[32] presented data from 32 patients with a history of resected bladder cancer who underwent an initial observation period after diagnosis of a new lesion.

Criteria for resection included significant growth, change in appearance suggesting grade or stage progression, or hematuria. Mean time observing tumors before operative intervention was 10 months and 3 of 45 observed tumors progressed to high-grade lesions. Eight tumors spontaneously regressed during observation. It is unreasonable to monitor small LG NMIBC lesions before office-based fulguration, but there is a risk that lesions could grow sufficiently to require management in an operating room.

COMPLICATIONS

No reports have specifically addressed complications of office-based fulguration. Rates of early postoperative complications after traditional operative TUR have been reported at 5.1% and include need for reoperation (2.7%), bleeding requiring transfusion (3.4%), bladder perforation (1.3%), and sepsis (<1%).[33] The authors' experience is that there is minimal postprocedure bleeding and they have not had any episodes requiring transfusion or operative/inpatient management for hematuria. Infection rates should approach those of similar endoscopic procedures, and the authors have not had any episodes of bladder perforation.

SUMMARY

LG non-muscle invasive bladder tumors recur frequently but typically have a low progression rate. Prior studies have shown that such tumors may be managed successfully with an office-based treatment approach rather than proceeding to an operating room for a formal TUR. Such an approach likely reduces operative and anesthetic-associated morbidity and cost. In carefully selected patients, office-based management of LG noninvasive bladder cancer is cost effective, well-tolerated, and represents a safe treatment strategy for recurrent LG-appearing bladder tumors.

REFERENCES

1. Siegel R, Ward E, Brawley O, et al. Cancer statistics, 2011: the impact of eliminating socioeconomic and racial disparities on premature cancer deaths. CA Cancer J Clin 2011;61:212–36. United States.
2. Fleshner NE, Herr HW, Stewart AK, et al. The national cancer data base report on bladder carcinoma. The American College of Surgeons Commission on Cancer and the American Cancer Society. Cancer 1996;78:1505–13. United States.
3. Sylvester RJ, van der Meijden AP, Oosterlinck W, et al. Predicting recurrence and progression in individual patients with stage Ta T1 bladder cancer using EORTC risk tables: a combined analysis of 2596 patients from seven EORTC trials. Eur Urol 2006;49(3):466–5 [discussion: 475–7].
4. Herr HW. Legacy of Edwin Beer: fulguration of papillary bladder tumors. J Urol 2005;173:1087–9. United States.
5. Epstein JI, Amin MB, Reuter VR, et al. The World Health Organization/International Society of Urological Pathology consensus classification of urothelial (transitional cell) neoplasms of the urinary bladder. Bladder Consensus Conference Committee. Am J Surg Pathol 1998;22(12):1435–48.
6. Herr HW, Donat SM, Reuter VE. Management of low grade papillary bladder tumors. J Urol 2007; 178(4 Pt 1):1201–5 [discussion: 1205].
7. Holmang S, Hedelin H, Anderstrom C, et al. Recurrence and progression in low grade papillary urothelial tumors. J Urol 1999;162(3 Pt 1):702–7.
8. Haukaas S, Daehlin L, Maartmann-Moe H, et al. The long-term outcome in patients with superficial transitional cell carcinoma of the bladder: a single-institutional experience. BJU Int 1999;83:957–63. England.
9. Schned AR, Andrew AS, Marsit CJ, et al. Survival following the diagnosis of noninvasive bladder cancer: WHO/International Society of Urological Pathology versus WHO classification systems. J Urol 2007;178(4 Pt 1):1196–200 [discussion: 1200].
10. Lamm D, Colombel M, Persad R, et al. Clinical practice recommendations for the management of non–muscle invasive bladder cancer. Eur Urol Suppl 2008;7(10):651–66.
11. Leblanc B, Duclos AJ, Benard F, et al. Long-term followup of initial Ta grade 1 transitional cell carcinoma of the bladder. J Urol 1999;162(6):1946–50.
12. Herr HW, Donat SM, Dalbagni G. Correlation of cystoscopy with histology of recurrent papillary tumors of the bladder. J Urol 2002;168(3):978–80.
13. Satoh E, Miyao N, Tachiki H, et al. Prediction of muscle invasion of bladder cancer by cystoscopy. Eur Urol 2002;41:178–81. Netherlands.
14. Botteman MF, Pashos CL, Hauser RS, et al. Quality of life aspects of bladder cancer: a review of the literature. Qual Life Res 2003;12(6):675–88.
15. Avritscher EB, Cooksley CD, Grossman HB, et al. Clinical model of lifetime cost of treating bladder cancer and associated complications. Urology 2006;68(3):549–53.
16. Noyes K, Singer EA, Messing EM. Healthcare economics of bladder cancer: cost-enhancing and cost-reducing factors. Curr Opin Urol 2008;18(5): 533–9.
17. Young MJ, Soloway MS. Office evaluation and management of bladder neoplasms. Urol Clin North Am 1998;25(4):603–11.
18. Schrag D, Hsieh LJ, Rabbani F, et al. Adherence to surveillance among patients with superficial bladder cancer. J Natl Cancer Inst 2003;95(8):588–97.

19. Hollenbeck BK, Ye Z, Dunn RL, et al. Provider treatment intensity and outcomes for patients with early-stage bladder cancer. J Natl Cancer Inst 2009; 101(8):571–80.
20. Hemani ML, Makarov DV, Huang WC, et al. The effect of changes in Medicare reimbursement on the practice of office and hospital-based endoscopic surgery for bladder cancer. Cancer 2010; 116(5):1264–71.
21. Klein FA, Whitmore WF Jr. Bladder papilloma: therapeutic and cost effect of outpatient department management. Urology 1981;18(3):247–9.
22. Herr HW. Outpatient flexible cystoscopy and fulguration of recurrent superficial bladder tumors. J Urol 1990;144(6):1365–6.
23. Wedderburn AW, Ratan P, Birch BR. A prospective trial of flexible cystodiathermy for recurrent transitional cell carcinoma of the bladder. J Urol 1999; 161(3):812–4.
24. Donat SM, North A, Dalbagni G, et al. Efficacy of office fulguration for recurrent low grade papillary bladder tumors less than 0.5 cm. J Urol 2004; 171(2 Pt 1):636–9.
25. Muraishi O, Mitsu S, Suzuki K, et al. A technique for resection of small bladder tumors using a flexible cystoscope on an outpatient basis: bladder tumor resection with newly designed hot cup forceps. J Urol 2001;166(5):1817–9.
26. Endo F, Shiga Y, Yashi M, et al. Office-based transurethral resection of multiple bladder tumors using blue dye-mixed local anesthesia: a descriptive cohort study. J Endourol 2010;24(2):267–70.
27. Jonler M, Lund L, Bisballe S. Holmium:YAG laser vaporization of recurrent papillary tumours of the bladder under local anaesthesia. BJU Int 2004; 94(3):322–5.
28. Syed HA, Biyani CS, Bryan N, et al. Holmium:YAG laser treatment of recurrent superficial bladder carcinoma: initial clinical experience. J Endourol 2001;15(6):625–7.
29. Soler-Martinez J, Vozmediano-Chicharro R, Morales-Jimenez P, et al. Holmium laser treatment for low grade, low stage, noninvasive bladder cancer with local anesthesia and early instillation of mitomycin C. J Urol 2007;178(6):2337–9.
30. Zhu Y, Jiang X, Zhang J, et al. Safety and efficacy of holmium laser resection for primary nonmuscle-invasive bladder cancer versus transurethral electroresection: single-center experience. Urology 2008;72:608–12.
31. Millan-Rodriguez F, Chechile-Toniolo G, Salvador-Bayarri J, et al. Primary superficial bladder cancer risk groups according to progression, mortality and recurrence. J Urol 2000;164(3 Pt 1):680–4.
32. Soloway MS, Bruck DS, Kim SS. Expectant management of small, recurrent, noninvasive papillary bladder tumors. J Urol 2003;170(2 Pt 1):438–41.
33. Collado A, Chechile GE, Salvador J, et al. Early complications of endoscopic treatment for superficial bladder tumors. J Urol 2000;164:1529–32.

Perioperative Chemotherapy
When to Use It, What to Use, and Why

David C. Johnson, MD, Raj S. Pruthi, MD*,
Michael E. Woods, MD

KEYWORDS

• Bladder cancer • Noninvasive • Chemotherapy • Intravesical • Perioperative

KEY POINTS

- Numerous intravesical chemotherapy agents are available for use in non-muscle invasive bladder cancer with different mechanisms of action and side-effect profiles.
- In the absence of suspected bladder perforation, immediate perioperative dose of intravesical chemotherapy reduces the risk of recurrence for low-grade disease.
- Induction and maintenance therapy is recommended in intermediate-risk disease.
- Intravesical chemotherapy is being investigated as a possible second-line treatment of high-risk non-muscle invasive bladder cancer in patients who are not operative candidates or who refuse cystectomy.

INTRODUCTION

Although transurethral resection of bladder tumor (TURBT) is the gold standard for initial diagnosis and primary treatment of non-muscle invasive bladder cancer (NMIBC),[1–6] up to 45% of patients will have a tumor recurrence within the first year after TURBT alone and 3% to 15% of patients will have tumor progression.[2] Tumor cells left in the bladder mucosa after incomplete TURBT as well as free tumor cells that reimplant immediately following TURBT are thought to contribute to the high rate of recurrence. Cytotoxic intravesical chemotherapy is a recommended adjunct to endoscopic resection to reduce the risk of post-TURBT tumor cell implantation and subsequent tumor recurrence, particularly in lower-risk tumors.[1–6] Instillation of antitumor agents into the bladder allows direct contact with the mucosa and tumor cells and minimizes systemic effects.

A variety of agents are available with distinct characteristics, mechanism of action, cost, and side-effect profile. These agents include mitomycin C (MMC); thiotepa; gemcitabine; and intercalating agents, such as doxorubicin, epirubicin, and valrubicin (**Table 1**). The cytotoxic ability of the chemotherapy agents is proportional to the concentration of the agent in the bladder and duration of exposure rather than the size of the dose administered.[7] Absorption, efficacy, and systemic toxicity depend on molecular characteristics, pH during instillation, and time to administration following resection.

Most chemotherapy agents are well tolerated, particularly a single perioperative dose. Local lower urinary tract symptoms, including frequency, urgency, and dysuria, are the most frequently reported side effects.[2,8] Hematuria, bladder pain, and prostatitis are encountered with similar frequency in all agents. Bladder contracture is a rare event with chemotherapy treatment; and systemic side effects (immunologic reactions, malaise/fatigue, nausea/vomiting, and neurologic, cardiovascular, or pulmonary complications) are less frequently seen than with immunotherapy regimens, such as bacilli Calmette-Guerin (BCG)

Disclosures: None.
Department of Urology, University of North Carolina, 2113 Physicians Office Building, CB 7235, 170 Manning Drive, Chapel Hill, NC 27599-7235, USA
* Corresponding author.
E-mail address: raj_pruthi@med.unc.edu

Urol Clin N Am 40 (2013) 183–195
http://dx.doi.org/10.1016/j.ucl.2013.01.001
0094-0143/13/$ – see front matter

Table 1
Intravesical chemotherapeutic agents

Agent	MW (kD)	Cystitis (%)	Other Toxicity	Dropout Rate (%)	Dose/Concentration	Cost ($)
Doxorubicin	580	20–40	Fever, allergy, bladder contraction (5%)	2–16	50 mg/50 mL	36
Epirubicin	580	10–30	Contracted bladder (rare)	3–6	50 mg/50 mL	595
Valrubicin	724	23–77	Rash (rare)	—	800 mg/55 mL	4400
MMC	328	30–40	Rash (8%–19%), contracted bladder (5%)	2–14	40 mg/20 mL	130
Thiotepa	189	10–30	Myelosuppression (8%–19%)	2–11	30 mg/30 mL	80
Gemcitabine	300	Minimal	Nausea (rare)	<10	1–2 g/50–100 mL	540–1080

Abbreviation: MW, molecular weight.

Data from Jones JS, Campbell SC. Non-muscle-invasive bladder cancer (ta, T1, and CIS). In: Wein AJ, Kavoussi LR, Novick AC, et al, editors. Campbell-Walsh Urology. 10th edition. Philadelphia: Elsevier; 2011. p. 2447–67; and O'Donnell MA. Practical applications of intravesical chemotherapy and immunotherapy in high-risk patients with superficial bladder cancer. Urol Clin North Am 2005;32(2):121–31.

and/or interferon. Side effects significantly increase with multiple doses of chemotherapy, which can make completing these regimens difficult.

In clinical practice, significant variations exist in treatment intensity and adherence to best-practice guidelines that tend toward underuse of intravesical therapy.[9–12] Physician self-reporting suggests that practice setting (private vs academic), years in practice, and tumor grade were associated with deviations from published guidelines.[13] These variations likely have significant economic as well as oncologic implications that warrant further study and efforts for quality improvement.[11,13] Clinicians should be informed on the most up-to-date evidence-based guidelines for intravesical chemotherapy for NMIBC.

CHEMOTHERAPY AGENTS: CHARACTERISTICS, DOSING, AND ADVERSE EVENTS

MMC

MMC is the most frequently used and thoroughly studied intravesical chemotherapy agent for NMIBC (see **Table 1**). It is a 328-kD DNA alkylating agent derived from *Streptomyces caespitosus*. It binds to DNA and causes a reductive activation reaction followed by 2 N-alkylations. This reaction results in DNA crosslinking, synthesis inhibition, and strand breakage. Although MMC is cell-cycle nonspecific, it seems to be more active during the G1 and S phases.

Optimal dosing and administration schedule continue to be debated.[14] Dosage varies between 20 to 80 mg per instillation.[7] Previously, the most commonly used dosing for multidose regimens was 40 mg in 40 mL of saline or sterile water administered weekly for 8 weeks followed by monthly for 1 year.[2] In 2001, Au and colleagues[15] studied measures to optimize the efficacy of MMC in a phase III randomized trial, which have largely been adopted as the standard of care. Higher drug dose (40 mg vs 20 mg), higher concentration (20 mL vs 40 mL) urinary alkalization (1.3 g $NaHCO_3$ by mouth the night prior, morning of, and 30 minutes before treatment), a period of dehydration before treatment (no fluids for 8 hours prior), and confirmed bladder emptying before instillation (<10 mL by ultrasound bladder scan) in the treatment arm resulted in increased recurrence-free survival. MMC is more stable in alkaline environments, yet its cytotoxic effect is greater in acidic urine. Whether its increased cytotoxic effect in lower pH outweighs its greater stability at a higher pH is unknown and a potential area for future study.[16] Other methods of optimizing drug delivery, including microwave hyperthermia and electromotive instillation to accelerate drug delivery into and across biologic membranes, have shown promise; but further confirmatory studies are required before becoming routinely used.[17–20]

Because of its moderately high molecular weight of 328 kD, transurothelial absorption of MMC is minimal. Therefore, systemic symptoms and life-threatening complications, such as myelosuppression, are rare. Bladder contraction and bladder wall calcification are also uncommon to

MMC. Primary complications include chemical cystitis, contact dermatitis, and allergic reactions, which resolve with discontinuation of therapy and topical steroid application if necessary.[8] A meta-analysis reveals that local complication rate after TURBT with single-dose MMC is approximately 2%, which is comparable with the rate after TURBT alone.[2] However, the rate of local cystitis increases to 20% to 40% of patients receiving multiple administrations and/or maintenance courses of MMC.[2,21]

Intercalating Agents

Doxorubicin (580 kD), epirubicin (580 kD), and valrubicin (724 kD) are 3 chemotherapy agents in the anthracycline antibiotic class and are derived from the bacterium *Streptomyces peucetius*. These drugs are DNA intercalating agents, acting primarily by binding to DNA and inhibiting the progression of the enzyme topoisomerase II during DNA replication. The topoisomerase II complex is unable to reseal the replicating DNA double helix, thus resulting in strand breaks and inhibition of essential cellular protein synthesis. The intercalating agents have a broad range of chemotherapy activity, disrupting the cell by several mechanisms, including cell membrane disruption through the production of free radicals. These agents are not cell-cycle specific but have maximal activity during the S phase.

Dosing of doxorubicin ranges from 10 to 100 mg, with a wide variety of administration schedules, from 3 times a week to monthly.[2]

Increased side effects with doxorubicin, including local symptoms of chemical cystitis in up to 50% of patients, hematuria, and reports of decreased bladder capacity, make this agent a less desirable choice.[7,8] Systemic side effects are rare because of the high molecular weight of this compound, but occasional reports of life-threatening myelosuppression have been reported.

Epirubicin is a derivative of doxorubicin (4′ carbon epimere), differing only in to the presence of a daunosamine side chain. Similar in terms of mechanism of action and efficacy, the different spatial orientation of the hydroxyl group at the 4′ carbon of the sugar moiety may account for faster elimination and potentially reduced toxicity. Although epirubicin is approved by the Food and Drug Administration (FDA) for use in various malignancies in the United States, it is only available for use in urothelial cancer in Europe.

Epirubicin has been evaluated as a single perioperative dose and a full 8-week course. Dosing ranges from 50 mg per instillation for weekly dosing to 100 mg per dose with single instillations.[22,23]

Multiple investigators have demonstrated efficacy of doxorubicin and epirubicin in reducing recurrence but not progression on NMIBC[22–27]; however, current guidelines make no clear recommendation on the use of these agents for prophylactic chemotherapy because of the side-effect profile, lack of long-term efficacy results, and controversial results.[1,3–7]

Valrubicin is a semisynthetic analogue of doxorubicin reserved for use in select BCG-refractory tumors.[28–30] Similar to the other intercalating agents, valrubicin inhibits nucleoside incorporation into nucleic acids resulting in cell-cycle arrest in G2. In addition, the principal metabolites of valrubicin inhibit DNA synthesis through inhibition of topoisomerase II.[30]

It has several molecular-level differences from doxorubicin, which allows for more rapid uptake and accumulation into cells.[31] These differences account for valrubicin's decreased contact and cardiac toxicity.[32] The fact that valrubicin is a macromolecule explains the lack of systemic absorption and toxicity.

It was previously removed from the market in 2002 because of impurities in the original formulation but reintroduced in 2009 and approved for the treatment of BCG-refractory carcinoma in situ (CIS) in patients who are not candidates for radical cystectomy. Valrubicin is typically administered weekly for 6 weeks at a dose of 800 mg per instillation.[33]

Thiotepa

N,N′,N′-triethylenethiophosphoramide (Thiotepa, thiotepa, 189 kD) is an organophosphorous compound that disrupts DNA synthesis and promotes strand breakage through its DNA alkylation activity. This agent is not cell-cycle specific.

Thiotepa is the first and only chemotherapeutic agent specifically approved for intravesical treatment of papillary bladder cancer.[34] Although efficacy has been proven through numerous clinical trials dating back to the 1970s,[34–38] its low molecular weight results in systemic absorption of up to half of the administered dose and a subsequent higher rate of systemic side effects, including myelosuppression and skin rash.[8] Consequently, the risk-benefit analysis of thiotepa is less favorable than other currently available agents and infrequently used in clinical practice.

Gemcitabine

Gemcitabine (300 kD) is a relatively novel chemotherapy agent. First approved in the United States for the treatment of pancreatic cancer, it is classified as an antimetabolite and has a broad range of anticancer activity.[2] Its structure mimics that of cytosine, one of the pyrimidine molecules of DNA.

Phosphorylation of gemcitabine by nucleoside kinases within the cancer cell forms active metabolites (gemcitabine diphosphate and gemcitabine triphosphate), which block DNA synthesis and lead to apoptosis.[39]

Several pharmacologic properties of gemcitabine are conducive to effective intravesical treatment and support utility in NMIBC. In vitro, researchers have demonstrated a robust cytotoxic effect against cultured bladder cancer cells.[40] In vivo, low molecular weight and high lipid solubility allows adequate uptake into malignant cells, whereas high plasma clearance reduces the risk of systemic side effects caused by absorption of the drug.[41]

Doses of 500 mg, 1000 mg, and 2000 mg in 50 mL saline, instilled for 1 to 2 hours, and administered weekly for 6 weeks have been studied.[2,42] Recent phase I trials demonstrate a favorable safety profile,[43] and several small phase II trials have subsequently reported good tolerability and potential efficacy in tumor response and disease-free survival in certain patient populations.[42,44–47] Systemic and local toxicities were generally minimal; these studies suggest that dose escalation may be possible, potentially increasing efficacy with a tolerable side-effect profile.[42]

Despite promising initial efficacy and tolerability data, recommendations on the use of intravesical gemcitabine cannot yet be made given the current available evidence. Variable clinical settings, patient population, trial objectives, and study design limit the current evidence base. Further evaluation by additional phase II and randomized phase III trials in an expanded patient population is warranted and ongoing.[2,48]

INDICATIONS

Risk Category Definitions

The major guidelines do not uniformly agree on the definition of low-, intermediate-, and high-risk disease.[1–5] For the remainder of this review, risk categories coincide with the following practical definitions outlined by the International Bladder Cancer Group: low risk is defined as solitary, primary low-grade Ta; intermediate risk as multiple or recurrent low-grade tumors; and high risk as any T1 and/or G3 and/or CIS.[6]

Single Perioperative Dose

A single perioperative dose of intravesical chemotherapy is recommended immediately after initial TURBT in suspected low-risk disease in the absence of concern for bladder perforation.[1–3,5,6] The National Cancer Control Network (NCCN) maintains that TURBT alone is the gold standard for low-risk patients but that an immediate postoperative chemotherapy dose should be considered based on the risk of recurrence and progression.[4] A single instillation at the time of TURBT reduces the rate of recurrence primarily in the first 2 years but does not reduce the risk of progression or survival. This benefit disappears in recurrent, large (>5 cm), high-grade or high-risk patients receiving BCG.[6] Studies have shown that the combination of negative urine cytology and cystoscopic expertise accurately identifies histologically confirmed low-grade tumors in greater than 90% of cases, which supports the ability of the urologist to predict which patients will benefit from a single instillation of perioperative chemotherapy preprocedurally.[49]

MMC is the most frequently administered single-dose agent and is the most widely investigated. Although optimal timing for post-TURBT MMC administration has not yet been determined, improved recurrence outcomes are found only in studies that administer MMC within 24 hours of TURBT.[50–53] Therefore, single-dose therapy should be administered immediately after TURBT, and ideally within 6 hours, when there is no suspicion of perforation.[1–6,54]

It is the authors' practice to administer MMC in the following manner. After resection and confirmation of absence of clinical perforation, place a 3-way catheter into the bladder and attach the inflow port to a saline infusion bag while still in the operating room. Administer MMC through the outflow port either in the operating room or in recovery and clamp the outflow tubing with a hemostat. After 1 hour, release the outflow tubing and allow irrigation and drainage to gravity for 30 to 60 minutes. The catheter may then be removed and discarded in a biohazard container. Gloves should be worn at all times when handling this agent.[54]

A 2004 meta-analysis of 7 randomized trials[22,23,26,38,55–57] compared a single perioperative instillation of intravesical chemotherapy following TURBT versus TURBT alone in patients with Ta or T1 bladder cancer.[50] Three trials included epirubicin (728 patients, 49.3%), 2 studied MMC (427 patients, 28.9%), and thiotepa (247 patients, 16.7%) and pirarubicin (160 patients, 10.8%) were evaluated in 1 trial each. Chemotherapy was instilled within 24 hours in all trials and generally immediately after or within 6 hours after TURBT. The trials were published between 1985 and 2002 and reported on patients who were accrued between 1981 and 1994. The mean follow-up was 3.4 years (range 2.0–10.7 years).

Recurrence occurred in 36.7% of patients receiving chemotherapy compared with 48.4% in the TURBT-only groups. This finding represented a 12% absolute reduction in risk of recurrence and a 39% decrease in the odds of recurrence within the study timeframe.[50]

There was no difference in the size of treatment effect in the epirubicin, MMC, and pirarubicin trials, although no benefit was observed in the trial using thiotepa, potentially because of the lower concentration used in the included study. It must be noted that this meta-analysis was not designed to determine superiority of a single agent.

Time to realization of treatment benefit varied between the studies, with 3 studies showing a benefit within 1 to 3 months, 1 study showing a benefit within 6 months, and 1 showing a benefit after 1 year. All studied that eventually showed reduced recurrence rate did so within the first 2 years, as previously suggested by Solsona and colleagues[56] in their trial of single-dose MMC.

The treatment effect was observed in patients with both solitary and multiple tumors; however, the recurrence rate was significantly higher in patients with multiple tumors after a single instillation (65.2% vs 35.8%). This finding suggests that a single instillation alone immediately after TURBT may be suboptimal in this patient population.

The number needed to treat based on this meta-analysis was 8.5 (11.7 TURBTs were avoided for every 100 patients treated with single-dose chemotherapy). The authors suggest that treatment is cost-effective because the cost of a TURBT, anesthesia, and possible hospitalization is greater than 8.5 times that of a single instillation of intravesical chemotherapy.[50]

Notably, in the absence of suspected perforation, a single dose of perioperative intravesical chemotherapy confers no additional morbidity to a TURBT alone.[2,8]

The American Urologic Association (AUA) Bladder Cancer Guideline Panel performed a meta-analysis focusing on the single-dose instillation of perioperative MMC after TURBT.[2,3] This analysis is comprised of the 2 studies on MMC included in the aforementioned meta-analysis but differs in that all risk groups are taken into account.[55,56] Tolley and colleagues[55] reported a 60% recurrence rate in patients treated with TURBT alone and a 45% recurrence rate in those treated with a single perioperative dose of MMC. Solsana and colleagues[56] found a statistically significant decrease in the recurrence rate in the MMC group up to 2 years; however, the benefit disappeared at the long-term follow-up of 8 years. A total of 427 patients were included in this meta-analysis. Single-dose MMC immediately after TURBT was found to decrease the recurrence rate by a statistically significant 17% (95% confidence interval [CI]: −28%, −8%).

Neither meta-analysis revealed a significant difference in disease progression or survival. Therefore, the benefit of a single instillation of perioperative intravesical MMC is limited to a reduction in the risk of tumor recurrence, predominantly in low-risk patients and primarily in the first 2 years.

Despite gemcitabine's encouraging efficacy and side-effect profile in certain applications, single perioperative instillations have not been found to reduce recurrence rates and currently should not be used for this purpose.[58]

Induction Therapy, With or Without Maintenance

Summary of guidelines

Although all guidelines recommend some form of adjuvant therapy for intermediate and high-risk bladder cancer, considerable controversy still exists as to the agent of choice for induction therapy (chemotherapy vs immunotherapy), the interval and duration of induction therapy, and the use and timing of maintenance therapy.[1–6] The varying definitions of risk stratification between the guideline organizations contribute to the controversy.[6]

The International Consultation on Bladder Tumors recommends a single immediate postoperative instillation of chemotherapy followed by further adjuvant intravesical chemotherapy for less than 6 months for intermediate-risk disease; however, the optimal schedule is not well defined.[1]

The AUA recommends an induction course of either MMC or BCG for intermediate-risk disease. Induction courses evaluated by the AUA ranged from a single perioperative dose to weekly instillations for 6 weeks, and no specific induction course was recommended. Despite acknowledging that maintenance therapy with MMC likely reduces the recurrence rate compared with induction MMC only, the AUA identified maintenance therapy as optional and does not define an optimal interval or duration.[2,3]

For low-grade Ta disease, the NCCN recommends observation, single-dose, or induction intravesical chemotherapy. For high-grade Ta disease, observation or intravesical therapy is recommended. BCG is the preferred intravesical agent; however, chemotherapy is also an acceptable alternative for high-grade Ta. The decision to administer intravesical therapy in patients with Ta pathology is based on factors such as tumor size and number of tumors, which may increase the risk of recurrence and progression. For T1 disease, adjuvant intravesical chemotherapy is only considered as a second-line treatment after BCG failure. Optimal dosing interval and duration for induction and maintenance therapies are not explicitly stated for either risk group.[4]

For low-risk disease, the European Association of Urology (EAU) recommends a single immediate postoperative instillation of chemotherapy. For patients with intermediate risk disease, the EAU recommends the addition of a minimum of 1 year of intravesical chemotherapy or BCG. Intravesical chemotherapy has no role as a first-line therapy in high-risk disease, including CIS.[5]

Evidence

Uniform superiority in terms of recurrence, progression, and/or survival of one particular intravesical agent has yet to be determined for the treatment of bladder cancer. MMC is widely considered to be the most active and effective of the available intravesical chemotherapy agents, but this perception has yet to be directly proven in a clinical trial. Rather, its superiority is inferred from a lack of any trials demonstrating superiority of any other chemotherapy agent when compared with BCG; a meta-analysis of 3 trials (1066 patients) that suggests MMC with maintenance was superior to BCG induction without maintenance for reducing the risk of recurrence.[2]

Historically, adjuvant BCG was found to be more effective in preventing recurrence when compared with thiotepa or doxorubicin.[2] However, subsequent meta-analyses comparing BCG with several different chemotherapeutic agents do not uniformly agree,[59–61] partly because of inconsistencies in patient populations, treatment schedules, tumor characteristics, and/or institutional variation in outcomes.[2] Recently, randomized controlled trials have proven equal efficacy between BCG and MMC in both short-term[62] and long-term[63] regimens. Notably, both of these studies include high-risk patients. In addition, no evidence exists to suggest superiority of BCG over MMC in reducing tumor progression in direct comparison analysis.[21,61,64,65] But a large meta-analysis of more than 4800 patients demonstrated a 27% reduction in progression with BCG plus maintenance versus MMC.[66]

Two randomized trials compared a 6-week course of intravesical gemcitabine with similar BCG schedules with or without maintenance.[66,67] In patients with primary Ta or T1 disease, gemcitabine was found to have equivalent efficacy in recurrence-free survival[67] but was inferior to BCG in high-risk groups.[66] Gemcitabine toxicity was consistently less than BCG and could potentially serve as an alternative to patients with high-risk disease who are unable to tolerate BCG. In conclusion, there is no direct evidence to suggest superiority of a single chemotherapeutic agent.

Similarly, controversy exists about the utility of additional intravesical chemotherapy as compared with a single perioperative instillation for patients with intermediate-risk bladder cancer.[1–6] A meta-analysis of 22 trials published in 1995 reported that maintenance chemotherapy was actually less effective than a single postoperative instillation.[68] Despite no randomized controlled trials directly comparing induction MMC with induction MMC plus maintenance, subsequent meta-analyses contradict this conclusion and suggest that maintenance therapy with MMC significantly enhances recurrence-free survival as compared with induction (either single-dose or short induction course) without maintenance therapy.[3] Notably, the decrease in recurrence rate was not observed until at least 2 years of maintenance therapy.[69] Furthermore, the analysis includes studies that had yet to incorporate modifications of the administration protocol of single-dose MMC that were shown to significantly improve efficacy and have largely been adopted as the standard of care.[15] A more recent randomized trial showed that a group of patients with intermediate- to high-risk bladder cancer undergoing a 6-week induction course with MMC plus monthly maintenance instillations for up to 3 years had significantly higher recurrence-free rates (86.1% [95% CI: 77.9%, 91.4%]) than the group undergoing the same induction course with no maintenance (65.5% [95% CI: 55.9%, 73.5%]).[62] Again, no studies comparing the effect on progression of maintenance MMC versus induction MMC alone are currently available for analysis; therefore, the effect on progression remains unclear.[3]

The optimal dosing interval and duration for induction and maintenance chemotherapy is not well defined. Only 2 of the 6 studies included in the 2007 AUA meta-analysis used identical induction and maintenance schedules.[70,71] The remaining 4 studies used widely variable schedules.[55,72–74] Results from studies, such as Friedrich and colleagues,[62] seem to support longer courses (greater than 12 months) of maintenance therapy and call into question the recommendations that limit maintenance chemotherapy to a maximum of 1 year.[5,75]

In conclusion, there is no consensus on the optimal maintenance dose, schedule, and duration due to lack of sufficient data, but more recent studies suggest an increased benefit to a more prolonged maintenance course.

Secondary/Salvage Therapies: Recurrent and/ or BCG-Refractory

Because of the high risk of progressing to muscle-invasive disease, early radical cystectomy is the recommended treatment of BCG-refractory bladder cancer.[1–6] However, intravesical chemotherapy may have a role in salvage therapy in certain patient populations who are either unable to tolerate or refuse cystectomy.

BCG failure is defined by the EAU as (1) detection of muscle-invasive tumor during follow-up; (2) high-grade NMIBC present at both 3- and 6-month follow-up; or (3) any worsening of disease under BCG treatment, such as a higher number of recurrences, higher T stage or grade, or appearance of CIS despite an initial response.[5] The International Bladder Cancer Group distinguishes recurrence (reappearance of disease after the completion of therapy) from treatment failure (any recurrence or progression of disease during therapy).[6]

In patients with recurrent disease, the management must take into account previous and current levels of risk as well as previous treatments received.[6] For select low- to intermediate-risk recurrences, treatment with repeat TURBT, single instillation of chemotherapy, and maintenance chemotherapy or BCG with a minimum of 1 year of maintenance may be considered.[4–6] Guidelines uniformly recommend cystectomy as the first-line treatment of patients with an intermediate to high risk of disease progression and a high risk of recurrence or treatment failure.[1–6] The following discussion outlines the existing data on the use of different intravesical agents in the BCG refractory setting.

MMC

Initial reports of secondary treatment with MMC for BCG-refractory bladder cancer demonstrate a minimal benefit. Only 19% (4 of 21 patients) who crossed over to receive MMC after BCG failure were disease free after 3 years.[76] A subsequent randomized trial evaluating only recurrent Ta and T1 disease reported more encouraging results with a 61% (33 of 55 patients) disease-free rate at a median follow-up of 3 years.[77] This trial also studied gemcitabine, however, and concluded that MMC was inferior in terms of both efficacy and tolerability; but it should be noted that only a 4-week induction course was used.

Valrubicin

Valrubicin is the only intravesical chemotherapy agent approved by the FDA for BCG-refractory bladder cancer in patients who are not candidates for radical cystectomy. An initial evaluation of 32 patients, 22 of whom had received prior BCG, reported a 42% complete response rate (negative biopsies and cytology) and a 22% partial response rate (negative biopsies but positive cytology), with a mean disease-free interval of 23 months. Five of the 8 patients (64%) who remained disease free at the time of last contact (12.1–38.5 months after treatment) had previously failed treatment that included BCG.[29]

A recent phase II/III trial designed to complement the pivotal phase III trial published in 2000[33] on valrubicin in BCG-refractory disease was conducted to further investigate the efficacy and tolerability of valrubicin as an alternative to cystectomy in patients with BCG-refractory CIS.[78] Although this earlier trial included only patients who had previously failed at least 2 intravesical therapies (including at least one BCG course), the supportive trial additionally included patients who were BCG intolerant or BCG naïve. Both trials, despite the dissimilarity in the patient population, reported an identical 18% complete response rate. This finding suggests that valrubicin may be equally effective in patients with less intensive prior intravesical courses and is consistent with the post hoc analysis of the 2000 trial, which concluded that the number of prior courses or instillations of intravesical therapy did not affect the response rate.[79]

Gemcitabine

Gemcitabine seems to be an increasingly viable option for salvage intravesical chemotherapy for both recurrent and BCG-refractory disease. Reported treatment regimens studied consisted of a 2000-mg dose in 50 mL saline once a week for 6 weeks,[46,77,80] whereas one trial treated patients with two 3-week courses of 2000 mg in 100 mL administered twice weekly.[47] Of note, no maintenance therapy was administered in any of these studies.

Addeo and colleagues[77] reported that a 6-week course of gemcitabine for recurrent Ta and T1 bladder tumors resulted in a 72% disease-free rate after 3 years of follow-up. The reduction in the recurrence rate was significantly higher, whereas toxicity, particularly chemical cystitis, was lower than in the group treated with a 4-week course of MMC. Mohanty and colleagues[80] reported a 60% (21 of 35 patients) tumor-free rate after 18 months in a similar cohort of patients with Ta or T1 BCG-refractory bladder cancer.

Several more observational studies have evaluated the efficacy and tolerability of gemcitabine as an alternative intravesical treatment in patients who are BCG refractory or BCG intolerant. Oosterlink and colleagues[81] reported a 12-month recurrence-free survival rate of 75% (18 of 24 patients) in the intermediate-risk subset (Ta-T1, G1-2, multifocal, >3 cm) and 46% (7 of 16 patients) in the high-risk (T1, G3, multifocal, highly recurrent, CIS) subset as defined by the EAU Working Group on Oncological Urology. The regimen was well tolerated, with less than 20% of patients experiencing local side effects.[46] Dalbagni and colleagues[47] studied 30 patients (14 with CIS, 14 with T1 ± CIS, and 2 with high-grade Ta) who were refractory or intolerant of BCG and refused cystectomy. Fifty percent (15 of 30 patients) had a complete response and 23% (7 of 30 patients) had a partial response. Recurrence-free survival was 21% after 1 year.

One recently published study reported on 20 patients with high-risk NMIBC with BCG-refractory disease who received a standard 6-week induction course and additional maintenance therapy of 2000 mg/50 mL weekly for 3 weeks at 3, 6, and 12 months. After 15 months, 45% (9 of 20 patients) were recurrence free with a mean time to the first recurrence of 3.5 months. In addition, 45% (5 of 11) of the patients who recurred had disease progression.[82]

In summary, recent data suggest that gemcitabine is well tolerated and has activity against BCG-refractory bladder cancer. It may also be considered in cases of higher-risk BCG-refractory bladder cancer in patients who are unable to tolerate BCG or who are not candidates for or refuse radical cystectomy. However, until further data are available, intravesical gemcitabine as a second-line agent for BCG-refractory NMIBC should continue to be considered experimental.[30]

ON-GOING TRIALS

MMC

The Memorial Sloan-Kettering Cancer Center is currently recruiting 220 patients to directly compare optimal doses of MMC (40 mg in 20 mL sterile water) and BCG (81 mg in 53 mL diluent and saline) on cancer recurrence after 2 years. Secondary outcomes include cancer progression and need for radical cystectomy. Both arms will receive an identical induction (weekly instillations for 6 weeks) and a maintenance course (3 weekly cycles at 3, 6, 12, 18, and 24 months) (Clinical Trials.gov ID: NCT00974818).

Studies to evaluate experimental methods for optimizing delivery of MMC, including preoperative instillation of electromotive MMC (Clinical Trials.gov ID: NCT01149174) and combined bladder wall hyperthermia with MMC (Clinical Trials.gov ID: NCT00384891), are ongoing.

Gemcitabine

The Southwest Oncology group has 2 ongoing trials involving gemcitabine. S0337 is designed to evaluate the efficacy of a single instillation of gemcitabine as primary treatment of patients with newly diagnosed or occasionally recurring grade I/II NMIBC and has reached its accrual goal of 340 subjects (ClinicalTrials.gov ID: NCT00445601). For BCG-refractory disease, S0353 is a multicenter phase II trial designed to evaluate the efficacy of an induction and maintenance regimen of gemcitabine. Eligibility requirements include stage Ta (grade III–IV or multifocal), T1 (grade II/III), or CIS and have failed at least 2 courses of BCG. The estimated enrollment is 45 subjects (ClinicalTrials.gov ID: NCT00234039).

Taxanes

Docetaxel and Paclitaxel are two members of the antimicrotubular taxane family that have an effective antiproliferative and apoptotic effect on bladder tumor cell lines in vitro.[83] Used in a variety of cancers, including metastatic bladder cancer,[84] phase I trials have recently demonstrated superior urothelial absorption relative to MMC, with minimal systemic concentrations and an excellent safety profile for intravesical administration.[85–87]

Efficacy in reducing recurrence and extending the durability of response to induction treatment of select patients with BCG-refractory NMIBC has been suggested by small phase I trials[88,89] and further investigation is warrented.[7] Columbia University is currently recruiting patients to a combined phase I and II trial to determine the safety and efficacy of a nanoparticle albumin-bound formulation of paclitaxel (ClinicalTrials.gov ID: NCT00583349).

Apaziquone

Apaziquone is a promising new chemical analogue of MMC approved in 2009 for fast track review status by the FDA for intravesical therapy of NMIBC. Apaziquone is a bioreductive prodrug that is converted into active metabolites by intracellular reductases, which are preferentially expressed in tumor cells. The active metabolites are alkylating agents that form DNA strand breaks, and interstrand cross-links resulting in direct damage to DNA synthesis, similar to MMC.[90]

Preclinical studies have shown this drug to be highly effective in bladder tumor cell lines with possible superiority over MMC and an acceptable toxicity profile, and results of phase II trials in patients with low-grade NMIBC have been encouraging.[91,92] Two identical, multicenter, prospective, randomized, phase III trials, each enrolling more than 800 patients with low-grade NMIBC, have been completed and results are pending (Clinical Trials.gov ID: NCT00598806 and NCT00461591). These trials will report on the effect on the recurrence rate of a single perioperative dose.

Two identical, randomized, placebo-controlled, phase III trials are actively recruiting to evaluate the safety and efficacy on the recurrence rate of 6 weekly instillations of apaziquone versus placebo after a single perioperative dose (Clinical Trials.gov ID: NCT01469221 and NCT01410565). The company Spectrum announced in early 2012 that the 2 trials did not meet the primary endpoint of statistically significant difference of tumor recurrence at 2 years, but other results of these trials are needed before coming to any conclusions about the role of apaziquone as an intravesical chemotherapeutic agent.[93]

SUMMARY

There are a multitude of different agents available for intravesical chemotherapy for NMIBC with variable chemical compositions, modes of action, and side-effect profiles. Although MMC is the most commonly used agent, no particular agent has been proven to be superior to other agents in randomized trials in terms of efficacy. For low-risk NMIBC, a single perioperative dose of intravesical chemotherapy within 24 hours of TURBT has been proven to be safe in the absence of obvious bladder rupture and effective in reducing the likelihood of recurrence by around 40%. The benefit on progression is yet unproven. Although perioperative intravesical chemotherapy is uniformly recommended for intermediate-risk NMIBC, considerable controversy remains about the agent of choice for induction therapy (chemotherapy vs immunotherapy), the interval and duration of induction therapy, and the optimal use and timing of maintenance therapy. Studies have suggested that additional long-term maintenance chemotherapy has been shown to significantly increase recurrence-free rates. Several new intravesical chemotherapy agents are showing early promise in patients who are BCG refractory and BCG intolerant and may serve as an alternative for patients who refuse or are unable to undergo cystectomy.

REFERENCES

1. Soloway MS. International consultation on bladder tumours. J Urol 2005;66(6):1–126.
2. American urological association: guideline for the management of nonmuscle invasive bladder cancer (stages ta, T1, and tis): 2007 update. 2007. Available at: www.auanet.org. Accessed December 1, 2012.
3. Hall MC, Chang SS, Dalbagni G, et al. Guideline for the management of nonmuscle invasive bladder cancer (stages ta, T1, and tis): 2007 update. J Urol 2007;178(6):2314–30.
4. National comprehensive cancer network: clinical practice guidelines in oncology: bladder cancer including upper tract tumors and urothelial carcinoma of the prostate. 2010. Available at: www.nccn.org. Accessed December 1, 2012.
5. Babjuk M, Oosterlinck W, Sylvester R, et al. EAU guidelines on non-muscle-invasive urothelial carcinoma of the bladder, the 2011 update. Eur Urol 2011;59(6):997–1008.
6. Brausi M, Witjes JA, Lamm D, et al. A review of current guidelines and best practice recommendations for the management of nonmuscle invasive bladder cancer by the international bladder cancer group. J Urol 2011;186(6):2158–67.
7. Williams SK, Hoenig DM, Ghavamian R, et al. Intravesical therapy for bladder cancer. Expert Opin Pharmacother 2010;11(6):947–58.
8. Thrasher JB, Crawford ED. Complications of intravesical chemotherapy. Urol Clin North Am 1992; 19(3):529–39.
9. Snyder C, Harlan L, Knopf K, et al. Patterns of care for the treatment of bladder cancer. J Urol 2003; 169(5):1697–701.
10. Hollenbeck BK, Ye Z, Dunn RL, et al. Provider treatment intensity and outcomes for patients with early-stage bladder cancer. J Natl Cancer Inst 2009; 101(8):571–80.
11. Madeb R, Golijanin D, Noyes K, et al. Treatment of nonmuscle invading bladder cancer: do physicians in the United States practice evidence based medicine? The use and economic implications of intravesical chemotherapy after transurethral resection of bladder tumors. Cancer 2009; 115(12):2660–70.
12. Chamie K, Saigal CS, Lai J, et al. Compliance with guidelines for patients with bladder cancer: variation in the delivery of care. Cancer 2011;117(23): 5392–401.
13. Nielsen ME, Smith AB, Pruthi RS, et al. Reported use of intravesical therapy for non-muscle-invasive bladder cancer (NMIBC): results from the Bladder Cancer Advocacy Network (BCAN) survey. BJU Int 2012;110(7):967–72.
14. Shelley MD, Mason MD, Kynaston H. Intravesical therapy for superficial bladder cancer: a systematic review of randomised trials and meta-analyses. Cancer Treat Rev 2010;36(3):195–205.
15. Au JL, Badalament RA, Wientjes MG, et al. Methods to improve efficacy of intravesical mitomycin C: results of a randomized phase III trial. J Natl Cancer Inst 2001;93(8):597–604.

16. Masters JR. Re: methods to improve efficacy of intravesical mitomycin C: results of a randomized phase III trial. J Natl Cancer Inst 2001;93(20):1574–5.
17. Lammers RJ, Witjes JA, Inman BA, et al. The role of a combined regimen with intravesical chemotherapy and hyperthermia in the management of non-muscle-invasive bladder cancer: a systematic review. Eur Urol 2011;60(1):81–93.
18. Kalsi J, Harland SJ, Feneley MR. Electromotive drug administration with mitomycin C for intravesical treatment of non-muscle invasive transitional cell carcinoma. Expert Opin Drug Deliv 2008;5(1):137–45.
19. Di Stasi SM, Valenti M, Verri C, et al. Electromotive instillation of mitomycin immediately before transurethral resection for patients with primary urothelial non-muscle invasive bladder cancer: a randomised controlled trial. Lancet Oncol 2011;12(9):871–9.
20. Oosterlinck W. Chemotherapy: electromotive mitomycin in superficial bladder cancer. Nat Rev Clin Oncol 2011;8(11):633–4.
21. Bohle A, Jocham D, Bock PR. Intravesical bacillus Calmette-Guerin versus mitomycin C for superficial bladder cancer: a formal meta-analysis of comparative studies on recurrence and toxicity. J Urol 2003;169(1):90–5.
22. Oosterlinck W, Kurth KH, Schroder F, et al. A prospective European Organization for Research and Treatment of Cancer genitourinary group randomized trial comparing transurethral resection followed by a single intravesical instillation of epirubicin or water in single stage ta, T1 papillary carcinoma of the bladder. J Urol 1993;149(4):749–52.
23. Rajala P, Kaasinen E, Raitanen M, et al. Perioperative single dose instillation of epirubicin or interferon-alpha after transurethral resection for the prophylaxis of primary superficial bladder cancer recurrence: a prospective randomized multicenter study–FinnBladder III long-term results. J Urol 2002;168(3):981–5.
24. Kurth K, Vijgh WJ, ten Kate F, et al. Phase 1/2 study of intravesical epirubicin in patients with carcinoma in situ of the bladder. J Urol 1991;146(6):1508–12 [discussion: 1512–3].
25. Kurth K, Tunn U, Ay R, et al. Adjuvant chemotherapy for superficial transitional cell bladder carcinoma: long-term results of a European Organization for Research and Treatment of Cancer randomized trial comparing doxorubicin, ethoglucid and transurethral resection alone. J Urol 1997;158(2):378–84.
26. Ali-el-Dein B, Nabeeh A, el-Baz M, et al. Single-dose versus multiple instillations of epirubicin as prophylaxis for recurrence after transurethral resection of pTa and pT1 transitional-cell bladder tumours: a prospective, randomized controlled study. Br J Urol 1997;79(5):731–5.
27. de Reijke TM, Kurth KH, Sylvester RJ, et al. Bacillus Calmette-Guerin versus epirubicin for primary, secondary or concurrent carcinoma in situ of the bladder: results of a European Organization for the Research and Treatment of Cancer genitourinary group phase III trial (30906). J Urol 2005;173(2):405–9.
28. Sweatman TW, Parker RF, Israel M. Pharmacologic rationale for intravesical N-trifluoroacetyladriamycin-14-valerate (AD 32): a preclinical study. Cancer Chemother Pharmacol 1991;28(1):1–6.
29. Greenberg RE, Bahnson RR, Wood D, et al. Initial report on intravesical administration of N-trifluoroacetyladriamycin-14-valerate (AD 32) to patients with refractory superficial transitional cell carcinoma of the urinary bladder. Urology 1997;49(3):471–5.
30. Patel T, Barlow LJ, McKiernan JM. Management of bacillus Calmette-Guerin refractory non-muscle invasive bladder cancer. AUA Update Series 2010;29(24):233–43.
31. Krishan A, Israel M, Modest EJ, et al. Differences in cellular uptake and cytofluorescence of Adriamycin and N-trifluoroacetyladriamycin-14-valerate. Cancer Res 1976;36(6):2108–9.
32. Israel M, Modest EJ, Frei E. N-trifluoroacetyladriamycin-14-valerate, an analog with greater experimental antitumor activity and less toxicity than Adriamycin. Cancer Res 1975;35(5):1365–8.
33. Steinberg G, Bahnson R, Brosman S, et al. Efficacy and safety of valrubicin for the treatment of bacillus Calmette-Guerin refractory carcinoma in situ of the bladder. The Valrubicin Study Group. J Urol 2000;163(3):761–7.
34. Jones JS, Campbell SC. Non-muscle-invasive bladder cancer (ta, T1, and CIS). In: Wein AJ, Kavoussi LR, Novick AC, et al, editors. Campbell-Walsh urology. 10th edition. Philadelphia: Elsevier; 2011. p. 2447–67.
35. Burnand KG, Boyd PJ, Mayo ME, et al. Single dose intravesical thiotepa as an adjuvant to cystodiathermy in the treatment of transitional cell bladder carcinoma. Br J Urol 1976;48(1):55–9.
36. Koontz WW Jr, Prout GR Jr, Smith W, et al. The use of intravesical thiotepa in the management of non-invasive carcinoma of the bladder. J Urol 1981;125(3):307–12.
37. Zincke H, Utz DC, Taylor WF, et al. Influence of thiotepa and doxorubicin instillation at time of transurethral surgical treatment of bladder cancer on tumor recurrence: a prospective, randomized, double-blind, controlled trial. J Urol 1983;129(3):505–9.
38. The effect of intravesical thiotepa on tumour recurrence after endoscopic treatment of newly diagnosed superficial bladder cancer. A further report with long-term follow-up of a medical research council randomized trial. Medical Research Council Working Party on Urological Cancer subgroup on

superficial bladder cancer. Br J Urol 1994;73(6): 632–8.
39. Mini E, Nobili S, Caciagli B, et al. Cellular pharmacology of gemcitabine. Ann Oncol 2006;17(Suppl 5): 7–12.
40. Kilani RT, Tamimi Y, Karmali S, et al. Selective cytotoxicity of gemcitabine in bladder cancer cell lines. Anticancer Drugs 2002;13(6):557–66.
41. Laufer M, Ramalingam S, Schoenberg MP, et al. Intravesical gemcitabine therapy for superficial transitional cell carcinoma of the bladder: a phase I and pharmacokinetic study. J Clin Oncol 2003;21(4): 697–703.
42. Serretta V, Galuffo A, Pavone C, et al. Gemcitabine in intravesical treatment of ta-T1 transitional cell carcinoma of bladder: phase I-II study on marker lesions. Urology 2005;65(1):65–9.
43. Raj G. Beyond BCG: gemcitabine. Current Clinical Urology. In: Lee CT, Wood DP, editors. Bladder cancer: diagnosis, therapeutics, and management. 1st edition. New York: Humana Press; 2009. p. 115–25.
44. Gontero P, Casetta G, Maso G, et al. Phase II study to investigate the ablative efficacy of intravesical administration of gemcitabine in intermediate-risk superficial bladder cancer (SBC). Eur Urol 2004; 46(3):339–43.
45. Mattioli F, Curotto A, Manfredi V, et al. Intravesical gemcitabine in superficial bladder cancer: a phase II safety, efficacy and pharmacokinetic study. Anticancer Res 2005;25(3c):2493–6.
46. Bartoletti R, Cai T, Gacci M, et al. Intravesical gemcitabine therapy for superficial transitional cell carcinoma: results of a phase II prospective multicenter study. Urology 2005;66(4):726–31.
47. Dalbagni G, Russo P, Bochner B, et al. Phase II trial of intravesical gemcitabine in bacille Calmette-Guerin-refractory transitional cell carcinoma of the bladder. J Clin Oncol 2006;24(18):2729–34.
48. Shelley MD, Jones G, Cleves A, et al. Intravesical gemcitabine therapy for non-muscle invasive bladder cancer (NMIBC): a systematic review. BJU Int 2012;109(4):496–505.
49. Herr HW, Donat SM, Dalbagni G. Correlation of cystoscopy with histology of recurrent papillary tumors of the bladder. J Urol 2002;168(3):978–80.
50. Sylvester RJ, Oosterlinck W, van der Meijden AP. A single immediate postoperative instillation of chemotherapy decreases the risk of recurrence in patients with stage ta T1 bladder cancer: a meta-analysis of published results of randomized clinical trials. J Urol 2004;171(6):2186–90.
51. Iborra JI, Ricos Torrent JV, Monros Lliso JL, et al. Results of a randomized, double blind prospective study of intravesical chemoprophylaxis with 2 drugs: adriamycin and mitomycin; and 2 ways of initiating the instillations: early and late. Effect on recurrence and progression. Arch Esp Urol 1992; 45(10):1001–7.
52. Bouffioux C, Kurth KH, Bono A, et al. Intravesical adjuvant chemotherapy for superficial transitional cell bladder carcinoma: results of 2 European Organization for Research and Treatment of Cancer randomized trials with mitomycin C and doxorubicin comparing early versus delayed instillations and short-term versus long-term treatment. European Organization for Research and Treatment of Cancer Genitourinary Group. J Urol 1995;153(3):934–41.
53. Kaasinen E, Rintala E, Hellstrom P, et al. Factors explaining recurrence in patients undergoing chemoimmunotherapy regimens for frequently recurring superficial bladder carcinoma. Eur Urol 2002;42(2): 167–74.
54. O'Donnell MA. Practical applications of intravesical chemotherapy and immunotherapy in high-risk patients with superficial bladder cancer. Urol Clin North Am 2005;32(2):121–31.
55. Tolley DA, Parmar MK, Grigor KM, et al. The effect of intravesical mitomycin C on recurrence of newly diagnosed superficial bladder cancer: a further report with 7 years of follow up. J Urol 1996; 155(4):1233–8.
56. Solsona E, Iborra I, Ricos JV, et al. Effectiveness of a single immediate mitomycin C instillation in patients with low risk superficial bladder cancer: short and long-term follow-up. J Urol 1999;161(4): 1120–3.
57. Okamura K, Ono Y, Kinukawa T, et al. Randomized study of single early instillation of (2"R)-4'-O-tetrahydropyranyl-doxorubicin for a single superficial bladder carcinoma. Cancer 2002;94(9):2363–8.
58. Bohle A, Leyh H, Frei C, et al. Single postoperative instillation of gemcitabine in patients with non-muscle-invasive transitional cell carcinoma of the bladder: a randomised, double-blind, placebo-controlled phase III multicentre study. Eur Urol 2009;56(3):495–503.
59. Huncharek M, Kupelnick B. Impact of intravesical chemotherapy versus BCG immunotherapy on recurrence of superficial transitional cell carcinoma of the bladder: metaanalytic reevaluation. Am J Clin Oncol 2003;26(4):402–7.
60. Huncharek M, Kupelnick B. The influence of intravesical therapy on progression of superficial transitional cell carcinoma of the bladder: a metaanalytic comparison of chemotherapy versus bacilli Calmette-Guerin immunotherapy. Am J Clin Oncol 2004;27(5):522–8.
61. Sylvester RJ, van der Meijden AP, Witjes JA, et al. Bacillus Calmette-Guerin versus chemotherapy for the intravesical treatment of patients with carcinoma in situ of the bladder: a meta-analysis of the published results of randomized clinical trials. J Urol 2005;174(1):86–91.

62. Friedrich MG, Pichlmeier U, Schwaibold H, et al. Long-term intravesical adjuvant chemotherapy further reduces recurrence rate compared with short-term intravesical chemotherapy and short-term therapy with bacillus Calmette-Guerin (BCG) in patients with non-muscle-invasive bladder carcinoma. Eur Urol 2007;52(4):1123–9.
63. Gardmark T, Jahnson S, Wahlquist R, et al. Analysis of progression and survival after 10 years of a randomized prospective study comparing mitomycin-C and bacillus Calmette-Guerin in patients with high-risk bladder cancer. BJU Int 2007;99(4):817–20.
64. Sylvester RJ, van der Meijden AP, Lamm DL. Intravesical bacillus Calmette-Guerin reduces the risk of progression in patients with superficial bladder cancer: a meta-analysis of the published results of randomized clinical trials. J Urol 2002;168(5): 1964–70.
65. Shelley MD, Wilt TJ, Court J, et al. Intravesical bacillus Calmette-Guerin is superior to mitomycin C in reducing tumour recurrence in high-risk superficial bladder cancer: a meta-analysis of randomized trials. BJU Int 2004;93(4):485–90.
66. Porena M, Del Zingaro M, Lazzeri M, et al. Bacillus Calmette-Guerin versus gemcitabine for intravesical therapy in high-risk superficial bladder cancer: a randomised prospective study. Urol Int 2010; 84(1):23–7.
67. Bendary L, Khalil S, Shahin A, et al. Intravesical gemcitabine versus bacillus Calmette-Guerin (BCG) in treatment of non-muscle invasive bladder cancer: short term comparative study. J Urol 2011; 185(Suppl 4):e664–5.
68. Lamm DL, Riggs DR, Traynelis CL, et al. Apparent failure of current intravesical chemotherapy prophylaxis to influence the long-term course of superficial transitional cell carcinoma of the bladder. J Urol 1995;153(5):1444–50.
69. Huncharek M, Geschwind JF, Witherspoon B, et al. Intravesical chemotherapy prophylaxis in primary superficial bladder cancer: a meta-analysis of 3703 patients from 11 randomized trials. J Clin Epidemiol 2000;53(7):676–80.
70. Hirao Y, Okajima E, Ohara S, et al. Prophylactic treatment for superficial bladder cancer following transurethral resection. Cancer Chemother Pharmacol 1987;20(Suppl):S85–90.
71. Akaza H, Koiso K, Kotake T, et al. Long-term results of intravesical chemoprophylaxis of superficial bladder cancer: experience of the Japanese urological cancer research group for Adriamycin. Cancer Chemother Pharmacol 1992;30(Suppl):S15–20.
72. Krege S, Giani G, Meyer R, et al. A randomized multicenter trial of adjuvant therapy in superficial bladder cancer: transurethral resection only versus transurethral resection plus mitomycin C versus transurethral resection plus bacillus Calmette-Guerin. Participating clinics. J Urol 1996;156(3): 962–6.
73. Tsushima T, Matsumura Y, Ozaki Y, et al. Prophylactic intravesical instillation therapy with Adriamycin and mitomycin C in patients with superficial bladder cancer. Cancer Chemother Pharmacol 1987; 20(Suppl):S72–6.
74. Huland H, Otto U. Mitomycin instillation to prevent recurrence of superficial bladder carcinoma. Results of a controlled, prospective study in 58 patients. Eur Urol 1983;9(2):84–6.
75. Sylvester RJ. Intravesical chemotherapy in non-muscle-invasive bladder cancer: what schedule and duration of treatment? Eur Urol 2007;52(4): 951–3.
76. Malmstrom PU, Wijkstrom H, Lundholm C, et al. 5-year follow-up of a randomized prospective study comparing mitomycin C and bacillus Calmette-Guerin in patients with superficial bladder carcinoma. Swedish-Norwegian bladder cancer study group. J Urol 1999;161(4):1124–7.
77. Addeo R, Caraglia M, Bellini S, et al. Randomized phase III trial on gemcitabine versus mytomicin in recurrent superficial bladder cancer: evaluation of efficacy and tolerance. J Clin Oncol 2010;28(4): 543–8.
78. Dinney CP, Greenberg RE, Steinberg GD. Intravesical valrubicin in patients with bladder carcinoma in situ and contraindication to or failure after bacillus Calmette-Guerin. Urol Oncol 2012. [Epub ahead of print].
79. Steinberg GD, Smith ND, Ryder K, et al. Factors affecting valrubicin response in patients with bacillus Calmette-Guerin-refractory bladder carcinoma in situ. Postgrad Med 2011;123(3):28–34.
80. Mohanty NK, Nayak RL, Vasudeva P, et al. Intravesicle gemcitabine in management of BCG refractory superficial TCC of urinary bladder-our experience. Urol Oncol 2008;26(6):616–9.
81. Oosterlinck W, Lobel B, Jakse G, et al. Guidelines on bladder cancer. Eur Urol 2002;41(2):105–12.
82. Perdona S, Di Lorenzo G, Cantiello F, et al. Is gemcitabine an option in BCG-refractory nonmuscle-invasive bladder cancer? A single-arm prospective trial. Anticancer Drugs 2010;21(1):101–6.
83. Kugler A, Haschemi R, Zoller G, et al. In vitro investigations of new therapeutic agents on bladder tumor cell lines. Urol Res 1997;25(4):247–50.
84. Calabro F, Sternberg CN. New drugs and new approaches for the treatment of metastatic urothelial cancer. World J Urol 2002;20(3):158–66.
85. Song D, Wientjes MG, Au JL. Bladder tissue pharmacokinetics of intravesical Taxol. Cancer Chemother Pharmacol 1997;40(4):285–92.
86. McKiernan JM, Masson P, Murphy AM, et al. Phase I trial of intravesical docetaxel in the management

of superficial bladder cancer refractory to standard intravesical therapy. J Clin Oncol 2006;24(19): 3075–80.

87. Hadaschik BA, ter Borg MG, Jackson J, et al. Paclitaxel and cisplatin as intravesical agents against non-muscle-invasive bladder cancer. BJU Int 2008; 101(11):1347–55.
88. Barlow L, McKiernan J, Sawczuk I, et al. A single-institution experience with induction and maintenance intravesical docetaxel in the management of non-muscle-invasive bladder cancer refractory to bacille Calmette-Guerin therapy. BJU Int 2009; 104(8):1098–102.
89. Laudano MA, Barlow LJ, Murphy AM, et al. Long-term clinical outcomes of a phase I trial of intravesical docetaxel in the management of non-muscle-invasive bladder cancer refractory to standard intravesical therapy. Urology 2010;75(1):134–7.
90. Bailey SM, Lewis AD, Knox RJ, et al. Reduction of the indoloquinone anticancer drug EO9 by purified DT-: a detailed kinetic study and analysis of metabolites. Biochem Pharmacol 1998;56(5):613–21.
91. Jain A, Phillips RM, Scally AJ, et al. Response of multiple recurrent TaT1 bladder cancer to intravesical apaziquone (EO9): comparative analysis of tumor recurrence rates. Urology 2009;73(5): 1083–6.
92. Hendricksen K, van der Heijden AG, Cornel EB, et al. Two-year follow-up of the phase II marker lesion study of intravesical apaziquone for patients with non-muscle invasive bladder cancer. World J Urol 2009;27(3):337–42.
93. Yutkin V, Chin J. Apaziquone as an intravesical therapeutic agent for urothelial non-muscle-invasive bladder cancer. Expert Opin Investig Drugs 2012; 21(2):251–60.

Side Effects of Perioperative Intravesical Treatment and Treatment Strategies for These Side Effects

Joshua G. Griffin, MD*, Jeff Holzbeierlein, MD

KEYWORDS

• Bladder • Superficial • Non-muscle invasive • Complications • Management
• Intravesical chemotherapy • Side effects • Toxicity

KEY POINTS

- Absorption of intravesical chemotherapy agents is dependent on molecular weight, concentration, and lipophilic properties. Absorption may also be influenced by surgical technique.
- Toxicity from perioperative intravesical chemotherapy includes both local and systemic effects. Chemical cystitis, manifesting as urgency, dysuria, and suprapubic discomfort is the most common reported side effect occurring in 3.5% to 25% of cases. Systemic complications are unusual, with rates of myelosuppression generally around 1%. The notable exception is thiotepa due to its small molecular weight.
- Severe local toxicity from perioperative intravesical chemotherapy includes bladder calcification, ulceration, or transmural necrosis, which can lead to perivesical fluid collections. These may occur in the setting of missed perforation or in deep resections.
- Skin eruptions are most common with mitomycin C but can occur with other agents. Although the exact cause has not been elicited, the condition usually resolves with removal of the agent and does not result in significant long-term morbidity.
- The most important measure to prevent complications from intravesical chemotherapy is to withhold the agent in the setting of known bladder perforation. In cases of deep resection or clinical suspicion, cystography should be performed to rule out extravasation before administration.
- Patients with peritoneal signs or severe abdominal pain during instillation should be evaluated and treated promptly for chemotherapy extravasation to prevent long-term complications associated with the necrotizing effects of these agents.

INTRODUCTION

Non-muscle invasive bladder cancer is the most common newly diagnosed urothelial bladder cancer with an extremely high propensity for recurrence. The use of perioperative intravesical chemotherapy is an important modality in the management of non-muscle invasive bladder cancer, particularly to help reduce the risk of recurrence. Immediate postoperative instillation of cytotoxic chemotherapy has been reported to result in greater than a 39% reduction in recurrence compared with transurethral resection (TUR) alone.[1] Both the American Urologic Association and European Association of Urology Guidelines recommend a single instillation of chemotherapy for patients with low-grade urothelial tumors.[2,3] These cytotoxic agents have minimal absorption

Department of Urology, University of Kansas Medical Center, 3901 Rainbow Boulevard, Mail Stop 3016, Kansas City, KS 66160, USA
* Corresponding author.
E-mail address: jgriffin3@kumc.edu

Urol Clin N Am 40 (2013) 197–210
http://dx.doi.org/10.1016/j.ucl.2013.01.005
0094-0143/13/$ – see front matter

when administered into the bladder, and therefore systemic side effects are low. Compared with immunotherapy, there is no demonstrable effect on disease progression but given the known risks of systemic absorption with immunotherapy agents such as Bacillus Calmette-Guérin (BCG), intravesical chemotherapy remains the agent of choice in the perioperative setting for non-muscle invasive urothelial tumors.

In this article, some of the side effects and complications that may be encountered with the administration of commonly used intravesical agents in the perioperative setting and strategies to help manage these toxicities are reviewed. Most of the published data obtained from previous reports have attempted to describe the toxicity associated with induction courses (typically 6 weeks); however, this article highlights the toxicity, side effects, and management of a single perioperative instillation of intravesical chemotherapy.

PROPERTIES AND CONSIDERATIONS OF CHEMOTHERAPIES USED INTRAVESICALLY IN THE PERIOPERATIVE SETTING

There is still ongoing debate with regard to the usefulness of perioperative chemotherapy. Some argue that the recurrences in this patient population are rarely invasive and in most cases they are amenable to office-based fulguration. Nonetheless, if a cytotoxic agent is to be administered in the perioperative setting, the benefits should outweigh the potential risks. With this in mind, there are several factors that may influence the urologists' choice of a chemotherapeutic agent for intravesical instillation.

One of the first factors to be considered is the risk of absorption of the chemotherapeutic agents, which may result in systemic toxicity. Although some factors affecting absorption may be under the control of the operating surgeon (such as surgical technique and depth of resection), others are strictly related to the physical properties of the agent. Such properties include molecular weight, concentration, and liphophilicity. Although concentration of cytotoxic agents in bladder tissue is necessary, too much absorption may result in toxic side effects. On the other hand, compounds with poor absorptive qualities achieve lower tissue concentrations, mostly working on the bladder surface. To better define the optimal qualities of cytotoxic compounds instilled in the bladder, Mishina and colleagues[4] determined that the ideal agent should have a pH between 6 and 7, a logP (partition coefficient) either between −0.4 and −1.2 or −7.5 and −8.0, and a molecular weight of at least 200.

Other factors that may increase absorption include agent dwell time, agent concentration, and bladder wall integrity (ie, bladder perforations).[5] Therefore, if an intravesical instillation is being considered perioperatively and there is any question of perforation, an intraoperative cystogram should be performed to rule out extravasation. Complications of bladder necrosis, inflammation, fibrosis, and peritonitis have all been reported in cases of missed perforation and are discussed later.

CHEMOTHERAPEUTIC AGENTS USED INTRAVESICALLY

As mentioned previously, there are several cytotoxic agents for use in the perioperative period, some of which remain in clinical trials (**Table 1**). Each has properties that help to explain its value as an intravesical agent and contribute to potential toxicities. Valrubicin is the only agent with US Food and Drug Administration (FDA) approval for intravesical use, although it is not routinely used in the immediate postoperative setting.

Mitomycin C (MMC) is an alkylating agent that has been used systemically to treat a variety of neoplasms. It has a molecular weight of 334 and

Table 1
Commonly used intravesical chemotherapy agents

Agent	Molecular Weight	Class	Dose (mg)
Mitomycin C	335	Antibiotic; inhibits DNA synthesis by crosslinking	20–60
Thiotepa	190	Alkylating agent; inhibits DNA synthesis by crosslinking	30–60
Doxorubicin	580	Anthracyline antibiotics; intercalate DNA and inhibit synthesis through several pathways	10–100
Epirubicin	580		
Pirarubicin	625		
Valrubicin	720		800
Gemcitabine	299	Cytidine analogue; inhibits DNA synthesis through several pathways	2000

is isolated from the bacterium *Streptomyces caespitosus*. There are several proposed mechanisms of action including inhibition of DNA synthesis by DNA crosslinking and superoxide free radical production.[6,7] FDA approval for systemic use in a variety of cancers was granted in 1974, although its use as an intravesical therapy is still considered off-label. Bone marrow suppression, manifesting as thrombocytopenia and leukopenia are the most common side effects reported when administered systemically.[8] Extravasation of mitomycin C when it is being administered intravenously is classically known to cause local tissue necrosis, which can be devastating and require surgical debridement in severe cases.[9–11] Other toxicities with systemic use include hemolytic uremic syndrome, and effects on cardiac, pulmonary, integumentary, and renal systems.[12–23]

MMC is the most extensively studied agent in terms of establishing an intravesical pharmacokinetic profile. In an experiment in which dog bladders were instilled with 20 mg in 40 mL saline, tissue concentrations decreased sharply with depth through the mucosal and submucosal layers (50% decrease for every 500 μm). Concentrations at depths less than 2000 μm were at the lowest levels of detection (0.1 μg/g) and the plasma concentrations were less than 100 μg/L.[24] This has also been shown in humans who were administered MMC before cystectomy; a logarithmic decrease in concentration of the agent with increasing depth up to 2000 μm was demonstrated.[25] In a study of 18 patients receiving 40 mg of MMC intravesically followed by serial plasma measurements, the maximum systemic concentration was approximately 36 ng/mL with no evidence of bone marrow suppression. The investigators noted that, based on other studies, this systemic concentration is much lower than that obtained when administering intravenous MMC with a concentration of 2.0 μg/mL immediately after injection.[26,27]

Doxorubicin and Derivatives

Doxorubicin is in the anthracycline class of cytotoxic agents, an antibiotic isolated from *Streptomyces peucetius*. Its proposed primary action is inhibition of DNA synthesis through intercalation, although the exact mechanism is not entirely clear.[28] With a molecular weight of 580, its absorption through the bladder wall is minimal. The acute side effects of doxorubicin when administered systemically include bone marrow suppression, gastrointestinal upset, and alopecia. Delayed effects include cardiomyopathy, secondary hematologic malignancies, and hepatic disease. The current recommended dose for intravesical use ranges from 30 to 50 mg. Previous studies demonstrated that a postoperative instillation of 40 mg in 20 mL of doxorubicin allowed to dwell for 2 hours resulted in 1% of the dose being absorbed and detectable in the plasma at very low levels (>0.2 μg/L) in 6 of 8 patients.[29]

Epirubicin is a derivative of doxorubicin, also with a molecular weight of 580 and minimal systemic absorption. When used systemically, it has been proposed to be as efficacious as doxorubicin but with less associated toxicity.[30] It is commonly used in Europe both as an immediate instillation after TUR as well as an induction course.[31] Detectable levels of epirubicin in plasma can be seen after immediate instillation. Tsushima and colleagues[32] obtained blood samples from 10 patients at 30, 60, and 120 minutes after a 1-hour intravesical instillation of either 20 mg/40 mL or 50 mg/100 mL epirubicin. At both concentrations there were detectable levels of epirubicin in plasma (20 mg/40 mL, <2.0 ng/mL at 1 hour, then undetectable; 50 mg/100 mL, 4.4 ng/dL at 1 hour, <3.0 ng/dL at 2 hours, then undetectable). The low circulating levels found with administration may cause some systemic side effects, although the incidence from previous trials is around 1.3%.[33]

Pararubicin and valrubicin are also derivatives of doxorubicin. Plasma pararubicin levels were studied in 20 patients who were given 30 mg of pararubicin intravesically at 2 concentrations for 1 hour after TUR. At all time points, pararubicin concentrations were less than detectable limits (2.5 ng/mL up to 120 minutes). The mean recovery percentage of the agent after draining the bladder was 73%.[34] Valrubicin is currently the only FDA approved intravesical agent for use in BCG refractory carcinoma in situ.[35] It has also been evaluated as an immediate instillation, although it is currently not approved for this use. Although its molecular weight of 723 is one of the largest of all the intravesical agents, it is highly lipophilic and rapidly absorbed into cell membranes, which could lead to increased absorption.[36] Studies evaluating the pharmacokinetics of valrubicin used as an induction course have revealed minimal detectable levels in plasma,[37] but in a pilot study of 22 patients in whom it was used in the perioperative setting, the systemic exposure was much higher, especially in cases of extensive resection and bladder perforation.[38]

Thiotepa

Thiotepa is the oldest agent used for intravesical instillation, with results of a series described as early as 1961.[39] As an alkylating agent, thiotepa produces a cytotoxic effect by DNA crosslinking. Its molecular weight of 189 makes thiotepa the smallest of all agents used intravesically. Previous investigators have shown significant systemic absorption of thiotepa when administered in the bladder. Jones and Swinney[39] found that up to one-third of the dose was absorbed in 16 patients treated with an induction course. Lunglmayr and Czech[40] demonstrated that approximately 20% of thiotepa was absorbed when given in patients with normal urothelium and this increased to near 100% in the setting of injured mucosa from fulguration or resection. Given these findings, thiotepa carries a more significant risk of absorption with resultant bone marrow suppression compared with some other contemporary agents used in the perioperative setting.[6,41]

Newer Intravesical Agents

Gemcitabine is the newest chemotherapy agent that has been investigated as an intravesical agent in the immediate postoperative and adjuvant settings. Commonly used systemically for invasive and metastatic bladder cancers, this agent has been proposed to be ideal for intravesical use. A cytidine analogue, it has several inhibitory effects on DNA synthesis, including inhibition of DNA polymerase.[42] It is typically administered in the immediate setting at a concentration of 20 to 40 mg/mL (2000 mg in 50 or 100 mL) with a dwell time of 30 to 40 minutes. In the only prospective randomized trial evaluating the effect of immediate intravesical gemcitabine on recurrence-free survival compared with placebo, patients were managed with continuous bladder irrigation for at least 20 hours after instillation.[43] At 12 months there was no difference in recurrence-free survival between the treatment and placebo groups.

Despite the ongoing evaluation of this agent in terms of efficacy, previous studies have shown gemcitabine to be well tolerated when administered in the perioperative setting. Maffezzini and colleagues[44] demonstrated detectable levels of gemcitabine in plasma after immediate instillation at a concentration of 40 mg/mL in a series of 15 patients. The degree of absorption was dependent on the extent of resection and peak levels were obtained at 15 minutes and were much less than the plasma concentration obtained with systemic administration. Toxicity was low with 1 patient developing grade 2 leukopenia (3000–3900/μL). A subsequent phase III trial of 358 patients randomized to placebo or immediate gemcitabine has also demonstrated a low risk of toxicity. Adverse events were similar in both groups (29.5% gemcitabine vs 26.5% placebo) and the investigators concluded that only about 6% of the adverse events in the treatment arm were likely attributed to intravesical instillation. Of these, postprocedural pain, pyrexia, and alopecia were reported in the treatment group (each 1.2%).[43] Cases of myelosuppression were not reported. Investigational studies using gemcitabine are ongoing, including the results of the Southwest Oncology trial, which recently completed accrual, and although the exact role for its use has not been defined, it seems to be safe as an immediate instillation.

Apaziquone is a synthetic analogue of MMC and is being studied in the perioperative period in patients with non-muscle invasive bladder cancer. It requires reduction by the intracellular enzyme deoxythymidine-diaphorase for cytotoxicity. Because this enzyme has been reported to be increased in bladder cancer cells, this may lead to selectivity and could prove advantageous in terms of efficacy and safety.[45] A pilot study evaluating the pharmacokinetics and side effect profile showed no detectable levels in plasma and similar toxicities to those reported in other series using MMC.[46] Docetaxel and paclitaxel are chemotherapy agents that inhibit microtubule depolymerization and are being investigated for intravesical use.

SIDE EFFECTS OF INTRAVESICAL CHEMOTHERAPY

Side effects from perioperative intravesical chemotherapy can be divided into 2 separate entities, local and systemic, both of which can further be described as minor or major. From the previous discussion, it is evident that systemic absorption of these agents is in general low and associated with minimal toxicity. However, local side effects are common but fortunately self-limiting in most cases. The following section discusses the local and systemic side effects that are associated with intravesical chemotherapy as well as treatment strategies to manage them.

The true incidence of both local and systemic side effects with intravesical chemotherapy when applied in the perioperative setting is difficult to assess. Much of the data describing adverse events with intravesical chemotherapy is limited to induction courses whereby patients undergo weekly instillations for variable lengths of time. **Table 2** shows local and systemic adverse events that have been reported in previous clinical trials using intravesical chemotherapy in the immediate postoperative setting. Although the overall toxicity is low, reporting on toxicity among these trials is inconsistent and therefore may be underestimated.

Table 2
Toxicities reported from previous trials using perioperative intravesical chemotherapy for superficial bladder cancer

Series	Agent/Dose	Design	No. of Patients Treated	Local Symptoms	Comments	Systemic Symptoms
Tolley et al,[47] 1996	MMC 40 mg	3 arms: (1) Immediate MMC (2) Immediate MMC + induction (3) Control	149	Very low	Delayed healing at resection site in a few cases	None reported
Solsona et al,[48] 1999	MMC 30 mg	2 arms: (1) Immediate MMC (2) Control	57	Chemical cystitis 3.5%	No difference in catheterization period or hospital stay between groups	None reported No hematologic changes
EORTC30831[49]	MMC 30 mg	2 arms: (1) Immediate treatment (2) Delayed treatment	228/229	Chemical cystitis 6% (both groups)	3.0% required delay or discontinuation in arm 1	Rash, dizziness, malaise 7% (severe 1.8%)
EORTC30832[49]	Doxorubicin 50 mg	2 arms: (1) Immediate treatment (2) Delayed treatment	189/188	Chemical cystitis 9% (both groups)	2.2% required delay or discontinuation in arm 1	Rash, dizziness, malaise 7.1% (severe 0.8%)
Mostafid et al,[50] 2006	MMC	Single arm	177	Pain 1%	Catheter malfunction in 1 patient resulting in MMC contamination on skin	None reported
Oosterlinck et al,[51] 1993	Epirubicin 80 mg/50 mL	2 arms: (1) Epirubicin (2) Control	205	Chemical cystitis 11.7%	Skin allergy 1%	No hematologic abnormalities
Ali-el-Dein et al,[52] 1997	Epirubicin 50 mg/50 mL	RCT, 3 arms: (1) Immediate treatment (2) Delayed treatment (3) Control	55	Chemical cystitis 22% (mild 16%, severe 6%)		None
Okamura et al,[53] 2002	Pirarubicin 30 mg	RCT, 2 arms: (1) Doxorubicin-THP (2) Control	84	Chemical cystitis 25%		No systemic or hematologic abnormalities
MRC Working Party on Urologic Cancer[54]	Thiotepa 30 mg/50 mL	RCT, 3 arms: (1) Control (2) Immediate treatment (3) Immediate and induction treatment	379	Chemical cystitis <1%		Fluid retention/edema in 1 patient

Abbreviation: THP, (2″R)-4′-O-tetrahydropyranyl.

Local Side Effects

Administration of cytotoxic chemotherapy into the bladder can induce an array of irritative voiding symptoms including dysuria, frequency, urgency, suprapubic discomfort, gross hematuria, and pelvic pain, which collectively are referred to as chemical cystitis. In some cases, the onset of symptoms is immediate and may necessitate removal of an agent for alleviation. All chemotherapeutic agents can produce 1 or a combination of these symptoms. In a meta-analysis published by Sylvester and colleagues,[1] that included perioperative instillations of epirubicin, thiotepa, MMC, or pirarubicin, the reported toxicity incidence of chemical cystitis was approximately 10%. The effects were described as mild and transient in nature. **Table 2** shows a list of previous clinical trials using immediate intravesical chemotherapy that have information regarding local toxicity.

It is evident from review of the studies that the prevalence of symptoms related to chemical cystitis ranges from 1% to 25%. However, these data should be interpreted with caution, because the different methods of reporting toxicity were inconsistent across these studies. Furthermore, some trials did not even address specific data on treatment toxicity (not shown) and true rates of side effects are likely unknown or underestimated. Nonetheless, no serious events were reported in any of these trials.

Management of Chemical Cystitis

Symptoms of chemical cystitis are usually self-limiting and require no further treatment in the perioperative setting. Agents such as phenazopyridine (pyridium) and anticholinergics can be used in more bothersome cases. Powdered opium and belladonna alkaloids in a suppository form can also be used during instillation to provide relief of spasms and discomfort, and to help with retention of the intravesical agent. Other strategies to help reduce discomfort during treatment include ensuring the bladder is empty before instillation of agent and ensuring meticulous hemostasis at the end of resection to prevent accumulation of blood clots that may occlude the catheter and further exacerbate these symptoms. It is difficult to know whether many of the symptoms of cystitis are related to the intravesical agent or the procedure itself; however, management is the same for both. In addition, anecdotal recommendations of a short course of oral steroids have been advocated as significantly beneficial in alleviating severe cystitis-type symptoms (Chang, unpublished data).

Stoehr and colleagues[55] described a novel technique in efforts to improve patient comfort during intravesical MMC instillation. They proposed that some of the pain associated with perioperative instillation resulted from the rigid resistance of a clamped catheter and proposed a technique of maintaining the agent in the bladder without clamping. By elevating the urine bag 1 m above the supine patient, MMC was retained in the bladder by hydrostatic pressure (**Fig. 1**). In a randomized trial comparing this technique with the more traditional method of catheter clamping, they found that pain levels scores were significantly lower with the clampless technique and the mean instillation time was significantly longer (110 min vs 83 min).

In our practice, we make every effort to leave the agent indwelling for 2 hours, although depending on the patient and the amount of resection performed, this is highly variable. Patients who experience intolerable side effects during this period are first examined to ensure there is no evidence of peritoneal signs indicating possible extravasation. If absent, an anticholinergic and an intravenous analgesic are administered for pain control as needed, and in our experience this often results in adequate symptom control. As long as this regimen results in sufficient symptom management, the catheter

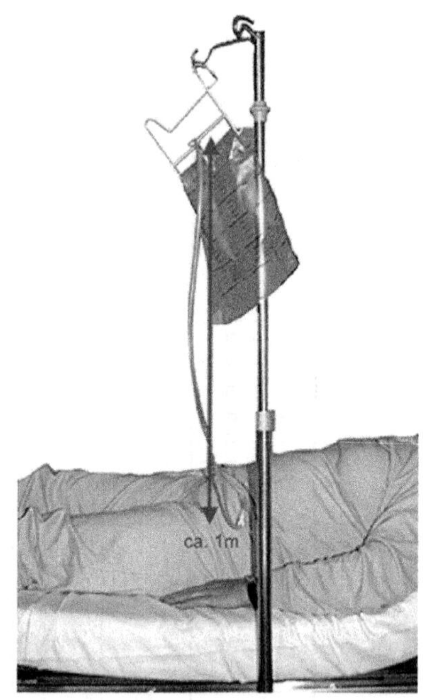

Fig. 1. Technique of maintaining a cytotoxic agent in the bladder through gravity. (*From* Stoehr B, Mueller T, Granig T, et al. Increasing patient comfort by optimized postoperative administration of intravesical mitomycin C. BJU Int 2008;102(11):1556–9; with permission.)

remains clamped with the agent in the bladder. If patient discomfort is not controlled by these measures, then the agent is carefully drained. If any evidence of a clot is present in the catheter at this time, the bladder is irrigated free of clots. In our experience, patients who have undergone large resections, patients with multiple previous resections or intravesical treatments, or patients who have had radiation therapy previously tend to have the most difficulty tolerating perioperative intravesical instillations.

Severe Local Side Effects of Intravesical Chemotherapy

Severe local complications from intravesical chemotherapy have been well described in several case reports. Although the cause is not entirely clear, it is likely that some of these complications occurred in cases of missed extravasation, as cystography was not performed. Examples of these complications include perivesical fat necrosis, bladder ulcerations, necrosis of the corpus spongiosum, fistula formation, perirectal fat necrosis with abscess, and pericystitis.

The necrotizing effects of MMC on the bladder have been described in several series. Doherty and colleagues[56] reported their findings from 12 patients who underwent radical cystectomy, 6 of whom had previous instillation of MMC or epirubicin. Median time between intravesical chemotherapy and cystectomy was 56 days. On pathologic examination, transmural and extravesical fat necrosis was significantly associated with intravesical chemotherapy supporting the fact that this treatment can lead to necrosis of the bladder wall (**Fig. 2**). Despite these findings, the investigators noted that no systemic or local side effects were encountered during the time of instillation. Branchereau and colleagues[57] described a case in which a patient developed full-thickness necrosis of the bladder after MMC instillation that ultimately required cystectomy. Thus, not all cases of bladder necrosis occur in the setting of suspected perforation. It has been suggested that cytotoxic agents may be capable of inducing a bladder perforation alone, especially if associated with deep resections of the anterior bladder wall.[58]

Bladder wall ulcerations and calcifications have been reported with intravesical chemotherapy use and may be present for months or years after treatment, and in our experience they are the most common local effect of intravesical MMC administration. In most cases these are asymptomatic; however, concomitant perivesical inflammation has also been reported and although rare, can cause pelvic pain that can be severe and prolonged in some cases.[59,60] Caution is advised against performing a biopsy or resection of these areas because they may not heal adequately and thus, as long as these ulcers or calcifications do not change during follow up, we usually do not perform a biopsy or repeat resection.

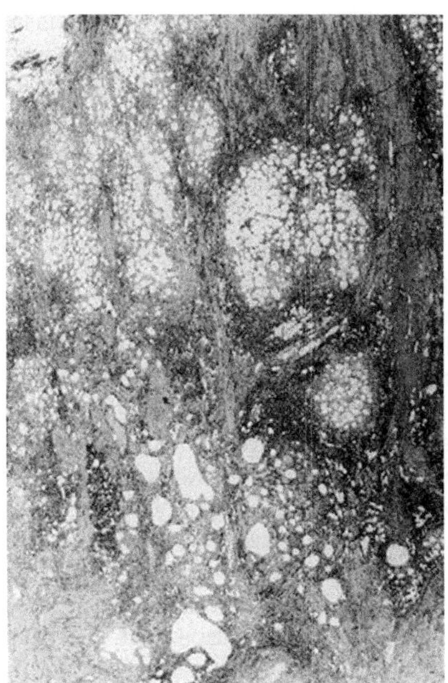

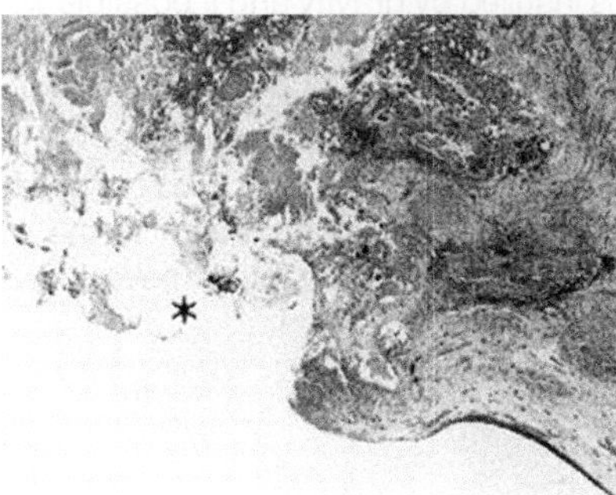

Fig. 2. Hematoxylin and eosin stain under low power magnification of a bladder specimen showing extravesical fat necrosis, fibrosis, and granulomatous inflammatory change. Asterisk indicates the site of TUR. (*From* Doherty AP, Trendell-Smith N, Stirling R, et al. Perivesical fat necrosis after adjuvant intravesical chemotherapy. BJU Int 1999;83(4):420–3; with permission.)

Treatment Strategies to Minimize Serious Local Toxicity

The risks of severe side effects are conceivably higher in the perioperative setting, due to the compromised integrity of the bladder wall, the possibility of catheter dislodgement or malfunction from blood clots as a result of recent resection. Extravasation of the agent into the submucosa or intraperitoneal/extraperitoneal space can cause significant damage to the bladder and surrounding tissue, resulting in necrosis, inflammation, and ulceration. Although the incidence of perforations is not entirely clear given the lack of routine cystography, Balbay and colleagues[61] found that extravasation was present in 60% of patients in a series of 35 undergoing tumor resection; larger tumor size was a significant predictor. Thus, the most important factors to reduce the incidence of these side effects is to establish meticulous hemostasis after tumor resection and to perform intraoperative cystography if there is any suspicion of bladder injury. We do not routinely perform cystograms in our patients unless there is clinical suspicion of perforation, but our threshold is extremely low when postoperative chemotherapy instillation is planned. It is also important that the agent is instilled by gravity and if possible while still under anesthesia to minimize patient discomfort with the filling. While the agent is indwelling, it is critical that the nursing staff be familiar with proper techniques for handling and disposing of these cytotoxic agents and remain alert to the warning signs of extravasation or other severe reactions to the agents.

Extravasation when it occurs in the acute setting can be either intraperitoneal or extraperitoneal and typically presents with pelvic pain or abdominal pain out of proportion to what is expected after TUR. If there is intraperitoneal extravasation, involuntary guarding, rigidity, and rebound tenderness consistent with an acute abdomen may be present. If extravasation is confirmed or suspected, the initial management is immediate evacuation of the agent followed by cystography for confirmation. Intraperitoneal perforations rarely heal with conservative measures and in cases where intravesical chemotherapy has been instilled, prompt exploratory laparotomy is required with evacuation of agent and repair of the defect. For extraperitoneal bladder perforations, catheter drainage until the bladder has healed is usually all that is required. We also recommend empirical use of an oral antibiotic for the duration of catheter use because a urinary tract infection in this setting could further complicate healing. A suggested algorithm for management is shown in **Fig. 3**.

In some instances, bladder extravasation can present in a delayed fashion, days to weeks after instillation (**Fig. 4**). Presenting complaints may include pelvic or abdominal pain, fever, signs of bowel obstruction, or ileus. Management in this setting involves catheter drainage, but it is also essential to perform imaging to evaluate for fluid

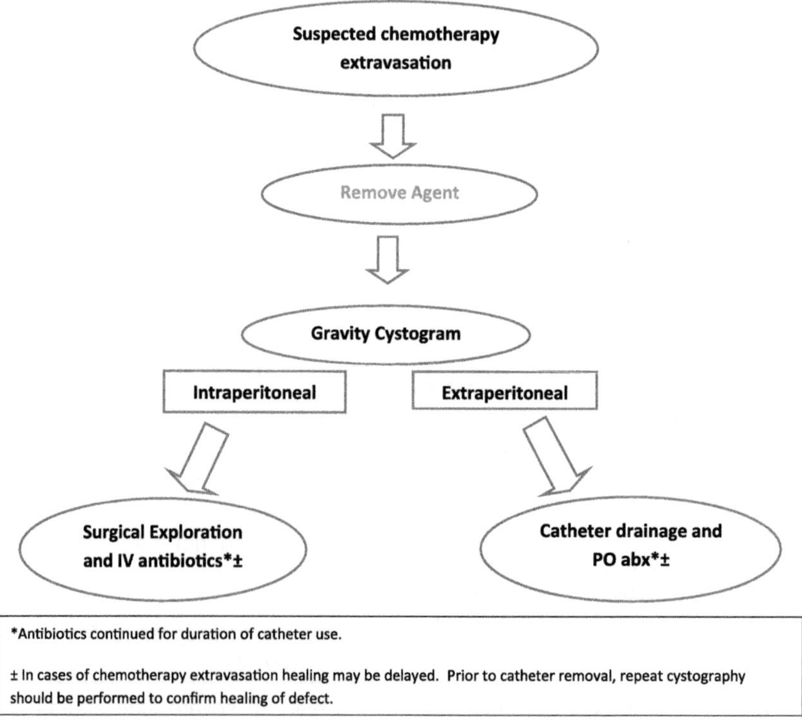

Fig. 3. Suggested algorithm for the management of suspected urinary extravasation during postoperative intravesical chemotherapy instillation.

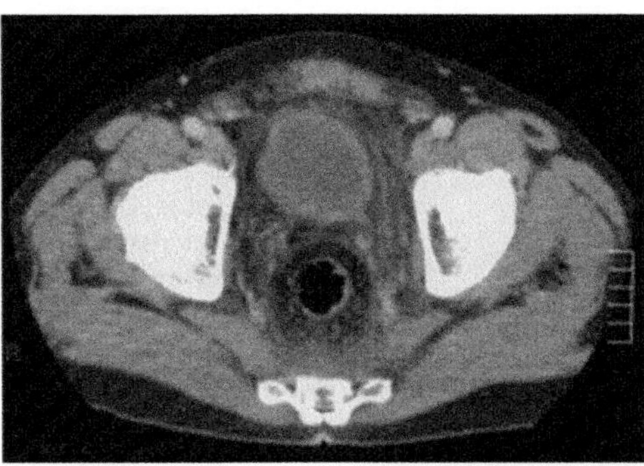
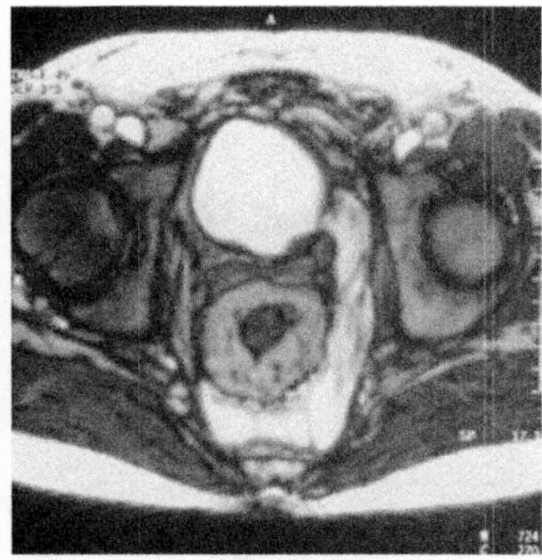

Fig. 4. Patient presenting with persistent pain 4 weeks after postoperative mitomycin C. Computed tomography scan shows bladder wall edema and perivesical stranding (*left*). Magnetic resonance imaging subsequently performed demonstrated left bladder wall perforation with extravasation (*right*). (*From* Nieuwenhuijzen JA, Bex A, Horenblas S. Unusual complication after immediate postoperative intravesical mitomycin C instillation. Eur Urol 2003;43(6):711–2; with permission.)

collection, abscess formation, fistula formation, or bowel obstruction. Several abnormalities have been described including perivesical stranding, extravasation, cutaneous, colovesical, and vesicovaginal fistulae, and the presence of a pelvic mass (typically at the bladder dome) adjacent to the small bowel have all been described.[62,63] Again, conservative management with catheter drainage of the bladder and percutaneous drainage of fluid collections is the treatment of choice in patients who are stable or do not present with peritoneal signs. When present, fluid collections should be drained and culture-directed antibiotics initiated. When conservative management fails, exploratory surgery is recommended, with excision of necrotic regions and bladder/fistula closure.[58,60,63] In rare cases, radical cystectomy with diversion may be necessary because of a lack of viable tissue or adequate bladder capacity.[63,64]

Skin Reactions

Intravesical chemotherapy can cause skin toxicity both by direct contact and by systemic exposure by absorption through bladder epithelium.[65,66] An estimated 9% of patients develop some type of cutaneous side effect from intravesical chemotherapy affecting both local and distant areas.[65,67] Although most case reports describing this side effect attribute it to mitomycin C, skin reactions caused by other agents such as epirubicin have also been described.[68]

The exact cause of this side effect is not entirely clear. Colver and colleagues[65] performed patch tests in 26 patients who had been previously exposed to MMC. They found a correlation between those who had strongly positive tests and those with cystitis (chemical) or skin eruption. Other series have performed patch tests to confirm reaction to MMC and epirubicin that support a delayed type IV mediated response.[58,59] Delayed hypersensitivity reactions from exposure to bladder epithelium seem to occur more frequently than direct contamination of skin.[67,69] Nonetheless, toxicity can develop from either direct spillage or systemic exposure, therefore the urologist must be diligent when using any intravesical agent in the perioperative setting.

Common manifestations of skin reactions include a generalized rash along with dermatitis of the hands and feet or genitalia. Other reported symptoms include eruptions of the face, trunk, or chest, vulvar dermatitis, and palpable purpura of the lower extremities (**Fig. 5**).[67] There have been 2 case reports describing severe necrotizing reactions involving the glans and ulceration of the penile shaft, which ultimately required total penectomy and perineal urethrostomy (**Fig. 6**).[70,71] In 1 case, spillage of MMC on the perineum after catheter removal[71] and suspicion of traumatic Foley catheter placement[70] were attributed as the possible inciting events.

Management of Skin Toxicity

In most cases, cutaneous side effects are self-limiting and resolve after removal of exposing agent. Antihistamines and corticosteroids are useful for those who develop generalized urticaria.[6] In most of the previous series describing skin toxicity, MMC was used as part of an induction course rather than as a single postoperative dose. If skin reactions develop after exposure in the perioperative setting and considerations are given to additional intravesical chemotherapy, a patch test may be helpful in distinguishing if there is an allergic mechanism present. In those cases, an alternative agent or immunotherapy may be considered in efforts to minimize recurrent reactions.

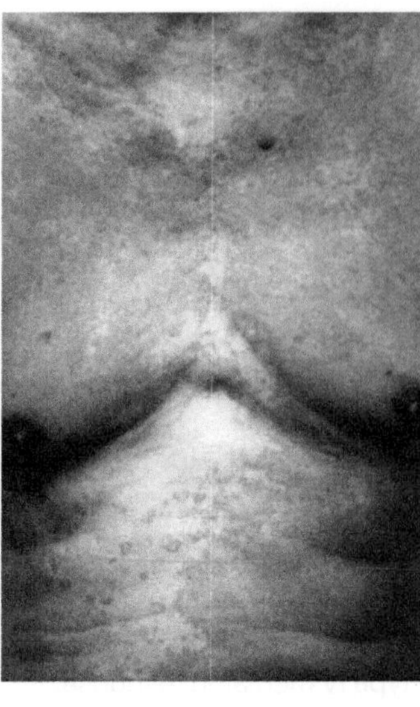
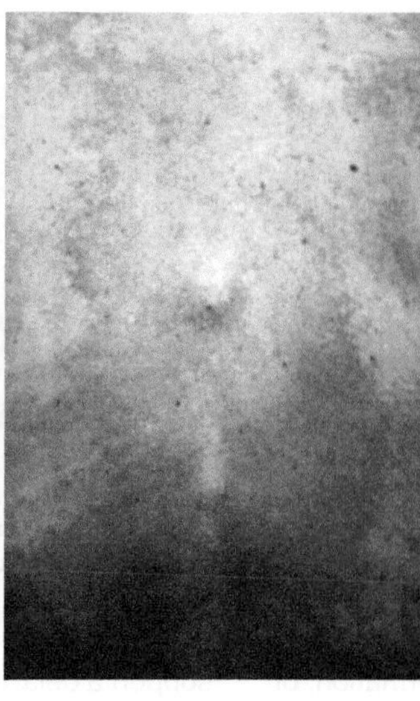

Fig. 5. Drug eruption affecting chest (*left*) and back (*right*) in a patient treated with epirubicin for non-muscle invasive bladder cancer. (*Reprinted from* Okumura A, Oishi N, Kaji K, et al. Drug eruption due to intravesical instillations of both epirubicin and mitomycin C. J Dermatol 2009;36(7):419–22; with permission.)

The patient and caregiver should use universal precautions when handling these agents. Specialized gloves for handling should be readily available and after use, the agents should be disposed of properly. The patient should be instructed to wash their hands and genitalia after the first several voids as residual chemotherapy could still be present. After discharge, it is important that the patient is counseled regarding signs of local and systemic skin reactions and to notify the physician if any of these unforeseen changes occur.

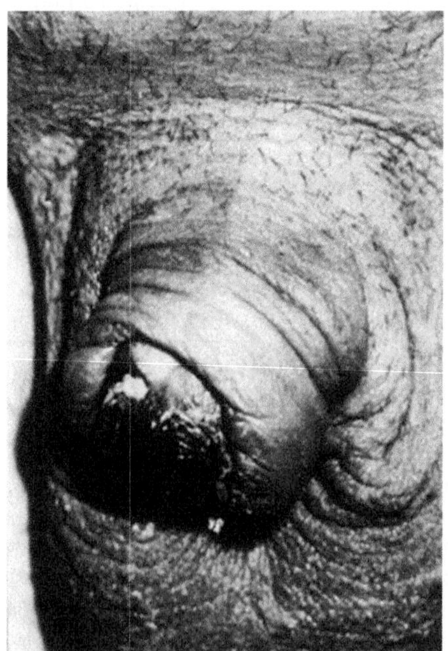

Fig. 6. Glans necrosis resulting from perioperative instillation of mitomycin C. (*From* Neulander EZ, Lismer L, Kaneti J. Necrosis of the glans penis: a rare complication of intravesical therapy with mitomycin c. J Urol 2000;164(4):1306; with permission.)

Systemic Toxicity

Systemic effects of intravesical chemotherapy are rare and primarily result in myelosuppression. Thiotepa is associated with the highest rates of myelosuppression, with leukopenia occurring in 8.4% to 54% and thrombocytopenia in 3.2% to 31% in previous reports.[6] The induction dose and frequency of administration varied among these series and not all included perioperative instillation.[6] Another trial using thiotepa in the perioperative setting did not report on rates of myelosuppression.[54] Soloway and Ford[41] reported their experience of more than 600 thiotepa instillations in 72 patients in both perioperative and induction settings. They found some form of myelosuppression in 18% of cases, which equated to 3.9% of total instillations, but there were no associated adverse outcomes.

MMC has the potential to cause myelosuppression when administered systemically. Given its higher molecular weight, however, systemic manifestations when it is given intravesically are fortunately rare. A review by Thrasher and Crawford[6] found myelosuppression reported in a total of 8 patients from 3 separate series including more than 150 patients. Multiple other series did not report any evidence of leukopenia or thrombocytopenia. Again, all of these studies involved induction courses after TUR in which patients had repeat instillations up to a year after treatment. Zein and colleagues,[72] using a single instillation of perioperative MMC at a dose of 80 mg, reported a fatal case of aplastic anemia that developed 2 weeks after instillation in a patient with a large resection. However, such reactions are isolated rather than consistent events across series.

The anthracyline agents (doxorubicin, epirubicin, pararubicin) have minimal absorption as previously discussed. Previous trials show the rate of systemic toxicity in the range of 1% (see **Table 2**). A pilot study evaluating tolerability and toxicity of valrubicin in the perioperative setting included 1 patient who developed grade IV neutropenia (<500/mm^3) along with mild anemia and thrombocytopenia.

Other systemic complaints occasionally reported with intravesical chemotherapy include malaise, fever, nausea, and vomiting. Whether these are more related to the procedure itself, the general anesthetic, or from the intravesical instillation is difficult to fully assess.

Management of Systemic Toxicity

Management is usually supportive. Blood products may be given in severe cases of myelosuppression, but the incidence of that is low. At present, the rarity of myelosuppression is such that routine use of laboratory evaluation is unjustified, and routine surveillance of counts is not recommend.[73]

Long-Term Complications

Intravesical chemotherapy may have long-term effects on the bladder, which may have significant implications. Benign chronic ulcers at the resection site have been described and are attributed to the effect of impaired healing from chemotherapy.[59,74] These ulcers can pose a diagnostic challenge at surveillance cystoscopy because they can be mistaken for recurrent disease. It is important to use ancillary tests such as urine cytology and fluorescence in situ hybridization in indeterminate situations. These lesions usually heal eventually and only if they change in character or size do we perform a biopsy to rule out recurrent disease.

Calcification or fibrosis of the bladder wall with resulting impaired capacity is another potential long-term complication, and the one most feared by urologists.[75–78] The incidence of bladder contracture with use of intravesical chemotherapy is approximately 5%.[2] Both MMC and epirubicin can cause a reduction of bladder volume and compliance. In a study by Michielsen and colleagues,[79] the urodynamic changes occurring after MMC and epirubicin instillations were studied in rats. They found a significant reduction in both bladder capacity and compliance that persisted for 3 weeks after treatment. Eijsten and colleagues[75] found that long-term results in a series of 75 patients treated with MMC at 2 doses resulted in 6 patients with bladder capacities less than 200 mL. The lasting effects of intravesical chemotherapy can therefore adversely affect urinary function and quality of life. Although prolonged changes of compliance resulting in frequency, urgency, and occasionally incontinence can occur, most patients can be managed with anticholinergic medications with ultimate resolution of these symptoms. In our experience, this may take up to 6 months but more commonly resolve in 3 months.

SUMMARY

Perioperative intravesical chemotherapy remains an important management option for patients with non-muscle invasive bladder cancer. Studies demonstrate consistent reductions in the risk of bladder tumor recurrence. However, the benefits must be carefully considered because patients can experience side effects some of which can be debilitating and even permanent. Many urologists use immediate postoperative intravesical chemotherapy in cases of recurrent tumor when the initial diagnosis is established, and this is certainly a reasonable approach. Proper counseling of patients regarding the risks of intravesical chemotherapy is crucial as well as proper education of operating room and nursing staff to reduce the potential risks associated with administration and handling. When adverse events do occur, early recognition, proper therapy and patient reassurance usually result in satisfactory outcomes.

REFERENCES

1. Sylvester RJ, Oosterlinck W, van der Meijden AP. A single immediate postoperative instillation of chemotherapy decreases the risk of recurrence in patients with stage Ta T1 bladder cancer: a meta-analysis of published results of randomized clinical trials. J Urol 2004;171(6):2186–90.
2. Hall MC, Chang SS, Dalbagni G, et al. Guideline for the management of nonmuscle invasive bladder cancer (stages Ta, T1, and Tis): 2007 update. J Urol 2007;178(6):2314–30.
3. Babjuk M, Oosterlinck W, Sylvester R, et al. EAU guidelines on non-muscle-invasive urothelial carcinoma of the bladder. Eur Urol 2008;54(2): 303–14.
4. Mishina T, Watanabe H, Kobayashi T, et al. Absorption of anticancer drugs through bladder epithelium. Urology 1986;27(2):148–57.
5. Lum BL. Intravesical chemotherapy of superficial bladder cancer. Recent Results Cancer Res 1983; 85:3–36.

6. Thrasher JB, Crawford ED. Complications of intravesical chemotherapy. Urol Clin North Am 1992; 19(3):529–39.
7. Paz MM, Zhang X, Lu J, et al. A new mechanism of action for the anticancer drug mitomycin C: mechanism-based inhibition of thioredoxin reductase. Chem Res Toxicol 2012;25(7):1502–11.
8. Bradner WT. Mitomycin C: a clinical update. Cancer Treat Rev 2001;27(1):35–50.
9. Zatkone Puskas G. Az extravazacio jelentosege az onkologiai apolasban. [The significance of extravasation in oncological care]. Magy Onkol 2008; 52(1):75–80 [in Hungarian].
10. Goolsby TV, Lombardo FA. Extravasation of chemotherapeutic agents: prevention and treatment. Semin Oncol 2006;33(1):139–43.
11. Albanell J, Baselga J. Systemic therapy emergencies. Semin Oncol 2000;27(3):347–61.
12. Bregman CL, Buroker RA, Bradner WT, et al. Cardiac, renal, and pulmonary toxicity of several mitomycin derivatives in rats. Fundam Appl Toxicol 1989;13(1):46–64.
13. Coetmeur D, Briens E, Le Breton-Belleguic C, et al. Pneumopathie interstitielle et mitomycine C. A propos d'un cas avec etude du lavage broncho-alveolaire. [Interstitial pneumonia and mitomycin C. Apropos of a case with analysis of the bronchoalveolar lavage]. Rev Pneumol Clin 1995;51(1):36–40 [in French].
14. Doll DC, Ringenberg QS, Yarbro JW. Vascular toxicity associated with antineoplastic agents. J Clin Oncol 1986;4(9):1405–17.
15. Janeiro Pais JM, Casas Agudo VP, Lopez Garcia D, et al. Mitomicina C endovesical y fibrosis pulmonar. [Pulmonary fibrosis and endovesical mitomycin C]. Actas Urol Esp 2009;33(7):822–5 [in Spanish].
16. Klein DS, Wilds PR. Pulmonary toxicity of antineoplastic agents: anaesthetic and postoperative implications. Can Anaesth Soc J 1983;30(4):399–405.
17. Linette DC, McGee KH, McFarland JA. Mitomycin-induced pulmonary toxicity: case report and review of the literature. Ann Pharmacother 1992;26(4): 481–4.
18. Liu K, Mittelman A, Sproul EE, et al. Renal toxicity in man treated with mitomycin C. Cancer 1971;28(5): 1314–20.
19. Simon P, Herve JP, Ramee MP, et al. La nephrotoxicite de la mitomycine C. Trois nouvelles observations et revue de la litterature. [Mytomycin C nephrotoxicity. 3 new cases and review of the literature]. Nephrologie 1982;3(4):152–7 [in French].
20. Crocker J, Jones EL. Haemolytic-uraemic syndrome complicating long-term mitomycin C and 5-fluorouracil therapy for gastric carcinoma. J Clin Pathol 1983;36(1):24–9.
21. Ravikumar TS, Sibley R, Reed K, et al. Renal toxicity of mitomycin-C. Am J Clin Oncol 1984;7(3):279–85.
22. Valavaara R, Nordman E. Renal complications of mitomycin C therapy with special reference to the total dose. Cancer 1985;55(1):47–50.
23. Verwey J, de Vries J, Pinedo HM. Mitomycin C-induced renal toxicity, a dose-dependent side effect? Eur J Cancer Clin Oncol 1987;23(2):195–9.
24. Wientjes MG, Dalton JT, Badalament RA, et al. Bladder wall penetration of intravesical mitomycin C in dogs. Cancer Res 1991;51(16):4347–54.
25. Wientjes MG, Badalament RA, Wang RC, et al. Penetration of mitomycin C in human bladder. Cancer Res 1993;53(14):3314–20.
26. Wajsman Z, Dhafir RA, Pfeffer M, et al. Studies of mitomycin C absorption after intravesical treatment of superficial bladder tumors. J Urol 1984;132(1): 30–3.
27. Sarna GP, Champlin R, Wells J, et al. Phase I study of high-dose mitomycin with autologous bone marrow support. Cancer Treat Rep 1982;66(2): 277–82.
28. Gewirtz DA. A critical evaluation of the mechanisms of action proposed for the antitumor effects of the anthracycline antibiotics adriamycin and daunorubicin. Biochem Pharmacol 1999;57(7):727–41.
29. Chai M, Wientjes MG, Badalament RA, et al. Pharmacokinetics of intravesical doxorubicin in superficial bladder cancer patients. J Urol 1994; 152(2 Pt 1):374–8.
30. Plosker GL, Faulds D. Epirubicin. A review of its pharmacodynamic and pharmacokinetic properties, and therapeutic use in cancer chemotherapy. Drugs 1993;45(5):788–856.
31. Koga H, Kuroiwa K, Yamaguchi A, et al. A randomized controlled trial of short-term versus long-term prophylactic intravesical instillation chemotherapy for recurrence after transurethral resection of Ta/T1 transitional cell carcinoma of the bladder. J Urol 2004;171(1):153–7.
32. Tsushima T, Miyaji Y, Noda M, et al. Absorption of epirubicin instilled intravesically immediately after transurethral resection of superficial bladder cancer. Urol Int 1998;60(3):161–4.
33. Shang PF, Kwong J, Wang ZP, et al. Intravesical Bacillus Calmette-Guerin versus epirubicin for Ta and T1 bladder cancer. Cochrane Database Syst Rev 2011;(5):CD006885.
34. Yamamoto Y, Nasu Y, Saika T, et al. The absorption of pirarubicin instilled intravesically immediately after transurethral resection of superficial bladder cancer. BJU Int 2000;86(7):802–4.
35. Dinney CP, Greenberg RE, Steinberg GD. Intravesical valrubicin in patients with bladder carcinoma in situ and contraindication to or failure after bacillus Calmette-Guerin. Urol Oncol 2012 [Epub ahead of print].
36. Niell HB, Hunter RF, Herrod HG, et al. Effects of N-trifluoroacetyladriamycin-14-valerate (AD-32) on

human bladder tumor cell lines. Cancer Chemother Pharmacol 1987;19(1):47–52.
37. Greenberg RE, Bahnson RR, Wood D, et al. Initial report on intravesical administration of N-trifluoroacetyladriamycin-14-valerate (AD 32) to patients with refractory superficial transitional cell carcinoma of the urinary bladder. Urology 1997;49(3):471–5.
38. Patterson AL, Greenberg RE, Weems L, et al. Pilot study of the tolerability and toxicity of intravesical valrubicin immediately after transurethral resection of superficial bladder cancer. Urology 2000;56(2): 232–5.
39. Jones HC, Swinney J. Thiotepa in the treatment of tumours of the bladder. Lancet 1961;2:615–8.
40. Lunglmayr G, Czech K. Absorption studies on intraluminal thio-tepa for topical cytostatic treatment of low-stage bladder tumors. J Urol 1971;106:72–4.
41. Soloway MS, Ford KS. Thiotepa-induced myelosuppression: review of 670 bladder instillations. J Urol 1983;130(5):889–91.
42. Mini E, Nobili S, Caciagli B, et al. Cellular pharmacology of gemcitabine. Ann Oncol 2006; 17(Suppl 5):v7–12.
43. Böhle A, Leyh H, Frei C, et al. Single postoperative instillation of gemcitabine in patients with non-muscle-invasive transitional cell carcinoma of the bladder: a randomised, double-blind, placebo-controlled phase III multicentre study. Eur Urol 2009;56(3):495–503.
44. Maffezzini M, Campodonico F, Puntoni M, et al. Systemic absorption and pharmacokinetics of single-dose intravesical gemcitabine after transurethral resection of the bladder in non-muscle-invasive bladder cancer. Urology 2009;74(5):1078–83.
45. Li D, Gan Y, Wientjes MG, et al. Distribution of DT-diaphorase and reduced nicotinamide adenine dinucleotide phosphate: cytochrome p450 oxidoreductase in bladder tissues and tumors. J Urol 2001;166(6):2500–5.
46. Hendricksen K, Gleason D, Young JM, et al. Safety and side effects of immediate instillation of apaziquone following transurethral resection in patients with nonmuscle invasive bladder cancer. J Urol 2008;180(1):116–20.
47. Tolley DA, Parmar MK, Grigor KM, et al. The effect of intravesical mitomycin C on recurrence of newly diagnosed superficial bladder cancer: a further report with 7 years of follow up. J Urol 1996; 155(4):1233–8.
48. Solsona E, Iborra I, Ricos JV, et al. Effectiveness of a single immediate mitomycin C instillation in patients with low risk superficial bladder cancer: short and long-term followup. J Urol 1999;161(4): 1120–3.
49. Bouffioux C, Kurth KH, Bono A, et al. Intravesical adjuvant chemotherapy for superficial transitional cell bladder carcinoma: results of 2 European Organization for Research and Treatment of Cancer randomized trials with mitomycin C and doxorubicin comparing early versus delayed instillations and short-term versus long-term treatment. European Organization for Research and Treatment of Cancer Genitourinary Group. J Urol 1995;153(3 Pt 2):934–41.
50. Mostafid AH, Rajkumar RG, Stewart AB, et al. Immediate administration of intravesical mitomycin C after tumour resection for superficial bladder cancer. BJU Int 2006;97(3):509–12.
51. Oosterlinck W, Kurth KH, Schroder F, et al. A prospective European Organization for Research and Treatment of Cancer Genitourinary Group randomized trial comparing transurethral resection followed by a single intravesical instillation of epirubicin or water in single stage Ta, T1 papillary carcinoma of the bladder. J Urol 1993;149(4):749–52.
52. Ali-el-Dein B, el-Baz M, Aly AN, et al. Intravesical epirubicin versus doxorubicin for superficial bladder tumors (stages pTa and pT1): a randomized prospective study. J Urol 1997;158(1):68–73 [discussion: 73–4].
53. Okamura K, Ono Y, Kinukawa T, et al. Randomized study of single early instillation of (2″R)-4′-O-tetrahydropyranyl-doxorubicin for a single superficial bladder carcinoma. Cancer 2002;94(9):2363–8.
54. The effect of intravesical thiotepa on the recurrence rate of newly diagnosed superficial bladder cancer. An MRC Study. MRC Working Party on Urological Cancer. Br J Urol 1985;57(6):680–5.
55. Stoehr B, Mueller T, Granig T, et al. Increasing patient comfort by optimized postoperative administration of intravesical mitomycin C. BJU Int 2008; 102(11):1556–9.
56. Doherty AP, Trendell-Smith N, Stirling R, et al. Perivesical fat necrosis after adjuvant intravesical chemotherapy. BJU Int 1999;83(4):420–3.
57. Branchereau J, Luyckx F, Hitier M, et al. Necrose vesicale dans les suites d'une instillation postoperatoire precoce (Ipop) de mitomycine C. [Bladder necrosis after an immediate post-operative mitomycin C instillation]. Prog Urol 2011;21(2):151–3 [in French].
58. Fazlioglu A, Tandogdu Z, Kurtulus FO, et al. Perivesical inflammation and necrosis due to mitomycin C instillation after transurethral resection of bladder tumor: we must be vigilant! Urol Int 2009;83(3): 362–3.
59. Cliff AM, Romaniuk CS, Parr NJ. Perivesical inflammation after early mitomycin C instillation. BJU Int 2000;85(4):556–7.
60. Nieuwenhuijzen JA, Bex A, Horenblas S. Unusual complication after immediate postoperative intravesical mitomycin C instillation. Eur Urol 2003; 43(6):711–2.
61. Balbay MD, Cimentepe E, Unsal A, et al. The actual incidence of bladder perforation following

transurethral bladder surgery. The Journal of Urology 2005;17(6):2260–2.

62. Oddens JR, van der Meijden AP, Sylvester R. One immediate postoperative instillation of chemotherapy in low risk Ta, T1 bladder cancer patients. Is it always safe? Eur Urol 2004;46(3):336–8.
63. Dangle PP, Wang WP, Pohar KS. Vesicoenteric, vesicovaginal, vesicocutaneous fistula -an unusual complication with intravesical mitomycin. Can J Urol 2008;15(5):4269–72.
64. Shapiro O, Jones K, Wang C, et al. Risk of postoperative intravesical mitomycin C instillation following transurethral bladder tumor resection. Can J Urol 2006;13(6):3317–20.
65. Colver GB, Inglis JA, McVittie E, et al. Dermatitis due to intravesical mitomycin C: a delayed-type hypersensitivity reaction? Br J Dermatol 1990;122(2):217–24.
66. de Groot AC, Conemans JM. Systemic allergic contact dermatitis from intravesical instillation of the antitumor antibiotic mitomycin C. Contact Dermatitis 1991;24(3):201–9.
67. Kunkeler L, Nieboer C, Bruynzeel DP. Type III and type IV hypersensitivity reactions due to mitomycin C. Contact Dermatitis 2000;42(2):74–6.
68. Okumura A, Oishi N, Kaji K, et al. Drug eruption due to intravesical instillations of both epirubicin and mitomycin C. J Dermatol 2009;36(7):419–22.
69. Bolenz C, Cao Y, Arancibia MF, et al. Intravesical mitomycin C for superficial transitional cell carcinoma. Expert Rev Anticancer Ther 2006;6(8): 1273–82.
70. Neulander EZ, Lismer L, Kaneti J. Necrosis of the glans penis: a rare complication of intravesical therapy with mitomycin c. J Urol 2000;164(4):1306.
71. Kureshi F, Kalaaji AN, Halvorson L, et al. Cutaneous complications of intravesical treatments for bladder cancer: granulomatous inflammation of the penis following BCG therapy and penile gangrene following mitomycin therapy. J Am Acad Dermatol 2006;55(2):328–31.
72. Zein TA, Friedberg N, Kim H. Bone marrow suppression after intravesical mitomycin C treatment. J Urol 1986;136(2):459–60.
73. Koya MP, Simon MA, Soloway MS. Complications of intravesical therapy for urothelial cancer of the bladder. J Urol 2006;175(6):2004–10.
74. Richards B, Tolley D. Benign ulcers after bladder instillation of mitomycin C. Lancet 1986;1(8471):45.
75. Eijsten A, Knonagel H, Hotz E, et al. Reduced bladder capacity in patients receiving intravesical chemoprophylaxis with mitomycin C. Br J Urol 1990;66(4):386–8.
76. Pouya M, Van Cangh PJ, Wese FX, et al. Calcification de la paroi vesicale apres instillation de la mitomycine C. A propos d'une observation. [Calcification of the bladder wall following instillation of mitomycin C. Apropos of a case report]. Acta Urol Belg 1995;63(4):19–21 [in French].
77. Drago PC, Badalament RA, Lucas J, et al. Bladder wall calcification after intravesical mitomycin C treatment of superficial bladder cancer. J Urol 1989; 142(4):1071–2.
78. Alter AJ, Malek GH. Bladder wall calcification after topical mitomycin C. J Urol 1987;138(5):1239–40.
79. Michielsen D, Amy JJ, Coomans D, et al. Mitomycin C and epirubicin: functional bladder damage in rats after repeat intravesical instillations. J Urol 2005; 173(6):2166–70.

Strategies for Optimizing Bacillus Calmette-Guérin

Jay B. Shah, MD, Ashish M. Kamat, MD*

KEYWORDS

• Superficial bladder cancer • Non-muscle invasive bladder cancer • Bacillus Calmette-Guérin

KEY POINTS

- Bacillus Calmette-Guérin (BCG) is arguably the most effective intravesical treatment option for patients with intermediate-to-high risk superficial bladder cancer.
- A poor understanding of how and when BCG should be used can lead to suboptimal outcomes.
- Careful attention to patient and tumor characteristics can help identify candidates most likely to respond to BCG.
- Specific technical strategies can be employed to optimize BCG outcomes.

INTRODUCTION

As discussed throughout this issue, bladder cancer represents a significant physical and emotional burden to patients as well as a substantial financial burden to society (see the article by James and colleagues elsewhere in this issue). For patients at the extremes of risk, treatment algorithms are relatively straightforward; yet the outcomes are variable. Within the spectrum of non-muscle invasive bladder cancer (NMIBC), for patients with the lowest-risk tumors, the mainstay of treatment is complete transurethral resection (TUR) followed by surveillance (see the article by O'Neil and colleagues elsewhere in this issue); for patients with the most advanced risk tumors, radical cystectomy may be the only viable option (see the article by Daneshmand elsewhere in this issue). Among the areas of greatest uncertainty within the discipline of bladder cancer is the management of patients with NMIBC thought to have a high risk of recurrence and/or intermediate-to-high risk of progression. In this setting, intravesical immunotherapy with bacillus Calmette-Guérin (BCG) is the current gold standard therapy with the highest response rates; however, despite its frequent use, it remains poorly understood, resulting in usage that is far from optimal.

In this article, the authors review the role that BCG has played in the management of bladder cancer over the last several decades and discuss specific approaches to optimize BCG. They focus on selection strategies to help practitioners identify candidates most likely to respond to BCG as well as on technical strategies to enhance the administration of the drug in such a way as to optimize the response rates, adverse effects, and outcomes (**Box 1**).

HISTORY OF BCG

The history of BCG dates back to the mid-1800s when scientists identified *Mycobacterium bovis* as the causative agent for bovine tuberculosis. Extrapolating from the successful use of the cowpox agent to develop a highly effective vaccine against smallpox in humans, clinical trials were performed in the late 19th century using *M bovis* to prevent tuberculosis in humans. Unfortunately, *M bovis* was proven to be highly virulent in people, and the approach was quickly abandoned.

Conflicts of Interest: Neither author has any relevant financial disclosures.

Department of Urology, MD Anderson Cancer Center, 1515 Holcombe Boulevard, Unit 1373, Houston, TX 77030, USA

* Corresponding author.

E-mail address: akamat@mdanderson.org

Urol Clin N Am 40 (2013) 211–218

http://dx.doi.org/10.1016/j.ucl.2013.01.012

0094-0143/13/$ – see front matter

Box 1
Strategies for practitioners

Tumor Characteristics

High-grade tumors with risk of recurrence/progression

No invasive component

No aberrant histology (micropapillary, small cell)

No T1 on prompt repeated TUR

Patient Characteristics

No active immunosuppression (eg, transplant)

Elderly okay

HIV (+) status okay

Personal history of tuberculosis okay

Technical Aspects

Give induction + maintenance (SWOG8507 protocol)

Minimize fluid intake in the hours before instillation

Start with empty bladder

Inspect voided urine for visible hematuria (routine urinalysis/dipstick not necessary)

Catheterize urethra atraumatically

Minimize lubricant (to avoid BCG clumping)

Avoid lidocaine (acidity degrades BCG)

No need for rotisserie-style turning

Statins/aspirin therapy okay to continue

Use antispasmodics for local symptoms

Use antipyretics for influenza-like symptoms

Give 1 dose of quinolone 6 hours after BCG

Admit suspected BCGosis/BCG sepsis for prompt workup and aggressive therapy

Several decades later, in 1908, a French bacteriologist, Albert Calmette and a veterinarian, Camille Guérin observed that incubation of *M bovis* in a glycerin-bile-potato medium rendered the bacteria slightly less virulent. Over the next 13 years, they serially passaged the bacteria 231 times, and in 1920 ultimately obtained a strain of *M bovis* that was avirulent in both animals and people.[1] This unique strain came to be known as bacillus of Calmette and Guérin (BCG).

Clinical trials using BCG as a vaccine against tuberculosis were initiated in 1921 but were not met with enthusiasm. Several early catastrophic events caused by cross-contamination with pathogenic strains led to public distrust of the agent. In one particularly disastrous situation in 1930 in Lübeck, Germany, 240 infants vaccinated shortly after birth all developed tuberculosis, and 72 of these newborns died.[2] After several decades of disuse, widespread BCG vaccination was once again implemented outside of North America to minimize the postwar increase in tuberculosis expected after World War II. In the United States, BCG vaccination has never been widely adopted.

In the last half century, there has been renewed interest in the application of BCG to the management of patients with various medical disorders. As a potent stimulus of the immune system, BCG has been studied as a treatment option for diabetes mellitus, multiple sclerosis, and Parkinson disease.[3–7]

In the field of oncology, the first hint that BCG may have a therapeutic role was present in 1929 when Pearl, a pathologist, observed that tuberculosis patients had fewer malignancies than patients who died of other diseases.[8] In the recent era, BCG has been studied to varying degrees in colorectal cancer, lung cancer, and melanoma.[9–11] Far and away, the most successful reapplication of BCG in the developed world has been in the field of bladder cancer.

The initial work suggesting a role for BCG within the bladder was performed in 1966 by Coe and Feldman, who demonstrated a consistent and potent T-helper type 1 immune response in pig bladders exposed to intravesical BCG.[12] 10 years later, Morales reported that 9 patients with superficial bladder cancer experienced a decrease in rate of tumor recurrence after intradermal and intravesical treatment with the Armand-Frappier strain of BCG.[13] This led to a prospective, randomized clinical trial in 1980 that confirmed the beneficial findings of the smaller initial report.[14] In this clinical trial, Lamm and colleagues demonstrated that treatment with a single percutaneous injection followed by 6 weekly intravesical administrations of BCG led to a decreased tumor recurrence rate at 1 year.

Since this initial trial, multiple investigators have undertaken larger trials aimed at more clearly identifying the optimal route, dosing, and scheduling parameters of BCG for patients with superficial bladder cancer.[15–18] These refinements form the basis of current guidelines concerning the optimal use of BCG in the management of bladder cancer and are discussed further in the following sections. In fact, when BCG is used optimally, it has a definite role in reducing progression and deaths from bladder cancer.[19,20]

OPTIMIZING PATIENT SELECTION FOR BCG THERAPY

As with all cancer therapies, successful use of BCG is critically dependent on careful patient selection.

For patients with NMIBC, the 2 main indications for the use of BCG are: adjunctive therapy to reduce the recurrence (and progression) of tumors after complete surgical resection of high-grade T_a or T_1 papillary tumors, and ii) primary treatment of carcinoma in situ (CIS).

Tumor Characteristics

For patients with low-grade papillary tumors, BCG therapy is typically not recommended, because, the most patients can be managed with surgical resection (plus or minus single-shot postoperative intravesical chemotherapy) alone. BCG has been used to treat residual tumor in patients with a high volume of disease within the bladder where surgical resection was deemed unachievable and/or for patients medically unfit for any operative procedures with complete response rates up to 66% and partial response rates up to 21%. In general, however, complete endoscopic control is recommended before BCG instillation.[15,21,22]

For patients with muscle-invasive disease, there is currently no standard role for BCG; the use of BCG or any other intravesical therapy limited to the mucosal surface should be considered insufficient. In 1 report of 13 patients with muscle invasive bladder cancer treated with BCG, only 1 of 13 patients had neither local nor systemic disease recurrence; 10 of 13 patients developed systemic disease, and 7 patients died from metastases.[23] The delay to removal of the bladder that these intravesical therapies impose can have disastrous consequences for patients.

Similarly, for patients with high-risk histologic variants of bladder cancer, BCG therapy may not be sufficient even if the tumors are superficial at diagnosis. For example, in patients found to have micropapillary architecture, the risk of early spread to regional lymph nodes or distant sites is sufficiently high to make conservative local therapy unsafe.[24,25] For patients with small cell histology or features of neuroendocrine differentiation, the propensity for early microscopic metastases also argues against the use of BCG and other conservative intravesical therapies.[26]

Given the efficacy of BCG in superficial urothelial tumors and the danger of BCG in muscle-invasive tumors and high-risk histologic variants, it is critical to accurately establish the true stage of any bladder tumor before deciding on therapy. Current guidelines recommend a repeat TUR for all patients with T_1 bladder cancer.[27,28] This is discussed in more detail by Ritch and colleagues elsewhere in this issue, but the guiding principle before intravesical therapy with BCG should be removal of all cancerous tissue, where feasible.

From the specific perspective of optimization of BCG, data from repeat TUR can help stratify patients into those at higher and lower risk of response to BCG. For example, data from Memorial Sloan Kettering Cancer Center (MSKCC) suggest that patients with initial T_1 disease found to have no tumor or stage less than or equal to T_a on repeat resection have a 19% chance of progression to muscle-invasive disease within 5 years, whereas those patients with evidence of continued T_1 disease at repeat TUR have an 80% chance of progression to muscle-invasive disease within 5 years.[29,30] While these data are colored with the particular referral biases (and no use of maintenance), it nonetheless provides an impetus to use the repeat TUR data as 1 variable in discussions with patients.

Given the important prognostic information that can be gained from a second TUR, the authors' practice is to perform repeat TUR at 4 to 6 weeks on all patients with T_1 bladder cancer being considered for intravesical therapy. In those patients who have had a complete TUR at the first setting and yet have T_1 disease at repeat TUR (ie, early recurrence of aggressive disease), the authors counsel the patients on the potential high failure rate of BCG and the benefit of early radical cystectomy. However, this does not apply to delayed repeat TUR or repeat TUR where the quality of initial TUR is suspect.

Location of tumor within the bladder may also help predict response to BCG. Tumors located in the prostatic urethra may not have adequate exposure to BCG during instillation and may thus have worse outcomes.[31] In these patients, it is the authors' practice to perform a limited TUR of prostate several weeks before initiation of BCG to facilitate surface contact of the medication with the urothelium of the prostatic urethra.

Patient Characteristics

Aside from staging and histologic concerns, patient selection must also be optimized. Because BCG is a live attenuated bacterium that exerts its effects primarily via a T_H1-driven response, the patient's immune status is highly relevant. Patients on active immunosuppressive medications following organ transplantation should be considered for BCG therapy only in select cases. Besides the risk from an infective viewpoint, the intense immunostimulatory cytotoxic response evoked by BCG may place the transplanted organ at risk of rejection.

Patients who are very elderly or have poor performance status may have weakened immune systems, but they are still eligible to receive BCG.[32,33] Although this immunosenescence is not a contraindication to BCG therapy, it may blunt the ability of BCG to evoke a sufficient immunostimulatory response. Patients with a history of human immunodeficiency virus (HIV) infection can usually also be safely treated with BCG. Given that most patients with HIV in the current era have intact immune systems, their bladder cancer can be managed the same as other patients, and similar outcomes can be expected.[34]

Lastly, some practioners mistakenly exclude patients with a personal history of tuberculosis from consideration for BCG therapy. Although there are no data specifically examining this, the authors and others have successfully treated these patients with BCG therapy. In fact, recent data suggest that pre-BCG priming enhances the response of patients.[35] However, given the prior exposure of these patients' immune systems to mycobacterial antigens, clinicians should be particularly vigilant about optimizing delivery with respect to the reduction of adverse effects.

OPTIMIZING ADMINISTRATION OF BCG

Although proper patient selection and use of maintenance therapy can improve overall outcomes with BCG therapy, there are also specific strategies in the administration of the drug that can increase the likelihood of successful intravesical treatment. The following paragraphs discuss aspects that can contribute to enhanced outcomes for patients treated with BCG therapy.

Strains

From the initial avirulent strain of *M bovis* cultured by Calmette and Guérin in 1920, multiple substrains of BCG have been isolated, and they have been used clinically to varying degrees. These BCG substrains are generally classified as either evolutionarily early (eg, Japan, Moreau, and Russian) or evolutionarily late (eg, Connaught, Danish, Glaxo, Phipps, and Tice). While the early and late substrains are known to be genetically distinct, the exact differences in antitumor activity, if any, remain unknown.

The wide geographic variation in success rates seen with large-scale clinical trials of BCG vaccination for tuberculosis has been postulated to be due at least in part to the variable clinical efficacy of different BCG substrains available locally around the world.[36–40] In bladder cancer, recent preclinical investigations suggest that immunomodulatory potential differs between the various BCG substrains, but the clinical impact of these differences remains undefined.[41,42] This should be kept in mind when comparing the results of clinical trials of BCG in bladder cancer that have used different substrains of BCG.

Dosing

As with other avirulent bacteria prepared for therapeutic use, the dosing measure of BCG is the colony-forming unit (CFU). CFU varies from strain to strain, and a vial of BCG may contain variable amounts of BCG CFU based on lot date, manufacturer, and other factors. Current data suggest that an intravesical dose between 10^8 and 10^9 CFU is effective, but response has been reported with doses as low as 10^6 CFU. These variations explain the differences in recommended milligram dose between different preparations of BCG (eg, Sanofi-Pasteur 81 mg; Tice, 50 mg; Tokyo, 40 mg; Dutch [RIVM], 120 mg).

Duration

The first randomized trial of BCG therapy for bladder cancer examined the efficacy of a treatment regimen that consisted of 6 weekly intravesical instillations of BCG.[14] Subsequent trials have investigated the effect of additional instillations given to boost the immune response. The initial 6-week treatment regimen is known as induction, and the subsequent instillations are referred to as maintenance therapy. In a large-scale cooperative group trial performed in the United States, Lamm and colleagues[18] demonstrated that routine use of BCG maintenance therapy given as 3 weekly instillations at the 3-, 6-, 12-, 18-, 24-, 30- and 36-month time points decreased both recurrence and progression rates for patients with NMIBC when compared with patients who received induction BCG therapy alone. A European intergroup trial published in 2010 found that routine use of this same 3-week BCG maintenance regimen resulted in improved time to recurrence, disease-specific survival, and overall survival when compared with patients receiving intravesical chemotherapy.[19] While future studies will likely continue to elucidate the specific details of the ideal maintenance regimen, the data currently available all suggest routine incorporation of maintenance therapy (using the SWOG 6+3 regimen) if BCG is to be used optimally.

Technique

It is important to optimize the administration of BCG in such a way that the bacterium has optimal propensity to adhere to the urothelium while at the same time causing the patients the least inconvenience/discomfort. In the authors' practice, patients presenting for treatment are instructed to minimize fluid intake in the hours before their scheduled BCG instillation and to empty their bladders immediately before BCG instillation. The voided urine specimen is visually inspected to confirm absence of gross hematuria (microscopic hematuria or positive dipstick is not a contraindication to BCG). BCG mixed in 50 mL normal saline is then instilled intravesically via a urethral catheter. Minimizing fluid intake and starting with an empty bladder increase the likelihood of successful retention of the medication for the recommended duration of 2 hours. Other technical tips include minimal use of lubricating jelly (to avoid clumping of bacteria), avoidance of lidocaine (the acidic composition can be deleterious), and, of course, to perform the instillation only in the setting of atraumatic catheterization.

An interesting practice among some urologists is to have patients lie recumbent during the instillation period and to have them rotate every 15 minutes in an attempt to evenly expose the entire bladder surface to BCG. Although well-intentioned, this rotisserie method does not seem to have any basis in the scientific literature. The elastic nature of the compliant bladder suggests that it changes size to accommodate the volume of fluid inside. Therefore, unless the instillation was incorrectly done and a large air pocket was introduced in the bladder, serial turning of the patient is not necessary. It is the authors' practice to have patients lie recumbent for several minutes after instillation of the BCG and then to allow them to ambulate normally during the 2-hour retention period.

Usage of certain medications has been suggested to be a relative contraindication for BCG therapy. Because of the increased propensity for hematuria while on antiplatelet agents such as aspirin or clopidogrel, patients taking these medications are sometimes not considered candidates for BCG therapy or are instructed to discontinue the medications during BCG therapy. Similarly, given the documented ability of statin medications to induce a T_H2 immune response (and therefore limit the ability of BCG to induce a T_H1 response), it has been suggested that patients discontinue statins during BCG therapy.[43]

The authors believe the risk of treatment-altering hematuria due to antiplatelet agents and the risk of immune steal due to statin therapy are both extremely low. There is even evidence to suggest that aspirin therapy may have a beneficial effect on the efficacy of BCG.[44] Similarly, since the initial report suggesting the negative effect of statin therapy on BCG efficacy, multiple authors have reported no impact of statin therapy on post-BCG outcomes.[45,46] It is the authors' practice to have patients continue their usual medications during BCG therapy. The authors generally do not initiate new medications or discontinue ongoing medications in most patients.

Reduction of Adverse Effects

A common misconception around the administration of BCG is that it is too toxic, and practitioners will often quote the data from the SWOG8507 study and cite that "less than 18% of patients finished 3 years of BCG."[18] Although this is true of that study, it must be recognized that these were results from 2 decades ago. and much has been learned since then about optimal administration of BCG. In fact, now, a diligent practitioner should be able to reduce the BCG discontinuation rate in their patients to less than 15%. This has been borne out by the large-scale study[47] in which less than 10% of patients receiving a full dose therapy for 3 years discontinued BCG because of toxicity. This section discusses the spectrum of adverse effects that may result from BCG and provides strategies to minimize these effects. Most of these side effects can be prevented or managed with minor interventions without the need for termination of BCG therapy. However, the most serious adverse effects demand immediate recognition and prompt initiation of aggressive measures.

Irritative voiding symptoms (dysuria, frequency, and urgency) and low-grade fever are the most commonly reported complaints immediately after BCG instillation.[48] In most cases, these resolve within 48 hours and do not need intervention. Many practitioners anecdotally regard the transient local symptoms and influenza-like symptoms as an encouraging sign of the intended immune activation effects of BCG therapy. Antispasmodic medications and over-the-counter antipyretics can be used with good effect to control the symptoms. In the authors' practice, patients who experience moderate or severe irritative voiding symptoms are prescribed antispasmodic medication for the acute episode, and they are also instructed to take the antispasmodic medication before subsequent BCG administrations.

The most serious adverse effects with BCG therapy are seen when the medication is inadvertently absorbed into the bloodstream. This allows the *M bovis* bacteria to access the systemic circulation. Depending on the amount of BCG absorbed and the extent of previous immune priming (eg, personal history of tuberculosis), the sequela of systemic BCG spread can range from prolonged pyrexia (BCGosis) to a severe systemic inflammatory response syndrome (BCG sepsis) to death.[48] Given these dangerous possibilities, it is imperative that practitioners employ all means to prevent systemic BCG absorption. For this reason, BCG administration should be postponed for any patient with visible hematuria. For patients with a history of tuberculosis, the authors also routinely perform urine dipstick to assess for microscopic hematuria, as absorption of even small amounts of BCG can incite a cytokine storm from the hypersensitized immune systems of these patients.

In all patients, urethral catheterization should be performed as atraumatically as possible, and BCG administration should be postponed if bleeding is triggered during catheterization. BCG should not be given in the presence of a urinary tract infection. During an episode of urinary tract infection, the risk for BCG intravasation is greater. This is because the urothelium is more permeable, and the surface vasculature is predisposed to bleeding more readily. For the treatment of urinary tract infections in patients receiving intravesical BCG, it was previously suggested that use of quinolone antibiotics was to be avoided because of their antimycobacterial activity.[49] More recently, several investigators have shown that short-term administration of a quinolone decreases the incidence of moderate-to-severe adverse events (especially grade 3 events) after BCG instillation.[50,51] For this reason, it is the authors' practice to instruct all patients to take 1 dose of a quinolone antibiotic 6 hours after BCG instillation. In the authors' experience, this practice increases patient comfort and decreases the likelihood of patient dropout from BCG therapy.

FUTURE DIRECTIONS

The integration of BCG into the management of patients with superficial bladder cancer has been among the most important advances in the field over the past several decades. Based on the results of multiple large-scale clinical trials conducted in the United States, Europe, and Asia, BCG therapy is now accepted as having a clear role in reducing recurrence, progression, and death from bladder cancer.

In the coming decades, the authors anticipate there will be increasing emphasis on developing accurate predictors of response to BCG therapy. Although several algorithms based on clinical parameters have been developed,[52,53] the recent acceleration in technologies for gene expression profiling suggests that future efforts will focus on developing molecular markers that predict BCG sensitivity and that allow for personalized cancer therapy. Multiple avenues are being investigated for use as potential molecular biomarkers of BCG sensitivity. These include tumor-associated markers (pRb, CD68, Bcl-2, Bax markers of gene expression and methylation), urinary markers (interleukin [IL]-2, IL-8, IL-18, tumor necrosis factor-α) and serum markers (single nucleotide polymorphisms in multiple DNA repair, inflammation, cell cycle, and apoptosis pathways).[54–57] At MD Anderson, the authors have recently performed a prospective clinical trial investigating the concept of molecular recurrence using fluorescence in situ hybridization to predict response to BCG therapy.[58] The authors are hopeful that this approach may help counsel patients undergoing BCG therapy, and it may also provide a role in future clinical trial design.

SUMMARY

For the treatment of patients with superficial bladder cancer and a moderate-to-high risk of tumor recurrence or progression, intravesical BCG has been the key development of the last generation because of its ability to decrease tumor recurrence, progression, and death from bladder cancer. However, because of its bacterial composition and its intravesical route of delivery, BCG has also brought with it a novel set of challenges that require thoughtful planning and vigilant monitoring. An understanding of when, to whom, and how BCG should be given is critical if optimal outcomes are to be achieved. As the ability to better select patients for BCG therapy continues to be refined in the future, outcomes with this unique treatment will only continue to improve.

REFERENCES

1. Guerin C. Early history of BCG. In: Rosenthal SR, editor. BCG vaccination against tuberculosis. Boston: Little Brown; 1957. p. 48–53.
2. Rosenthal SR. BCG vaccination against tuberculosis. Boston: Little, Brown & Company; 1957.
3. Faustman DL, Wang L, Okubo Y, et al. Proof-of-concept, randomized, controlled clinical trial of bacillus-Calmette-Guerin for treatment of long-term type 1 diabetes. PLoS One 2012;7(8):e41756. http://dx.doi.org/10.1371/journal.pone.0041756.
4. Ristori G, Buzzi MG, Sabatini U, et al. Use of Bacille Calmette-Guèrin (BCG) in multiple sclerosis. Neurology 1999;53(7):1588–9.
5. Paolillo A, Buzzi MG, Giugni E, et al. The effect of Bacille Calmette-Guérin on the evolution of new enhancing lesions to hypointense T1 lesions in relapsing remitting MS. J Neurol 2003;250(2):247–8.
6. Rutschmann OT, McCrory DC, Matchar DB. Immunization Panel of the Multiple Sclerosis Council for Clinical Practice Guidelines: Immunization and MS: a summary of published evidence and recommendations. Neurology 2002;59(12):1837–43.

7. Yong J, Lacan G, Dang H, et al. BCG Vaccine-induced neuroprotection in a mouse model of parkinson's disease. PLoS One 2011;6(1):e16610. http://dx.doi.org/10.1371/journal.pone.0016610.
8. Pearl R. Cancer and tuberculosis. Am J Hyg 1929;9:97–159.
9. Mosolits S, Nilsson B, Mellstedt H. Towards therapeutic vaccines for colorectal carcinoma: a review of clinical trials. Expert Rev Vaccines 2005;4(3):329–50.
10. Miyazawa N, Suemasu K, Ogata T, et al. BCG immunotherapy as an adjuvant to surgery in lung cancer: a randomized prospective clinical trial. Jpn J Clin Oncol 1979;9(1):19–26.
11. Lu CY, Lin GC, Gu JZ, et al. A preliminary study of BCG adjuvant therapy in oral and maxillofacial malignant melanoma. Shanghai Kou Qiang Yi Xue 1994;3(3):144–5 [in Chinese].
12. Coe JE, Feldman JD. Extracutaneous delayed hypersensitivity, particularly in the guinea-pig bladder. Immunology 1966;10(2):127–36.
13. Morales A, Eidinger D, Bruce AW. Intracavitary bacillus Calmette-Guerin in the treatment of superficial bladder tumors. J Urol 1976;116(2):180–3.
14. Lamm DL, Thor DE, Harris SC, et al. BCG immunotherapy of superficial bladder cancer. J Urol 1980;124:38–40.
15. Brosman SA. Experience with bacillus Calmette-Guerin in patients with superficial bladder carcinoma. J Urol 1982;128(1):27–30.
16. Bretton PR, Herr HW, Kimmel M, et al. The response of patients with superficial bladder cancer to a second course of intravesical BCG. J Urol 1990;143:710–3.
17. Catalona WJ, Hudson MA, Gillen DP, et al. Risks and benefits of repeated courses of intravesical BCG for superficial bladder cancer. J Urol 1987;137:220–4.
18. Lamm DL, Blumenstein BA, Crismon JD, et al. Maintenance BCG immunotherapy for recurrent TA, T1 and CIS TCC of the bladder: a randomised Southwest Oncology Group Study. J Urol 2000;163:1124–9.
19. Sylvester RJ, Brausi MA, Kirkels WJ, et al. Long-term efficacy results of EORTC genito-urinary group randomized phase 3 study 30911 comparing intravesical instillations of epirubicin, bacillus Calmette-Guérin, and bacillus Calmette-Guérin plus isoniazid in patients with intermediate- and high-risk stage Ta T1 urothelial carcinoma of the bladder. Eur Urol 2010;57(5):766–73.
20. Herr HW, Schwalb DM, Zhang ZF, et al. Intravesical bacillus Calmette-Guérin therapy prevents tumor progression and death from superficial bladder cancer: ten-year follow-up of a prospective randomized trial. J Clin Oncol 1995;13(6):1404–8.
21. Schellhammer PF, Ladaga LE, Fillion MB. Bacillus Calmette-Guerin for superficial transitional cell carcinoma of the bladder. J Urol 1986;135(2):261–4.
22. Akaza H, Hinotsu S, Aso Y, et al. BCG treatment of existing papillary cancer and carcinoma in situ of the bladder. Cancer 1995;75:552–9.
23. Rosenbaum RS, Park MC, Fleischmann J. Intravesical bacille Calmette-Guérin therapy for muscle invasive bladder cancer. Urology 1996;47(2):208–11.
24. Kamat AM, Gee JR, Dinney CP, et al. The case for early cystectomy in the treatment of nonmuscle invasive micropapillary bladder carcinoma. J Urol 2006;175(3 Pt 1):881–5.
25. Kamat AM, Dinney CP, Gee JR, et al. Micropapillary bladder cancer: a review of the University of Texas M. D. Anderson Cancer Center experience with 100 consecutive patients. Cancer 2007;110(1):62–7.
26. Lynch SP, Shen Y, Kamat A, et al. Neoadjuvant chemotherapy in small cell urothelial cancer improves pathologic downstaging and long-term outcomes: results from a retrospective study at the MD Anderson Cancer Center. Eur Urol 2012 Apr 17. [Epub ahead of print].
27. American Urologic Association. The Management of Bladder Cancer: Diagnosis and treatment recommendations. Available at: http://www.auanet.org/content/clinical-practice-guidelines/clinical-guidelines/main-reports/bladcan07/chapter1.pdf. Accessed January 23, 2012.
28. Babjuk M, Oosterlinck W, Sylvester R, et al. European Association of Urology (EAU): EAU guidelines on nonmuscle-invasive urothelial carcinoma of the bladder, the 2011 update. Eur Urol 2011;59(6):997–1008.
29. Herr HW. The value of a second transurethral resection in evaluating patients with bladder tumors. J Urol 1999;162:74.
30. Dalbagni G, Herr HW, Reuter VE. Impact of a second transurethral resection on the staging of T1 bladder cancer. Urology 2002;60:822.
31. Gofrit ON, Pode D, Pizov G, et al. Prostatic urothelial carcinoma: is transurethral prostatectomy necessary before bacillus Calmette-Guérin immunotherapy? BJU Int 2009;103(7):905–8.
32. Joudi FN, Smith BJ, O'Donnell MA, et al. The impact of age on the response of patients with superficial bladder cancer to intravesical immunotherapy. J Urol 2006;175(5):1634–9.
33. Shariat SF, Milowsky M, Droller MJ. Bladder cancer in the elderly. Urol Oncol 2009;27(6):653–67.
34. Gaughan EM, Dezube BJ, Bower M, et al. HIV-associated bladder cancer: a case series evaluating difficulties in diagnosis and management. BMC Urol 2009;31:9–10.
35. Biot C, Rentsch CA, Gsponer JR, et al. Pre-existing BCG-specific T cells improve intravesical immunotherapy for bladder cancer. Sci Transl Med 2012;4(137):137ra72.
36. Colditz GA, Brewer TF, Berkey CS. Efficacy of BCG vaccine in the prevention of tuberculosis. J Am Med Assoc 1994;271(9):698–702.

37. Fine PE. Variation in protection by BCG: implications of and for heterologous immunity. Lancet 1995; 346(8986):1339–45.
38. Hart PD, Sutherland I. BCG and vole bacillus vaccines in the prevention of tuberculosis in adolescence and early adult life. Final report of the Medical Research Council. Br Med J 1977;2(6082):293–5.
39. Comstock GW, Palmer CE. Long-term results of BCG in the southern United States. Am Rev Respir Dis 1966;93(2):171–83.
40. Tuberculosis Prevention Trial. Trial of BCG vaccines in south India for tuberculosis prevention. Indian J Med Res 1979;70:349–63.
41. Secanella-Fandos S, Luquin M, Julián E. Connaught and Russian showed the highest direct antitumoral effects among different BCG substrains. J Urol 2012. http://dx.doi.org/10.1016/j.juro.2012.09.049. pii: S0022-5347(12)04880-X.
42. Gsponer JR, Biot C, Bisiaux A, et al. Immunotherapy of bladder cancer using bacillus Calmette Guerin (BCG): generation of cytotoxic T-cells is BCG strain dependent. American Association for Cancer Research 2012 Meeting (abstract # 5386).
43. Hoffman P, Roumeguere T, van Velthoven R. Use of statins and outcome of BCG treatment for bladder cancer. N Engl J Med 2006;355:2705–7.
44. Gee JR, Jarrard DF, Bruskewitz RC, et al. Reduced bladder cancer recurrence rate with cardioprotective aspirin after intravesical bacille Calmette-Guérin. BJU Int 2009;103(6):736–9.
45. Skolarus TA, Lee EW, Virgo KS, et al. Intravesical bacille Calmette-Guérin therapy for nonmuscle-invasive bladder cancer: effects of concurrent statin therapy. J Am Coll Surg 2009;209(2):248–53.
46. Berglund RK, Savage CJ, Vora KC, et al. An analysis of the effect of statin use on the efficacy of bacillus calmette-guerin treatment for transitional cell carcinoma of the bladder. J Urol 2008;180(4):1297–300.
47. Oddens J, Brausi M, Sylvester R, et al. Final results of an EORTC-GU cancers group randomized study of maintenance bacillus Calmette-Guérin in intermediate- and high-risk Ta, T1 papillary carcinoma of the urinary bladder: one-third dose versus full dose and 1 year versus 3 years of maintenance. Eur Urol 2013;63(3):462–72.
48. Rischmann P, Desgrandchamps F, Malavaud B, et al. BCG intravesical installations: recommendations for side-effects management. Eur Urol 2000; 37(Suppl 1):33–6.
49. Durek C, Rusch-Gerdes S, Jocham D, et al. Interference of modern antibacterials with bacillus Calmette-Guérin viability. J Urol 1999;163:1959–62.
50. Colombel M, Saint F, Chopin D, et al. The effect of ofloxacin on bacillus Calmette-Guerin induced toxicity in patients with superficial bladder cancer: results of a randomized, prospective, double-blind, placebo controlled, multicenter study. J Urol 2006; 176(3):935–9.
51. Damiano R, De Sio M, Quarto G, et al. Short-term administration of prulifloxacin in patients with nonmuscle-invasive bladder cancer: an effective option for the prevention of bacillus Calmette-Guérin-induced toxicity? BJU Int 2009;104(5):633–9.
52. Sylvester RJ, van der Meijden AP, Oosterlinck W, et al. Predicting recurrence and progression in individual patients with stage Ta T1 bladder cancer using EORTC risk tables: a combined analysis of 2596 patients from seven EORTC trials. Eur Urol 2006;49(3):466–77.
53. Fernandez-Gomez J, Madero R, Solsona E, et al. Predicting nonmuscle-invasive bladder cancer recurrence and progression in patients treated with bacillus Calmette-Guerin: the CUETO scoring model. J Urol 2009;182(5):2195–203.
54. Thalmann GN, Sermier A, Rentsch C, et al. Urinary Interleukin-8 and 18 predict the response of superficial bladder cancer to intravesical therapy with bacillus Calmette-Guerin. J Urol 2000;164(6): 2129–33.
55. Saint F, Salomon L, Quintela R, et al. Do prognostic parameters of remission versus relapse after bacillus Calmette-Guérin (BCG) immunotherapy exist? Analysis of a quarter century of literature. Eur Urol 2003;43(4):351–60 [discussion: 360–1].
56. Ajili F, Kaabi B, Darouiche A, et al. Prognostic value of Bcl-2 and Bax tumor cell expression in patients with non-muscle invasive bladder cancer receiving bacillus Calmette-Guerin immunotherapy. Ultrastruct Pathol 2012;36(1):31–9.
57. Lima L, Dinis-Ribeiro M, Longatto-Filho A, et al. Predictive biomarkers of bacillus Calmette-Guérin immunotherapy response in bladder cancer: where are we now? Adv Urol 2012;2012:232609.
58. Kamat AM, Dickstein RJ, Messetti F, et al. Use of fluorescence in situ hybridization to predict response to bacillus Calmette-Guérin therapy for bladder cancer: results of a prospective trial. J Urol 2012; 187(3):862–7.

New Agents for Bacillus Calmette-Guérin–Refractory Bladder Cancer

Jennifer J. Ahn, MD, James M. McKiernan, MD*

KEYWORDS

• Non-muscle invasive bladder cancer • Bacillus Calmette-Guérin failure
• Bacillus Calmette-Guérin refractory • Intravesical therapy • Salvage agents

KEY POINTS

- BCG is the most effective treatment for non-muscle invasive bladder cancer, yet roughly 50% of patients still experience tumor recurrence (BCG failures).
- Radical cystectomy is recommended for BCG failure by the AUA and EAU, because no other local therapy has proved as effective at providing oncologic cure.
- Multiple salvage agents have been or are currently under investigation, including intravesical chemotherapy, drug delivery enhancement technology, immunotherapy, and targeted therapies, with varying success rates.
- Despite ongoing research on promising therapeutic approaches, it remains difficult to counsel and treat patients with BCG failure, particularly those who cannot tolerate or refuse radical cystectomy.

INTRODUCTION

An estimated 73,510 individuals will be diagnosed with bladder cancer in the United States in 2012.[1] Roughly 70% will initially be diagnosed with non-muscle invasive cancer (Ta, T1, or carcinoma in situ [CIS]) at presentation; treatment includes transurethral resection (TUR) and possible adjuvant intravesical therapy. The remaining 30% with muscle-invasive disease have a worse prognosis, and a different treatment course, which may include radical cystectomy, systemic chemotherapy, radiation, or any combination of the above. For patients with non-muscle invasive bladder cancer (NMIBC), the aim is to prevent tumor recurrence, which occurs in 50% to 90% of patients at 5 years, and most importantly, disease progression to muscle invasion, which occurs in up to 20% of patients.[2] The risk of recurrence and progression is related to multiple factors, including tumor grade, stage, presence of CIS, and multifocality.[3,4]

Intravesical bacillus Calmette-Guérin (BCG) treatment was first described in 1976, and is currently the standard of care for patients with high-grade NMIBC and CIS.[5,6] BCG reduces cancer recurrence by 40%, compared with TUR alone, and also reduces progression, unlike other intravesical agents.[7] Although BCG is the most effective treatment, roughly 50% of patients still experience a recurrence within 5 years.[8] With each BCG failure, the risk of progression rises; failing two or more courses of BCG increases the risk of developing MIBC from 7% to 30%.[9]

Funding Sources: Dr McKiernan: Celgene, and the Prostate Cancer Foundation; Dr Ahn: None.
Conflict of Interest: None.
Department of Urology, Columbia University Medical Center, Herbert Irving Pavilion, 11th Floor, 161 Fort Washington Avenue, New York, NY 10032, USA
* Corresponding author.
E-mail address: jmm23@columbia.edu

Urol Clin N Am 40 (2013) 219–232
http://dx.doi.org/10.1016/j.ucl.2013.01.008
0094-0143/13/$ – see front matter

DEFINING BCG FAILURE

Currently, there is no standardization of terminology for defining BCG failure. In 2003, Herr and Dalbagni[10] published data from a prior trial evaluating the use of BCG maintenance, and analyzed 93 BCG-naive patients with high-grade NMIBC who then underwent BCG induction. Fifty-one percent of patients were randomized to receive monthly maintenance BCG. At 3-month follow-up, 43% had presence of tumor; by 6 months, only 20% had persistent or recurrent tumor, suggesting a possible prolonged or delayed immunotherapeutic effect of BCG. Long-term tumor recurrence rates correlated only with the presence of tumor at 6-month evaluation, and not with the presence of tumor at 3 months, nor the use of maintenance therapy. As a result, they proposed that patients should not be considered BCG refractory until at least 6 months of follow-up.

In 2005, the International Consensus Panel on T1 bladder cancer aimed to better describe BCG failure by offering four classifications.[11] "BCG-refractory disease" was defined as persistent or rapidly recurrent disease at 6 months after induction, despite maintenance or repeat induction at 3 months. Any worsening of stage, grade, or tumor burden at 3 months was also included in this definition. If disease is persistent or recurrent at 3 months, but is nonexistent at 6 months, regardless of TUR status, the patient is considered "BCG-resistant," indicating that they do respond to BCG, but not as robustly as a complete, immediate responder. The third category is "BCG-relapsing disease," describing patients who are disease-free at 6 months, but ultimately recur, either early (before 12 months), intermediate (12–24 months), or late (>24 months). The fourth and final classification is "BCG-intolerant disease." This refers to those who cannot tolerate a full course of BCG, secondary to drug toxicity or a serious adverse event, and have recurrent disease in the face of incomplete treatment. These four definitions encompass all patients for whom BCG does not provide a complete cure, yet unfortunately these categories can overlap, because a given patient could have BCG-resistant disease, but then ultimately have a late recurrence, thus classifying the individual as a BCG-relapser. There are also variables in how patients are managed, particularly in the use of maintenance, dose reduction, follow-up, and preference in the use of salvage therapies and timing of cystectomy. In addition, the thoroughness of cystoscopic surgical resection is difficult to control for across all these categories and can contribute substantially to disease-free status in patients with high-grade Ta, or T1 bladder cancer.[12] Therefore, standardizing this complicated group of patients would be valuable for assessing prognosis and treatment outcomes.

To this end, Shirakawa and colleagues[13] retrospectively applied the previously mentioned BCG failure definitions to a cohort of 173 patients who failed BCG as treatment of NMIBC to assess their prognostic validity. Significant risk factors for stage progression (defined as muscle invasion or distant metastases) included BCG-refractory disease versus the other three subtypes, and grade 3 histology at time of BCG failure. BCG-refractory patients also had significantly lower disease-specific survival as compared with the BCG-relapsing and BCG-intolerant groups. Interestingly, only 3 of 173 patients were classified as BCG-resistant. Fourteen percent of patients experienced stage progression, at a mean time of 2.4 years from BCG failure. Intuitively, it seems that BCG-refractory disease should have worse outcomes than BCG-relapsing disease, but validating this is important, as this group attempted to do. The retrospective nature of the paper, along with different treatment protocols, including various other intravesical agents, and a significant number of Grade 1 to 2 Ta tumors, makes it difficult to interpret and to generalize. This investigation does further clarify that standardization of subtypes in this disease state and validation of the outcome research in this population are still needed to better assist clinicians in making appropriate treatment decisions in this group of high-risk patients.

STANDARD TREATMENT OPTIONS

Repeat Induction

On failing one course of BCG, a second BCG induction course can result in a significant response rate.[14] Brake and colleagues[14] examined 126 patients with T1 disease who underwent induction BCG, 37 (29%) of whom recurred at a median of 16 months. The 24 subjects with non-muscle invasive recurrence underwent a second 6-week induction course of BCG, with a 79% response rate (19 of 24) at a median of 24 months, displaying the benefit of repeat induction at time of recurrence. However, 13% of patients (17 of 126) developed progression to MIBC, either after one course (N = 13) or two courses (N = 4) of BCG. There was no placebo group in this study, so it is impossible to know the true effect of second BCG induction as compared with TUR alone. In addition, patients with residual tumor after repeat induction went on to cystectomy; thus, it is unknown if they would have achieved a delayed response, as is seen with primary BCG induction.

Maintenance

Another form of additional BCG is maintenance therapy, as reported in the pivotal randomized trial conducted by the Southwest Oncology Group (SWOG) in 2000.[15] Patients with BCG-naive NMIBC were randomized to receive intravesical and percutaneous BCG for a 6-week induction course, or induction plus 3 weeks of maintenance at 3, 6, 12, 18, 24, 30, and 36 months. Five-year recurrence-free survival was significantly higher in the maintenance group (60% vs 41%), although there was no significant difference in overall survival. A subset analysis of patients with CIS also showed an improved response rate with maintenance. However, only 16% of patients randomized to maintenance received all 3 years of therapy because of a combination of recurrence and adverse events.

A more recent follow-up review of the SWOG BCG maintenance trial evaluated potential risk factors for recurrence and progression.[16] Early and late (>12 months) recurrence were associated with increased risk of death, compared with no recurrence, but the timing of recurrence was not found to significantly correlate with survival. Of the 394 patients who were disease-free after induction BCG and thus randomized, 185 ultimately recurred and 37 went on to cystectomy, with a 5-year survival rate of 56% for greater than or equal to T2 disease, and 95% for less than or equal to T2 disease. Patients in the maintenance arm were more likely to undergo early cystectomy, at a median time of 11 months versus 24 months, although the rates of cystectomy for MIBC were similar (45% vs 49%). These data provide further evidence that those who recur after BCG, whether early or late, have worse survival than patients who have complete responses (CRs).

Cystectomy

It is difficult to determine exactly when and how to treat a patient who fails BCG. Guzzo and colleagues[17] examined a cohort of 184 patients with cT1 or CIS who underwent cystectomy (64% with prior BCG). Nineteen percent (35 of 184) of patients were upstaged to pT2, and when compared with a group of cT2 who underwent cystectomy (and found also to be pT2), recurrence-free survival rates were lower at 3 and 5 years (64% and 61% vs 83% and 74%). Prior BCG therapy with subsequent upstaging was found to be a risk factor for long-term recurrence compared with patients with known MIBC, highlighting that BCG failure portends poor outcomes, even despite cystectomy.

Delaying radical cystectomy has been shown to increase the risk of death, which can be disconcerting to those receiving BCG, because several weeks of treatment typically elapse before response to therapy is assessed.[18–20] Herr and Sogani[21] showed that in BCG-failure patients, cystectomy within 2 years of initial BCG provided improved 15-year disease-specific survival compared with patients who had cystectomy at least 2 years after BCG (69% vs 26%; $P = .003$). Reviewing two historical cohorts in which different treatment paradigms were used, Raj and colleagues[22] compared early (at T1 recurrence) with late cystectomy (at progression to MIBC) in BCG-failure patients. Although retrospective and not randomized, it showed a trend toward improved progression-free and cancer-specific survival in the early cystectomy cohort.

Conversely, Badalato and colleagues[23] reviewed a more contemporary series of 349 patients with high-grade T1 bladder cancer, and showed that immediate cystectomy (within 90 days of diagnosis and without further TUR or intravesical therapy) did not offer a benefit in cancer-specific survival, as compared with conservative therapy. In the more recent subgroup (2000–2010), only 56.7% went on to cystectomy after attempted conservative treatment. Although retrospective in nature, this analysis suggests that delaying cystectomy may be a feasible option to consider.

The American Urological Association guidelines currently recommend radical cystectomy as first-line therapy in patients who fail BCG. The European Association of Urology guidelines state that a patient has failed BCG when a patient develops MIBC, or when high-grade NMIBC is present at both 3 and 6 months.[24] They also recommend cystectomy as the next line of treatment in early BCG failures (in patients who can tolerate it) because of the increased risk of developing MIBC. National Comprehensive Cancer Network guidelines also recommend early cystectomy for patients with recurrence after BCG, although these guidelines do not clearly define BCG failure. Early cystectomy is widely recommended because it is superior in the oncologic control of BCG-refractory bladder cancer. However, in the patient who is not fit for cystectomy, refuses cystectomy, or has a late or low-grade recurrence after BCG, there are multiple agents for salvage therapy, which are examined in the remainder of this article.

SALVAGE AGENTS

Mitomycin C

Mitomycin C (MMC) is an alkylating agent that causes DNA cross-linking and inhibition of DNA synthesis (**Table 1**).[25] It is widely used in NMIBC as an adjunct to TUR in preventing tumor recurrence, and can be used postoperatively and with

Table 1
Generalized dosing schedules based on phase I-III trials

Agent	Mechanism of Action	Dose	Duration	Frequency	Maintenance	Notes	References
Mitomycin C	Alkylating agent, cross-links DNA, inhibits DNA synthesis	40 mg in 20 mL sterile water				Can administer immediately after TURBT × 1 Can cause chemical cystitis	
Thermochemotherapy	Local microwave hyperthermia by catheter improves drug penetration, causes local cytotoxicity	20–40 mg in 50 mL sterile water	Two consecutive 30-min instillations	Weekly × 6 wk	Monthly × 6 mo	Administer 20–40 d after TURBT	29–33
Electromotive Drug Administration	Electric current by catheter enhances membrane permeability	40 mg in 100 mL sterile water	30 min at 23–25 mA	Weekly × 6 wk	None	Must wash bladder before administration Start 3 wk after TURBT May also give preoperatively ×1	27,36–39
BCG-IFN	Stimulates immune response	BCG + 50 million units IFN-α in 50 mL sterile saline	1–2 h	Weekly × 6 wk	3 weekly instillations at 3, 6, 12, 18, 24 mo	If BCG-naive, use full-strength BCG If BCG-refractory, use one-third strength BCG Dose reduction as needed	42–44
Gemcitabine	Nucleoside analog, inhibits DNA synthesis	2000 mg in 50–100 mL sterile saline	1–2 h	Weekly × 6 wk	Monthly × 10 mo	Maintain urine pH 5.5–7.0	50–54

Valrubicin	Semisynthetic anthracycline, inhibits nucleic acid synthesis and topoisomerase II	800 mg in 75 mL sterile saline	2 h	Weekly × 6 wk	None	Administer 2 wk after TURBT Food and Drug Administration approved for BCG refractory CIS	55–57
Docetaxel	Microtubule stabilizer, inhibits mitosis and induces apoptosis	75 mg in 100 mL sterile saline	2 h	Weekly × 6 wk	Monthly × 9 mo	Administer 1–6 wk after TURBT	60,61
Paclitaxel	Microtubule stabilizer, inhibits mitosis and induces apoptosis						
Nanoparticle albumin-bound	Nanoparticle albumin-bound formulation improves solubility and uptake by urothelium	500 mg in 100 mL sterile saline	2 h	Weekly × 6 wk	Monthly × 9 mo		66
Hyaluronic Acid	Conjugation to HA improves solubility and uptake by urothelium	600 mg in 50 mL isotonic solution	2 h	Weekly × 6 wk	None		69
Mycobacterial cell wall-DNA complex	Mycobacterial cell wall stimulates immune response without live vaccine	8 mg in 50 mL sterile saline	2 h	Weekly × 6 wk	3 weekly instillations at 3, 6, 12, 18, 24 mo	Administer within 60 d of TURBT	72,73
Gemcitabine plus Mitomycin C	Combination therapy to maximize cytotoxic effects	1000 mg gemcitabine in 50 mL sterile water; 40 mg MMC in 20 mL sterile water	90 min for gemcitabine 90 min for MMC	Weekly × 6 wk	Monthly × 12 mo		74

maintenance. However, it can cause significant chemical cystitis, and has not proved effective in the setting of BCG failure. A randomized prospective study of BCG versus MMC showed a recurrence-free rate of only 19% (4 of 21) in the group that crossed over to MMC (median follow-up, 64 months).[26] These low success rates have been attributed in part to inadequate drug delivery and tissue penetration, leading to assistive devices that use hyperthermia and electric current, allowing for more effective uptake of drug into the urothelial cells.[27,28] Both modalities have been used in patients after BCG failure with improved results.

Thermochemotherapy

Thermochemotherapy (TCT) uses local microwave-hyperthermia to the bladder, by way of a specialized catheter, to a temperature of 42C $\pm$ 2°C (Synergo, Medical Enterprises, Amsterdam, the Netherlands).[29] The heat improves drug penetration into the urothelium, and is also cytotoxic, damaging DNA and inducing apoptosis.[30–32] Nativ and colleagues[33] reported their retrospective view of 111 patients with prior BCG failure who had undergone TCT-MMC treatment with six weekly treatments of 20 mg MMC with two consecutive 30-minute cycles of TCT, followed by maintenance therapy as warranted. Recurrence-free rates were 85% (1 year) and 56% (2 years), and the average time to recurrence was 16 months. Patients were stratified by BCG failure categories (refractory, recurrent, resistant, intolerant),[11] and there was no significant difference in response rates. The 2-year recurrence rate for the BCG-refractory group was 56% versus 44% in the other groups. Completion of maintenance was the only factor found to correlate with lower recurrence rates. Forty-five percent of patients experienced adverse events, mostly local urinary toxicities, and 5.4% patients withdrew because of significant side effects. There is no comparison group in this retrospective review; however, a significant 2-year recurrence-free rate was seen in a high-risk group of patients.

Electromotive MMC

Another mechanism of enhancing intravesical drug efficacy is electromotive delivery.[34] Electromotive drug administration (EMDA) involves enhancing membrane permeability and drug transport by way of electric current. MMC is not ionic at urinary pH states, and thus requires a salt-containing solution to aid with transport across urothelial membranes.[35] Physionizer 30 (Physion, Mirandola, Italy) allows for a gradual increase in the current by a transurethral catheter, to a maximum of 23 to 25 mA, with a total treatment time of 30 minutes. EMDA-MMC has shown superiority over MMC in a randomized trial of 108 patients with CIS (solitary or concurrent T1) with response rates of 58% (EMDA-MMC) and 31% (MMC) at 6 months, and median time to recurrence of 35 versus 19.5 months.[27] A third arm in this study received induction BCG with recurrence rates similar to that of EMDA-MMC. Long-term follow-up of 82 months showed similar equivalence of EMDA-MMC to BCG, and superiority to MMC alone with regards to recurrence, but no significant difference with overall survival or disease-specific survival.[36]

The previously mentioned trial did not include BCG-failure patients, and so Sockett and colleagues[37] reported on 13 BCG-failure patients who received a 6-week course of EMDA-MMC, with a 31% recurrence-free rate at 15-month follow-up. EMDA-MMC has also been evaluated in conjunction with BCG in a randomized trial of 212 patients, and was shown to be more effective in reducing recurrence, progression, and all-cause and cancer-specific mortality than BCG alone.[38] Additionally, it has been shown to be safe and effective immediately before transurethral resection of bladder tumor (TURBT) in a BCG-naive population.[39]

MMC's activity in preventing tumor recurrence seems to be enhanced by TCT and EDMA technology, and is relatively well-tolerated. However, these tools have not been widely studied in the BCG-failure population, aside from Colombo and colleagues[28] prospective trial, nor have the two modalities been directly compared with each other. There are currently no known ongoing trials evaluating enhanced MMC after BCG failure, and these treatments will likely be targeted more toward incident NMIBC.

BCG and Interferon

Because BCG acts by eliciting an immune response, the immunostimulant interferon (IFN)-α2b was introduced as another intravesical agent, showing some short-term efficacy alone.[40,41] O'Donnell and colleagues[42] published their experience in using BCG-IFN in patients with BCG failure, hypothesizing that patients failed because of an incomplete immune response, and that the addition of IFN would enhance the immunotherapeutic effect. Forty patients were given 6 to 8 weeks of induction BCG (one-third strength) and IFN, with further BCG dose reduction for patients with treatment intolerance. CR rates of 63% and 53% were seen at 12 and 24 months, respectively, and at 30-month median follow-up, 22 (55%) of 40 of patients were disease free. Initial induction treatments were well-tolerated, but treatment discontinuation was encountered with progressive maintenance treatments, and 40% of patients ended therapy early because of intolerance.

Given these promising results, a multicenter phase II trial enrolled 1106 patients to receive BCG-IFN, inclusive of all types of NMIBC, regardless of prior treatment status.[43] BCG-naive patients received full-strength BCG-IFN, whereas reduced strength BCG was given to BCG-recurrent or BCG-intolerant subjects, with maintenance given to responders as tolerated. Of the 467 BCG-failure patients enrolled, 39% had received at least two courses of prior BCG, and 47% had recurred or persisted at 6 months, indicating a BCG-refractory state, whereas the remaining 53% were BCG-relapsing. At 24 months, 45% of prior BCG-failure patients were disease-free, and on multivariate analysis, patients with at least two prior courses of BCG had a significantly worse outcome than those with none or one courses.

Rosevear and colleagues[44] re-examined the 231 subjects in the previously mentioned phase II trial who had CIS immediately before enrollment (63% CIS alone, 37% concurrent with Ta or T1), 52% of whom were BCG failures. Response rates at 24 months were 23% (failed $\geq$2 courses BCG); 57% (failed one course); and 60% (BCG-naive). On multivariate analysis, having two or more courses of BCG was a significant risk factor for BCG-IFN failure, as compared with less than or equal to one course (hazard ratio, 2.003), as was BCG refractory disease, compared with intermediate BCG recurrence (>12 months) with a hazard ratio of 1.547. BCG-IFN seems to be an effective and safe salvage therapy, displaying acceptable response rates at 2 years. However, individuals who have failed multiple courses of BCG and those with early failure are less responsive to BCG-IFN combination therapy, and should consider early cystectomy if deemed appropriate.

Gemcitabine

Gemcitabine (Gemzar) is another antineoplastic agent used systemically in many cancers and has proved effective in combination with cisplatin (with or without paclitaxel) for treating metastatic urothelial cancer, and in the neoadjuvant setting before cystectomy.[45–49] Gemcitabine is a nucleoside analog and is incorporated into DNA, halting DNA synthesis, thus leading to cell death.[50] It also irreversibly inhibits ribonucleotide reductase, preventing deoxyribonucleotide production, subsequent DNA synthesis, and repair, thereby inducing apoptosis.

A phase II trial by Dalbagni and colleagues[50] at Memorial Sloan Kettering Cancer Center evaluated 30 patients who had failed BCG and were refusing cystectomy; 23 had CIS only. Gemcitabine was administered twice weekly for two 3-week periods with 1 week of rest in between, at a dose of 2000 mg (the highest soluble dose). At 3-month assessment, 50% (15 of 30) of patients achieved a CR, whereas 23% (7 of 30) had a partial response, defined as a negative cystoscopy and biopsy, but positive cytology. Of the 15 initial complete responders, 12 recurred at a median of 3.6 months, with one case of progression. Half of all nonresponders underwent cystectomy, whereas the other half (N = 4) had not shown disease progression at a median follow-up of 19 months. Ultimately, 10% of all patients were recurrence-free at 1 year. Eight grade 3 toxicities were reported, 75% of which were dysuria or frequency, one requiring cystectomy despite no evidence of disease.

This phase II trial enrolled a very high-risk population, with most patients being truly BCG-refractory after two prior induction cycles. A significant initial response rate was seen (50%); however, the response was not durable in most patients. Maintenance therapy was not evaluated in this trial, and many patients went on to cystectomy, making it difficult to determine the long-term rates of recurrence and progression.

Gacci and colleagues[51] reported on a group of nine patients who had failed two BCG induction courses. This cohort received 6 weeks of intravesical gemcitabine, followed by a maintenance schedule of 3 weekly instillations at 3, 6, 12, 18, and 24 months. Again, it was well-tolerated, but six (67%) of nine patients recurred, anywhere from 4 to 19 months after onset of treatment. Two of those patients recurred with cT2 disease, and subsequently underwent cystectomy, and were alive without recurrence at last follow-up. Three patients remained recurrence-free at 13, 17, and 21 months of follow-up. Although this is a small pilot study, it confirms the tolerability of gemcitabine, and raises the possibility of using maintenance therapy for initial responders.

A larger multicenter phase II trial was conducted by Bartoletti and colleagues[52] using intravesical gemcitabine, treating 116 patients with Ta, T1, or CIS, 40 (35%) of whom had failed BCG treatment, using the definition of persistent disease at 6 months postinduction. A total of 17.5% of patients reported adverse effects, requiring cessation of treatment in two cases. In the absence of maintenance therapy, at 1-year follow-up, 25.4% recurred at a median of 7 months. The subset analysis of the BCG failure group indicated that recurrence rates may be slightly higher, although it did not reach statistical significance. Overall, gemcitabine was more effective in patients with superficial disease and with no prior history of intravesical treatment.

In 2010, Addeo and colleagues[53] reported results of a randomized phase III trial, comparing intravesical gemcitabine with MMC for recurrent NMIBC. The gemcitabine treatment course consisted of a 6-week induction course, followed by 10 monthly maintenance treatments for initial responders. Of 120 enrolled patients, 109 were ultimately randomized with 54 and 55 patients in each treatment arm, respectively. A total of 91 patients had prior BCG treatment, although definitions of failure were not provided. At a median follow-up of 36 months, disease-free survival was superior in the gemcitabine arm, which was a consistent finding in the pretrial grade 3 histology group. Tumor progression occurred in 10 (18%) of 55 MMC patients, and in 6 (11%) of 54 of gemcitabine patients. With regards to adverse effects, MMC had a significantly higher rate (72.2% vs 38.8%), particularly with chemical cystitis (21.1% vs 5.5%) and dysuria frequency (20% vs 9.2%). Treatment delay occurred 10% of the time with MMC, and only 5% of the time for gemcitabine. In this phase III trial with many high-risk BCG-failure patients, gemcitabine proved slightly better at preventing recurrence, and had fewer adverse effects compared with MMC.

Recently, a national phase II nonrandomized study of monthly maintenance for intravesical gemcitabine (SWOG S0353) was completed.[54] Forty-seven patients who had failed two or more courses of BCG were treated, including patients with CIS (60%). At 3-month evaluation, 21 (45%) were disease-free, and 13 of those were continuously disease-free at the 12 months (28% of all evaluable patients). Three grade 3 toxicities were reported, whereas 30 patients had grade 1 to 2 toxicities, most of which were dysuria and urinary frequency. These data for gemcitabine maintenance therapy in a high-risk BCG-failure group indicate that a sizable portion of patients respond to therapy with a tolerable side effect profile, consistent with prior studies. However, it remains to be seen whether or not maintenance therapy adds benefit in preventing long-term progression and recurrence.

Although its efficacy has been illustrated in systemic disease, gemcitabine's role as an intravesical agent is still being evaluated. Phase I and II trials have shown it to be safe and somewhat effective in the treatment of recurrent NMIBC. The study populations have been somewhat heterogeneous, but have included many patients who have previously failed two induction courses of BCG and are thus at highest risk of recurrence and progression. Initial response rates of up to 50% have been reported and durable responses (disease free at $\geq$1 year) in 28% of patients, with the addition of maintenance therapy.

Valrubicin

Valrubicin (Valstar) is the only intravesical agent currently approved by the Food and Drug Administration for the treatment of BCG-refractory NMIBC. Valrubicin was developed as a lipid-soluble semisynthetic analog of doxorubicin (adriamycin), with modifications allowing for more rapid uptake into cells, and less potential for cardiac toxicity.[55] It interferes with nucleoside incorporation into nucleic acids, causing chromosomal damage. It is also converted in the cytoplasm to *N*-trifluoroacetyladriamycin, which then binds to topoisomerase II, inhibiting DNA repair and replication, RNA and protein synthesis, and ultimately results in cell cycle arrest during the G2 phase.

Greenberg and colleagues[55] reported the first experience with intravesical valrubicin in 1997, in a trial of 32 patients, 22 (69%) of whom had CIS after BCG treatment. Most patients experienced adverse effects, mostly limited to grade 1 to 2 urinary toxicity. In short-term follow-up, a CR rate of 41% was seen. A phase I trial enrolling 22 patients evaluated the safety of immediate post-TUR administration of valrubicin.[56] This modality was found to be well-tolerated, with minimal systemic absorption, significant only in a patient who experienced bladder perforation. Response rates were not reported.

This led to a multi-institutional study reported by Steinberg and colleagues[57] enrolling 90 patients with CIS who had received at least one prior course of BCG. Six weekly doses of 800-mg valrubicin were administered intravesically, based on prior dose escalation studies. A CR rate of 21% (19 of 90) was observed, defined as no disease at 3- or 6-month follow-up. For these 19 patients, median time to failure or last evaluation was more than 18 months, with seven patients (8%) still disease-free at a mean of 30 months of follow-up. Forty-four patients had cystectomy, with median time to cystectomy of 24 months for the nonresponders. Six cystectomy patients had greater than or equal to pT3a disease, and two had pN+ disease. Four patients have died of bladder cancer, none of whom was a complete responder. Treatment was well-tolerated, with local urinary toxicity as the primary complaint. Based on these data, valrubicin was approved by the Food and Drug Administration for intravesical treatment of BCG-refractory bladder cancer in patients who cannot tolerate the morbidity and mortality associated with cystectomy.

Docetaxel

Taxanes are chemotherapeutic agents that stabilize microtubules, preventing cell division and subsequently cause M-phase cell cycle arrest. They are used widely in oncology, and have shown efficacy in metastatic bladder cancer.[58,59] Intravesical docetaxel (Taxotere) was first studied in a phase I trial in which 18 patients with NMIBC who had failed BCG or BCG-IFN received 6 weekly instillations.[60] Eight patients (44%) reported grade 1 to 2 toxicity, including hematuria, urgency, and dysuria, whereas none experienced grade 3 to 4 toxicity, and a maximum tolerated dose was not reached. All patients completed six treatments, and there was no drug detected on serum measurements. Results of the original cohort of patients have been recently reported with a median follow-up of 48 months.[61] No delayed toxicity was reported, and 4 (22%) of 18 had a durable CR without maintenance or any other therapy, whereas 3 (17%) of 18 had a durable partial response, meaning a non-muscle invasive recurrence treated by local resection.

Paclitaxel

Because intravesical docetaxel was shown to be well-tolerated in patients with BCG-refractory NMIBC[60] another taxane was investigated in a phase I trial of *nab*-paclitaxel (Abraxane), a nanoparticle albumin-bound formulation that facilitates drug delivery into cells.[62–65] The *nab* technology also allows for higher concentrations of taxane to be administered, which is important to note, because the maximum tolerated dose was never reached with docetaxel.[60] Eighteen patients with NMIBC were enrolled in this phase I dose escalation study in 2008 to 2009, all of whom had had at least one course of BCG induction, with a mean of 2.8 prior courses.[66] Twelve of the eighteen had also received BCG-IFN therapy, and three had received MMC, whereas three had received other experimental intravesical agents. No grade 2 or higher toxicities were noted, whereas 10 of 18 patients experienced grade 1 local toxicity, none of which required cessation of treatment. There was only one instance of detectable serum levels of paclitaxel, which resolved within a week. At first follow-up assessment, 5 (28%) of 18 patients demonstrated a CR. The efficacy of *nab*-paclitaxel is currently being evaluated in an ongoing phase II trial (clinicaltrials.gov ID NCT00583349).

An alternative drug delivery platform is hyaluronic acid (HA), a glycosaminoglycan abundant in human connective tissues. Binding HA to paclitaxel was shown to increase solubility and to increase in vitro antitumor activity, without systemic absorption in animal models.[67,68] Bassi and colleagues[69] published a phase I study of intravesical paclitaxel-HA (ONCOFID-P-B), enrolling 16 patients with BCG-refractory CIS, with 15 of 16 receiving all 6 weekly instillations. A total of seven patients reported 11 adverse events, three of which were serious, including exacerbation of pre-existing atrial fibrillation, resultant heart failure, and significant hematuria after a bladder biopsy 40 days after drug administration. At post-treatment assessment, 9 (60%) of 16 exhibited a CR. This phase I study indicates that a different formulation of paclitaxel may also be safe to administer intravesically in patients with BCG-refractory CIS; it is not clear if the significant adverse events were treatment-related. A phase II study using paclitaxel-HA for patients with G1-G2 Ta urothelial cancer is currently enrolling patients in Europe, but it excludes patients with CIS or T1 lesions, and does not require prior BCG failure, making it less applicable for patients seeking salvage therapy after BCG failure. It is hoped that it will shed more light on the overall efficacy of intravesical taxanes.

Mycobacterial Cell Wall Extract

BCG has been proved as the most effective agent in high-risk NMIBC, but carries the risk of BCG sepsis, because it is a live attenuated vaccine. To retain antitumor efficacy but reduce toxicity, the concept of using mycobacterial cell wall extract came about, and was first reported in 2001 as intravesical treatment in patients with CIS.[70,71] However, the emulsion contained thimerosal, which has its own toxicities. Subsequently, a mycobacterial cell wall-DNA complex (MCC) was developed, and a multi-institutional open label study with 55 patients was conducted.[72] MCC was administered weekly for 6 weeks, and then for 3 weeks at Weeks 12 and 24 as maintenance therapy. Twenty-eight patients in this cohort had had prior BCG therapy, whereas eight patients had no history of intravesical therapy. In the intention-to-treat analysis, response rates of 27% (4 mg) and 46% (8 mg) were seen at 12 weeks with identical rates at 26 weeks. At 18 months, disease-free rates of 23% (4 mg) and 29% (8 mg) were noted. Serious adverse events occurred at rates of 32% and 33% in the 4-mg and 8-mg of MCC groups, respectively, one of which necessitated treatment cessation.

Currently, a phase III trial is ongoing (clinicaltrials.gov ID: NCT00406068) using MCC in patients with BCG-refractory disease, or recurrent high-grade NMIBC less than or equal to 2 years after initial BCG success.[73] Eight milligrams of MCC was administered as a 6-week induction course, followed by 3 weekly instillations at 3, 6,

12, 18, and 24 months as maintenance. Interim results of 129 patients in this multi-institutional trial show a 1-year disease-free survival rate of 25%, with recurrence at a median of 177 days. Eighty-six percent of patients reported a treatment-related adverse event, mostly urinary. Two patients had to cease treatment based on adverse effects (asthenia, vomiting). These interim results show some efficacy of MCC in patients who have failed BCG, although not as effective as repeat BCG induction.[14] Again, there is no standard control agent for this population against which to compare these agents, but MCC does seem to elicit a response in a select group of patients. MCC was recently being evaluated in a phase III open-label, randomized trial as compared with MMC for BCG-failure patients (clinicaltrials.gov ID: NCT01200992). However, the trial was closed early because of poor accrual. Ultimately, MCC may be better suited as an alternative to BCG in primary treatment of NMIBC, provided it has similar efficacy and less toxicity.

COMBINATION THERAPY

Each salvage agent discussed has yielded clinical responses in certain patients, but none with any appreciable superiority at this point in time. In addition, it is not clear which patients will respond. BCG-refractory status and two or more prior courses of BCG have been associated with worse outcomes in some studies,[15,43,44] but not all of these individuals fail salvage therapy. A more recent strategy to address the relative lack of efficacy of single-agent intravesical salvage regimens has been the pursuit of multidrug combination intravesical therapy.

Breyer and colleagues[74] used a combination of MMC and gemcitabine in 10 patients with BCG-intolerant or BCG-refractory disease, defined as a positive biopsy after two induction courses. One gram of gemcitabine was given and retained for 90 minutes, drained from the bladder, followed by 40 mg of MMC. This continued for 6 weeks, with monthly maintenance given to responders. Six patients (60%) had a CR at 3 months, and are recurrence-free at a median of 14 months (4–34 months). No significant adverse events were reported.

In 2012, Chen and colleagues[75] provided a retrospective report of 114 patients with BCG-naive NMIBC who received a cocktail of intravesical MMC-doxorubicin-cisplatin.

In a nonrandomized comparison with a group that received BCG, recurrence rates were similar between the two groups, with fewer adverse effects reported in the MMC-doxorubicin-cisplatin group. Although this did not include a BCG-failure group, it suggests that a multidrug regimen is a tolerable and feasible option for intravesical treatment. Well-designed prospective trials using multiagent therapy have yet to be conducted, but it seems

Table 2
Ongoing and pending clinical trials

Drug	Trial Number	Phase	Description
rAd-IFN/Syn3 (Instiladrin)	NCT01687244	II	Interferon-α2b transfected into urothelial cells by adenovirus vector
RAD001 (Everolimus)	NCT01259063	I/II	Intravesical gemcitabine plus oral everolimus (mTOR inhibitor)
Dovitinib	NCT01732107	II	Oral dovitinib (tyrosine kinase inhibitor) for patients with FGFR3 overexpression or mutation
Sunitinib	NCT01118351	II	Oral sunitinib (tyrosine kinase inhibitor)
EN3348	NCT01200992	III	Mycobacterial cell wall-DNA complex vs mitomycin C
ALT-801	NCT01625260	I/II	Recombinant protein–interleukin-2 plus anti-p53-receptor
DTA-H19/PEI	NCT00595088	II	dsDNA plasmid, diphtheria toxin gene under H19 regulation (upregulated in tumor cells)
CG0070	Pending	II	Granulocyte-macrophage colony–stimulating factor transfected into urothelial cells by adenovirus vector
nab-rapamycin	Pending	I/II	Intravesical nanoparticle albumin-bound rapamycin (mTOR inhibitor)

logical that multiple agents would be more effective in the intravesical setting, as has been shown through the use of multidrug systemic chemotherapy, such as methotrexate-vinblastine-doxorubicin-cisplatin and gemcitabine-cisplatin.

FUTURE THERAPIES

Each salvage agent used is based on prior systemic chemotherapy experience (eg, gemcitabine, taxanes), or builds on knowledge of existing intravesical agents (eg, TCT-MMC, EMDA-MMC, MCC). Many current trials (**Table 2**) focus on targeted therapies, guided by knowledge of bladder cancer pathogenesis, and by technology advances in drug development. CG0070 and oportuzumab monatox are two such intravesical drugs whose phase I and II trial results have recently been published.[76,77] CG0070 is an oncolytic adenovirus that preferentially replicates in cells with defective retinoblastoma (Rb) pathways (typically seen in bladder cancer), and also encodes human granulocyte-macrophage colony–stimulating factor, resulting in targeted cytotoxicity. Oportuzumab monatox uses recombinant fusion protein technology to combine anti-EpCAM antibody with *Pseudomonas* exotoxin A, enabling preferential binding to urothelial cancer cells, and inducing apoptosis. Additionally, mammalian target of rapamycin (mTOR) inhibitors and tyrosine kinase inhibitors are under investigation, because those pathways have been linked to urothelial cancer pathogenesis, and provide a clear target for treatment.

Another important avenue of future research is to continue to elucidate molecular markers that predict sensitivity and resistance to systemic chemotherapeutic agents[78–80] and other intravesical agents.[81] A better understanding of this may enable treatment choices to be tailored to individual risk profiles. Despite ongoing efforts, there is currently no superior alternative for BCG-failure patients. However, it is hoped that advances in understanding genomic alterations of urothelial cancer and in drug development technology will result in effective targeted therapies and individualized treatment as an effective method of addressing BCG failure.

SUMMARY

BCG has been established as the primary treatment of high-risk NMIBC. However, if patients do not respond or later recur, the most reliable treatment option is cystectomy. For those who are unwilling or unable to undergo this significant procedure, there is a multitude of alternative intravesical therapies. Each has been shown to have some degree of efficacy and has provided durable CRs for certain patients. However, with the existing evidence, it is difficult to recommend one agent over another, or over cystectomy, because none has proved itself as reliably effective. Further work needs to be done to determine the risk profile of each BCG-failure patient, and to establish durable and successful treatments for this high-risk group.

REFERENCES

1. Howlader N, Noone AM, Krapcho M, et al, editors. SEER cancer statistics review, 1975-2009 (Vintage 2009 Populations). Bethesda (MD): National Cancer Institute; 2012. Available at: http://seer.cancer.gov/csr/1975_2009_pops09/. Accessed August 8, 2012, based on November 2011 SEER data submission, posted to the SEER web site.
2. Rubben H, Lutzeyer W, Fischer N, et al. Natural history and treatment of low and high risk superficial bladder tumors. J Urol 1988;139(2):283–5.
3. Millan-Rodriguez F, Chechile-Toniolo G, Salvador-Bayarri J, et al. Primary superficial bladder cancer risk groups according to progression, mortality and recurrence. J Urol 2000;164(3 Pt 1):680–4.
4. Pasin E, Josephson DY, Mitra AP, et al. Superficial bladder cancer: an update on etiology, molecular development, classification, and natural history. Rev Urol 2008;10(1):31–43.
5. Morales A, Eidinger D. Bacillus Calmette-Guerin in the treatment of adenocarcinoma of the kidney. J Urol 1976;115(4):377–80.
6. Brausi M, Witjes JA, Lamm D, et al. A review of current guidelines and best practice recommendations for the management of nonmuscle invasive bladder cancer by the International Bladder Cancer Group. J Urol 2011;186(6):2158–67.
7. Sylvester RJ, van der MA, Lamm DL. Intravesical bacillus Calmette-Guerin reduces the risk of progression in patients with superficial bladder cancer: a meta-analysis of the published results of randomized clinical trials. J Urol 2002;168(5):1964–70.
8. Morales A. Long-term results and complications of intracavitary bacillus Calmette-Guerin therapy for bladder cancer. J Urol 1984;132(3):457–9.
9. Catalona WJ, Hudson MA, Gillen DP, et al. Risks and benefits of repeated courses of intravesical bacillus Calmette-Guerin therapy for superficial bladder cancer. J Urol 1987;137(2):220–4.
10. Herr HW, Dalbagni G. Defining bacillus Calmette-Guerin refractory superficial bladder tumors. J Urol 2003;169(5):1706–8.
11. Nieder AM, Brausi M, Lamm D, et al. Management of stage T1 tumors of the bladder: international consensus panel. Urology 2005;66(6 Suppl 1):108–25.

12. Herr HW. The value of a second transurethral resection in evaluating patients with bladder tumors. J Urol 1999;162(1):74–6.
13. Shirakawa H, Kikuchi E, Tanaka N, et al. Prognostic significance of bacillus Calmette-Guerin failure classification in non-muscle-invasive bladder cancer. BJU Int 2012;110(6 Pt B):E216–21.
14. Brake M, Loertzer H, Horsch R, et al. Long-term results of intravesical bacillus Calmette-Guerin therapy for stage T1 superficial bladder cancer. Urology 2000;55(5):673–8.
15. Lamm DL, Blumenstein BA, Crissman JD, et al. Maintenance bacillus Calmette-Guerin immunotherapy for recurrent TA, T1 and carcinoma in situ transitional cell carcinoma of the bladder: a randomized Southwest Oncology Group Study. J Urol 2000; 163(4):1124–9.
16. Lerner SP, Tangen CM, Sucharew H, et al. Patterns of recurrence and outcomes following induction bacillus Calmette-Guerin for high risk Ta, T1 bladder cancer. J Urol 2007;177(5):1727–31.
17. Guzzo TJ, Magheli A, Bivalacqua TJ, et al. Pathological upstaging during radical cystectomy is associated with worse recurrence-free survival in patients with bacillus Calmette-Guerin-refractory bladder cancer. Urology 2009;74(6):1276–80.
18. Mahmud SM, Fong B, Fahmy N, et al. Effect of preoperative delay on survival in patients with bladder cancer undergoing cystectomy in Quebec: a population based study. J Urol 2006;175(1):78–83 [discussion: 83].
19. Chang SS, Hassan JM, Cookson MS, et al. Delaying radical cystectomy for muscle invasive bladder cancer results in worse pathological stage. J Urol 2003;170(4 Pt 1):1085–7.
20. Kulkarni GS, Urbach DR, Austin PC, et al. Longer wait times increase overall mortality in patients with bladder cancer. J Urol 2009;182(4):1318–24.
21. Herr HW, Sogani PC. Does early cystectomy improve the survival of patients with high risk superficial bladder tumors? J Urol 2001;166(4):1296–9.
22. Raj GV, Herr H, Serio AM, et al. Treatment paradigm shift may improve survival of patients with high risk superficial bladder cancer. J Urol 2007;177(4): 1283–6 [discussion: 1286].
23. Badalato GM, Gaya JM, Hruby G, et al. Immediate radical cystectomy vs conservative management for high grade cT1 bladder cancer: is there a survival difference? BJU Int 2012;110(10):1471–7.
24. Babjuk M, Oosterlinck W, Sylvester R, et al. EAU guidelines on non-muscle-invasive urothelial carcinoma of the bladder, the 2011 update. Eur Urol 2011;59(6):997–1008.
25. Kamat AM, Lamm DL. Intravesical therapy for bladder cancer. Urology 2000;55(2):161–8.
26. Malmstrom PU, Wijkstrom H, Lundholm C, et al. 5-year followup of a randomized prospective study comparing mitomycin C and bacillus Calmette-Guerin in patients with superficial bladder carcinoma. Swedish-Norwegian Bladder Cancer Study Group. J Urol 1999;161(4):1124–7.
27. Di Stasi SM, Giannantoni A, Stephen RL, et al. Intravesical electromotive mitomycin C versus passive transport mitomycin C for high risk superficial bladder cancer: a prospective randomized study. J Urol 2003;170(3):777–82.
28. Colombo R, Da Pozzo LF, Salonia A, et al. Multicentric study comparing intravesical chemotherapy alone and with local microwave hyperthermia for prophylaxis of recurrence of superficial transitional cell carcinoma. J Clin Oncol 2003;21(23):4270–6.
29. Colombo R, Lev A, Da Pozzo LF, et al. A new approach using local combined microwave hyperthermia and chemotherapy in superficial transitional bladder carcinoma treatment. J Urol 1995;153(3 Pt 2):959–63.
30. van der Heijden AG, Verhaegh G, Jansen CF, et al. Effect of hyperthermia on the cytotoxicity of 4 chemotherapeutic agents currently used for the treatment of transitional cell carcinoma of the bladder: an in vitro study. J Urol 2005;173(4):1375–80.
31. Paroni R, Salonia A, Lev A, et al. Effect of local hyperthermia of the bladder on mitomycin C pharmacokinetics during intravesical chemotherapy for the treatment of superficial transitional cell carcinoma. Br J Clin Pharmacol 2001;52(3):273–8.
32. Alfred Witjes J, Hendricksen K, Gofrit O, et al. Intravesical hyperthermia and mitomycin-C for carcinoma in situ of the urinary bladder: experience of the European Synergo working party. World J Urol 2009;27(3):319–24.
33. Nativ O, Witjes JA, Hendricksen K, et al. Combined thermo-chemotherapy for recurrent bladder cancer after bacillus Calmette-Guerin. J Urol 2009;182(4): 1313–7.
34. Au JL, Badalament RA, Wientjes MG, et al. Methods to improve efficacy of intravesical mitomycin C: results of a randomized phase III trial. J Natl Cancer Inst 2001;93(8):597–604.
35. Di Stasi SM, Riedl C. Updates in intravesical electromotive drug administration of mitomycin-C for non-muscle invasive bladder cancer. World J Urol 2009;27(3):325–30.
36. Di Stasi SM, Storti L, Giurioli A, et al. Carcinoma in situ of the bladder: long-term results of a randomized prospective study comparing intravesical electromotive mitomycin-C, passive diffusion mitomycin-C and Bacillus Calmette-Guerin [abstract 439]. Eur Urol Suppl 2008;7(3):180.
37. Sockett LJ, Borwell J, Symes A, et al. Electro-motive drug administration (EMDA) of intravesical mitomycin-C in patients with high-risk non-invasive bladder cancer and failure of BCG immunotherapy [abstract U17]. BJU Int 2008;101(Suppl 5):50.

38. Di Stasi SM, Giannantoni A, Giurioli A, et al. Sequential BCG and electromotive mitomycin versus BCG alone for high-risk superficial bladder cancer: a randomised controlled trial. Lancet Oncol 2006; 7(1):43–51.
39. Di Stasi SM, Valenti M, Verri C, et al. Electromotive instillation of mitomycin immediately before transurethral resection for patients with primary urothelial non-muscle invasive bladder cancer: a randomised controlled trial. Lancet Oncol 2011;12(9):871–9.
40. Glashan RW. A randomized controlled study of intravesical alpha-2b-interferon in carcinoma in situ of the bladder. J Urol 1990;144(3):658–61.
41. Belldegrun AS, Franklin JR, O'Donnell MA, et al. Superficial bladder cancer: the role of interferon-alpha. J Urol 1998;159(6):1793–801.
42. O'Donnell MA, Krohn J, DeWolf WC. Salvage intravesical therapy with interferon-alpha 2b plus low dose bacillus Calmette-Guerin is effective in patients with superficial bladder cancer in whom bacillus Calmette-Guerin alone previously failed. J Urol 2001;166(4):1300–4 [discussion: 1304–5].
43. Joudi FN, Smith BJ, O'Donnell MA, National BCG-Interferon Phase 2 Investigator Group. Final results from a national multicenter phase II trial of combination bacillus Calmette-Guerin plus interferon alpha-2B for reducing recurrence of superficial bladder cancer. Urol Oncol 2006;24(4):344–8.
44. Rosevear HM, Lightfoot AJ, Birusingh KK, et al. Factors affecting response to bacillus Calmette-Guerin plus interferon for urothelial carcinoma in situ. J Urol 2011;186(3):817–23.
45. Lorusso V, Manzione L, De Vita F, et al. Gemcitabine plus cisplatin for advanced transitional cell carcinoma of the urinary tract: a phase II multicenter trial. J Urol 2000;164(1):53–6.
46. Lorusso V, Pollera CF, Antimi M, et al. A phase II study of gemcitabine in patients with transitional cell carcinoma of the urinary tract previously treated with platinum. Italian Co-operative Group on Bladder Cancer. Eur J Cancer 1998;34(8):1208–12.
47. Moore MJ, Tannock IF, Ernst DS, et al. Gemcitabine: a promising new agent in the treatment of advanced urothelial cancer. J Clin Oncol 1997; 15(12):3441–5.
48. Stadler WM, Kuzel T, Roth B, et al. Phase II study of single-agent gemcitabine in previously untreated patients with metastatic urothelial cancer. J Clin Oncol 1997;15(11):3394–8.
49. Dash A, Pettus JA IV, Herr HW, et al. A role for neoadjuvant gemcitabine plus cisplatin in muscle-invasive urothelial carcinoma of the bladder: a retrospective experience. Cancer 2008;113(9):2471–7.
50. Dalbagni G, Russo P, Sheinfeld J, et al. Phase I trial of intravesical gemcitabine in bacillus Calmette-Guerin-refractory transitional-cell carcinoma of the bladder. J Clin Oncol 2002;20(15):3193–8.
51. Gacci M, Bartoletti R, Cai T, et al. Intravesical gemcitabine in BCG-refractory T1G3 transitional cell carcinoma of the bladder: a pilot study. Urol Int 2006;76(2):106–11.
52. Bartoletti R, Cai T, Gacci M, et al. Intravesical gemcitabine therapy for superficial transitional cell carcinoma: results of a Phase II prospective multicenter study. Urology 2005;66(4):726–31.
53. Addeo R, Caraglia M, Bellini S, et al. Randomized phase III trial on gemcitabine versus mytomicin in recurrent superficial bladder cancer: evaluation of efficacy and tolerance. J Clin Oncol 2010;28(4): 543–8.
54. Skinner EC, Goldman B, Sakr WA, et al. 1666 SWOG S0353 phase II trial of intravesical gemcitabine in patients with non-muscle invasive bladder cancer who recurred following at least two prior courses of BCG. J Urol 2012;187(Suppl 4):e673.
55. Greenberg RE, Bahnson RR, Wood D, et al. Initial report on intravesical administration of N-trifluoroacetyladriamycin-14-valerate (AD 32) to patients with refractory superficial transitional cell carcinoma of the urinary bladder. Urology 1997;49(3):471–5.
56. Patterson AL, Greenberg RE, Weems L, et al. Pilot study of the tolerability and toxicity of intravesical valrubicin immediately after transurethral resection of superficial bladder cancer. Urology 2000;56(2): 232–5.
57. Steinberg G, Bahnson R, Brosman S, et al. Efficacy and safety of valrubicin for the treatment of bacillus Calmette-Guerin refractory carcinoma in situ of the bladder. The Valrubicin Study Group. J Urol 2000; 163(3):761–7.
58. Calabro F, Sternberg CN. New drugs and new approaches for the treatment of metastatic urothelial cancer. World J Urol 2002;20(3):158–66.
59. Rangel C, Niell H, Miller A, et al. Taxol and taxotere in bladder cancer: in vitro activity and urine stability. Cancer Chemother Pharmacol 1994;33(6):460–4.
60. McKiernan JM, Masson P, Murphy AM, et al. Phase I trial of intravesical docetaxel in the management of superficial bladder cancer refractory to standard intravesical therapy. J Clin Oncol 2006;24(19): 3075–80.
61. Laudano MA, Barlow LJ, Murphy AM, et al. Long-term clinical outcomes of a phase I trial of intravesical docetaxel in the management of non-muscle-invasive bladder cancer refractory to standard intravesical therapy. Urology 2010;75(1):134–7.
62. Sparreboom A, Scripture CD, Trieu V, et al. Comparative preclinical and clinical pharmacokinetics of a cremophor-free, nanoparticle albumin-bound paclitaxel (ABI-007) and paclitaxel formulated in Cremophor (Taxol). Clin Cancer Res 2005;11(11): 4136–43.
63. Desai NP, Trieu V, Hwang LY, et al. Improved effectiveness of nanoparticle albumin-bound (nab) paclitaxel

versus polysorbate-based docetaxel in multiple xenografts as a function of HER2 and SPARC status. Anticancer Drugs 2008;19(9):899–909.
64. Gradishar WJ. Albumin-bound paclitaxel: a next-generation taxane. Expert Opin Pharmacother 2006;7(8):1041–53.
65. Gradishar WJ, Tjulandin S, Davidson N, et al. Phase III trial of nanoparticle albumin-bound paclitaxel compared with polyethylated castor oil-based paclitaxel in women with breast cancer. J Clin Oncol 2005;23(31):7794–803.
66. McKiernan JM, Barlow LJ, Laudano MA, et al. A phase I trial of intravesical nanoparticle albumin-bound paclitaxel in the treatment of bacillus Calmette-Guerin refractory nonmuscle invasive bladder cancer. J Urol 2011;186(2):448–51.
67. Tringali G, Lisi L, Bettella F, et al. The in vitro rabbit whole bladder as a model to investigate the urothelial transport of anticancer agents The ONCOFID-P paradigm. Pharmacol Res 2008;58(5–6):340–3.
68. Rosato A, Banzato A, De Luca G, et al. HYTAD1-p20: a new paclitaxel-hyaluronic acid hydrosoluble bioconjugate for treatment of superficial bladder cancer. Urol Oncol 2006;24(3):207–15.
69. Bassi PF, Volpe A, D'Agostino D, et al. Paclitaxel-hyaluronic acid for intravesical therapy of bacillus Calmette-Guerin refractory carcinoma in situ of the bladder: results of a phase I study. J Urol 2011; 185(2):445–9.
70. Meyer TJ, Ribi EE, Azuma I, et al. Biologically active components from mycobacterial cell walls. II. Suppression and regression of strain-2 guinea pig hepatoma. J Natl Cancer Inst 1974;52(1):103–11.
71. Morales A, Chin JL, Ramsey EW. Mycobacterial cell wall extract for treatment of carcinoma in situ of the bladder. J Urol 2001;166(5):1633–7 [discussion: 1637–8].
72. Morales A, Phadke K, Steinhoff G. Intravesical mycobacterial cell wall-DNA complex in the treatment of carcinoma in situ of the bladder after standard intravesical therapy has failed. J Urol 2009; 181(3):1040–5.
73. Cohen Z. Efficacy and safety of mycobacterial cell wall DNA complex in the treatment of patients with non-muscle invasive bladder cancer at high risk of progression and who are refractory to BCG. Vienna (Austria): 26th annual EAU Congress 2011.
74. Breyer BN, Whitson JM, Carroll PR, et al. Sequential intravesical gemcitabine and mitomycin C chemotherapy regimen in patients with non-muscle invasive bladder cancer. Urol Oncol 2010;28(5):510–4.
75. Chen CH, Yang HJ, Shun CT, et al. A cocktail regimen of intravesical mitomycin-C, doxorubicin, and cisplatin (MDP) for non-muscle-invasive bladder cancer. Urol Oncol 2012;30(4):421–7.
76. Burke JM, Lamm DL, Meng MV, et al. A first in human phase 1 study of CG0070, a GM-CSF expressing oncolytic adenovirus, for the treatment of nonmuscle invasive bladder cancer. J Urol 2012; 188(6):2391–7.
77. Kowalski M, Guindon J, Brazas L, et al. A phase II study of oportuzumab monatox: an immunotoxin therapy for patients with noninvasive urothelial carcinoma in situ previously treated with bacillus Calmette-Guerin. J Urol 2012;188(5):1712–8.
78. Paik S, Shak S, Tang G, et al. A multigene assay to predict recurrence of tamoxifen-treated, node-negative breast cancer. N Engl J Med 2004;351(27): 2817–26.
79. Bellmunt J, Paz-Ares L, Cuello M, et al. Gene expression of ERCC1 as a novel prognostic marker in advanced bladder cancer patients receiving cisplatin-based chemotherapy. Ann Oncol 2007; 18(3):522–8.
80. Smith SC, Baras AS, Lee JK, et al. The COXEN principle: translating signatures of in vitro chemosensitivity into tools for clinical outcome prediction and drug discovery in cancer. Cancer Res 2010;70(5):1753–8.
81. Wosnitzer MS, Domingo-Domenech J, Castillo-Martin M, et al. Predictive value of microtubule associated proteins tau and stathmin in patients with nonmuscle invasive bladder cancer receiving adjuvant intravesical taxane therapy. J Urol 2011; 186(5):2094–100.

Determining the Role of Cystectomy for High-grade T1 Urothelial Carcinoma

Siamak Daneshmand, MD

KEYWORDS

• Bladder cancer • T1 • High grade • T1G3 • BCG • Cystectomy • Treatment

KEY POINTS

- Pathologic upstaging from initial high-grade T1 to muscle-invasive disease (≥T2) from either repeat resection or cystectomy ranges from 25% to 50% depending on whether muscle was present at initial resection.
- Long-term studies show progression rates of up to 50% for high-grade T1 urothelial carcinoma of the bladder with up to 30% cancer-specific death.
- Although there has been significant effort in identifying factors associated with aggressive behavior, molecular markers are not in routine clinical use and need further validation.
- Presence of concomitant carcinoma in situ, tumor multifocality, hydronephrosis, tumor size (greater than 3 cm), stage T1b, and presence of residual T1 at repeat resection deem a patient high risk and immediate cystectomy should be strongly considered.
- The incidence of lymph node involvement in patients treated with radical cystectomy for HGT1 bladder cancer is 12% to 15%.
- Immediate radical cystectomy can provide a cancer-specific survival of greater than 80% in properly staged patients.

INTRODUCTION

High-grade T1 (HGT1) urothelial carcinoma of the bladder is a potentially lethal disease that requires meticulous attention. The HGT1 group represents about 20% of the patients who present with non-muscle invasive bladder cancer (NMIBC).[1] These tumors have a high propensity to recur and progress to muscle invasion with associated risk of metastasis and death. Long-term studies show progression rates as high as 50% with more than 30% of patients succumbing to the disease.[2] As opposed to noninvasive disease (Ta or carcinoma in situ [CIS]) or muscle-invasive disease (≥T2), treatment guidelines are not concrete and considerable variation exists in treatment modalities. Most studies have short-term follow-up, making it difficult to assess the true long-term efficacy of proposed treatment regimens. There are no randomized trials comparing intravesical therapy with up-front cystectomy for HGT1 bladder cancer, making valid conclusions more difficult. The few long-term studies of intravesical therapy for initial diagnosis of HGT1disease show a discouraging rate of progression and disease-specific mortality. Further confounding the issue is the often considerable heterogeneity in the HGT1 patient population, depending on the presence or absence of CIS, multifocality, tumor differentiation, tumor within a diverticulum, and, most importantly, whether there is muscle present in the resected specimen. Although there is a refined understanding of some of the molecular mechanisms and biology of high-grade bladder cancer, the currently available tools cannot adequately

USC Institute of Urology, Norris Comprehensive Cancer Center, 1441 Eastlake Avenue, Suite 7416, Los Angeles, CA 90089, USA
E-mail address: daneshma@usc.edu

Urol Clin N Am 40 (2013) 233–247
http://dx.doi.org/10.1016/j.ucl.2013.01.003
0094-0143/13/$ – see front matter

differentiate patients who are best suited for aggressive initial management (ie, cystectomy).

Transurethral resection (TUR) of the bladder tumor (TURBT) alone has long been recognized as inadequate treatment, with 40% to 50% of patients progressing to stage T2 or greater disease in just 3 years.[3] The addition of intravesical bacillus Calmette-Guérin (BCG) immunotherapy following TURBT has been shown in randomized trials to significantly improve the 10-year tumor progression-free and disease-specific survival rates compared with TURBT alone.[4] This combination now constitutes the current standard first-line therapy. Patients who fail induction BCG therapy and/or have recurrent disease shortly following treatment are at significant risk of progression to muscle-invasive disease and radical cystectomy should be seriously considered.[5–7] Second-line treatments for bladder preservation are generally not very effective. Additional intravesical agents in patients who develop a recurrence following BCG therapy include BCG plus interferon, mitomycin C, gemcitabine, Doxorubicin, docetaxel, apaziquone, various combinations of these agents, and newer investigational therapies. The outcomes of trials investigating salvage intravesical therapies are generally poor and have short follow-up.[8–10] Because effective second-line bladder-sparing therapy using intravesical agents is not well established, many experts consider the standard treatment in this setting to be radical cystectomy. This article reviews the clinical and pathologic features that characterize HGT1 disease, with special emphasis on the role of early radical cystectomy.

PATHOLOGY

Optimal management of bladder cancer relies heavily on information garnered from TUR of the tumor. Grade, stage, and depth of tumor invasion play a fundamental role in subsequent prognostication and treatment strategies. In addition, depth of tumor invasion within the lamina propria, associated CIS, lymphovascular invasion (LVI), and aberrant differentiation all have been shown to be important risk factors for progression of HGT1 disease. Interpretation of lamina propria invasion may be difficult in TUR specimens, especially when there is a high degree of cautery artifact. In a study of centralized pathologic review of 1400 patients treated in 5 European Organization for Research and Treatment of Cancer (EORTC) randomized phase III trials comparing various adjuvant treatments for NMIBC, the investigators found significant variation in grade and stage. More than half the tumors (53%) were downstaged to Ta, whereas 10% of the cases were upstaged to muscle-invasive (T2) disease. There was agreement on the diagnosis of HGT1 disease in only 50% of the cases.[11] In addition, there is considerable understaging of the disease, particularly when there is no muscle included in the resected specimen. The goal of TUR is eradication of the tumor whenever possible with adequate sampling of the muscularis propria. Fluorescence cystoscopy (blue light) using hexaminolevulinate (HAL) has recently been shown to improve the detection and complete resection of NMIBCs.[12] Numerous studies have now documented up to 50% understaging when muscle is absent from the TURBT specimen.[13,14] Even when muscle is present in the resected specimen, adequate staging cannot be presumed since studies have shown that, even in that setting, there is still a 10% to 15% chance of upstaging to muscle-invasive disease. These patients are destined to fail with conservative therapy because intravesical agents are ineffective in this setting. The presence of muscle in a resected specimen does not automatically imply that it was derived from the tumor base. Jancke and colleagues[15] investigated the presence of residual tumor in what they called the 'marginal resection' following complete TURBT for Ta/T1 disease. A marginal resection of 7 mm was removed following macroscopic resection of all visible tumors. Of the 94 patients evaluated, 24 (26%) had residual tumor in the marginal resection, which had a significant impact on recurrence. Incomplete tumor resection not only leads to early recurrence but, more importantly, is probably the source for tumor progression and dissemination. Cystectomy series for clinical T1 disease also reflect similar understaging with 30% to 40% of patients being upstaged to muscle-invasive disease. In the series from Vanderbilt University including 78 patients, 31 patients (40%) were upstaged to T2 disease. Final pathologic stage had a significant impact on survival, with 98% of patients with pathologic stage T1 being disease free during follow-up compared with 65% with stage pT2 or greater disease (P<.01).[13]

SUBSTAGING

The existence of muscularis mucosae within the subepithelial connective tissue has been well described and used for prognostication.[16] However, the degree of development of this layer is variable.[17] The depth of tumor invasion into the lamina propria has been proved to be associated with outcome.[18–20] Angulo and colleagues[21] examined a series of 170 patients with HGT1 disease and differentiated 98 of them (58%) into those with tumor invasion confined to the lamina propria (pT1a) and those with tumor infiltrating into the submucosa (pT1b). Cox regression analysis of pT1 subcategory showed the depth of subepithelial connective tissue invasion to be an independent prognostic factor (*P*<.05). Five-year recurrence-free survival (RFS) was 86% for patients with stage pT1a tumors compared with 52% of those with pT1b tumors. Several other investigators have replicated similar results corroborating the feasibility of substaging of T1 tumors. Other researchers have studied this concept with further granularity. Orsola and colleagues[16] reported on 97 patients with T1 disease substaged according to invasion superficial to (T1a), into (T1b), or beyond the muscularis mucosae (T1c). They were able to subclassify 87% of the cases and, although the recurrence rate was similar for all groups, progression rate for deep lamina propria invasion (T1b and T1c) was significantly higher than for T1a tumors (34% vs 8%, *P* = .016). Multivariate analysis revealed depth of invasion and CIS to be the independent prognostic factors, with a hazard ratio (HR) of 4.47 and 3.19, respectively. However, a recent study by van Rhijn and colleagues[22] found no association between depth of invasion and progression or disease-specific survival. However, they did introduce a novel substaging system of pT1 bladder cancer differentiating tumors into T1 microinvasive (T1m) and T1 extensive (T1e) tumors. They then determined the invasion of the muscularis mucosae–vascular plexus into T1a/b/c categories according to invasion above, into, or beyond the muscularis mucosae. They found substage (T1m/T1e) to be significant for progression and disease-specific survival but not substage according to depth of invasion (T1a/b/c). More significantly they were able to classify all 134 cases into the new substaging system (T1m/T1e). Others have corroborated the significance of microinvasive versus extensive-invasive T1 to be prognostic for recurrence, progression, and survival in the largest series of initial pT1 tumors (n = 209) reported thus far.[23] In their study, depth of invasion into the lamina propria was also not significant. Not all patients had a restaging TURBT. The finding that extensive invasion of the lamina propria is highly prognostic can help identify patients better suited for upfront cystectomy.

OTHER PROGNOSTIC FACTORS

Numerous other factors have been studied in an attempt to further substratify patients into low versus high risk of progression. Although there is generally limited information obtained from a TURBT specimen, various clinicopathologic features are present that can help differentiate patients into risk categories. LVI and tumor location have been correlated with outcomes in cystectomy performed for clinical or pathologic T1 disease.[24,25] In one study, nontrigonal tumor location was one of the factors significantly associated with prolonged RFS.[26] In addition, the specimen can be submitted for molecular marker analysis, which may elucidate the underlying biologic behavior of the tumors. van Rhijn and colleagues[27] performed a head-to-head comparison of the EORTC risk scores with 4 molecular markers in HGT1 bladder cancers treated conservatively with BCG. Their subclassification into the new system of T1m (microinvasive) versus T1e (extensive-invasive) was found to be the most important clinical variable in predicting progression to muscle-invasive disease. The study included 129 patients from two universities, and T1 substaging was performed using the new system (T1m/T1e), as well as according to depth of invasion within the lamina propria (T1a/b/c). The molecular markers studied were fibroblast growth factor receptor 3 (FGFR3) gene mutation and Ki-67, P53, P27 expression, all of which have significant prognostic value in predicting bladder cancer outcomes. Factors significant for progression were female gender, substage (T1m/T1e), and presence of CIS. Molecular markers were significant for progression in a multivariable model; however, its value was only modest.[27] Acikalin and colleagues[28] studied the clinical significance of maspin and Ki-67 expression in TURBT specimens from 68 patients with newly diagnosed T1 bladder cancer. Maspin expression was an independent predictor of recurrence and progression, with negative maspin expression having a 4.3 times higher risk of progression compared with maspin-positive patients. However, Ki-67 expression had no correlation with recurrence, progression, or cancer-specific mortality. Other studies of molecular markers including p53, Ki-67, Cox-2, and NMP-22 and cell cycle analysis (S phase fraction) have identified an association with increased progression risk.[29–34] Although considerable effort has gone into identifying factors associated with aggressive behavior, these markers are not in routine clinical use and need validation in large series to establish whether they offer any additional information compared with routine histopathologic evaluation.

RESTAGING TURBT

As previously mentioned, there is significant understaging in patients with HGT1 disease. If muscle is absent from the initial resection, repeat resection to include muscularis propria at the base of the tumor resection is mandatory because there is more than 50% probability of finding muscle-invasive disease.[14,35] Over the past decade or so, it has become clear that, in all patients with HGT1 disease, reresection of the tumor base is important not only from a prognostic standpoint but also as a potential therapeutic strategy. Even when muscle is present in the specimen, repeat resection can uncover occult muscle-invasive disease in at least 10% of cases, which has a profound impact on decision making.[36–38]

The advantages of the restaging have been well documented and include not only better stage and risk stratification but also eradication of residual noninvasive disease for improved therapeutic response to intravesical therapy. When patients have undergone restaging TURBT, the risk of upstaging following cystectomy theoretically should be very low. This was shown in at least 1 small study from Memorial Sloan Kettering on a cohort of 71 patients with HGT1 disease of whom 15 underwent immediate cystectomy. Although 12 patients had residual disease found at cystectomy, only 2 were upstaged to muscle-invasive disease.[39] Herr and colleagues,[40] from the same institution, also showed that the presence of residual T1 disease on repeat TUR is associated with a significantly increased risk of progression to muscle-invasive disease. Of the 92 patients with T1 disease at reresection, 82% progressed to muscle-invasive disease at 5 years as opposed to 19% of patients with less than T1 disease (pT0, pTa, CIS). This finding is strong evidence in favor of immediate cystectomy for patients who have residual HGT1 disease on restaging TURBT. Patients should be counseled accordingly when considering conservative management. Young patients and those with life expectancy of more than 10 to 15 years should almost certainly be advised against having intravesical treatment because the risk of recurrence and progression remains well beyond 5 years. This risk is continuous in patients treated conservatively, in contrast with patients who have a cystectomy, for which relapse is rare beyond 3 years.

In addition to providing critical assessment of pathologic features of the tumor, restaging TUR also seems to improve the response to BCG therapy. Herr and colleagues[41] compared 132 patients who underwent a single TUR before BCG therapy with 215 patients who had undergone restaging TUR. Notwithstanding the limitations of a nonrandomized comparison, 75 (57%) of the single TUR group had recurrent tumor at the first cystoscopy versus 62 (29%) of the restaging TUR group. More importantly, 45 (34%) in the former group later progressed to higher stage disease, compared with 16 (7%), respectively (P = .001). One of the most convincing studies supporting restaging TURBT came from a randomized trial reported by Divrik and colleagues[42] in 2010. In this trial, 210 newly diagnosed patients with HGT1 disease were randomized between a single TUR versus a restaging TUR 2 to 6 weeks following initial resection. With an adequate median follow-up of more than 5 years, recurrence (71% vs 40%), progression (24% vs 7%), and cystectomy rates (24% vs 13%) were significantly higher in the single TUR group. There were 11 deaths caused by bladder cancer in the single TUR group compared with only 5 in the second TUR group (P = .04). This study was criticized for methodological flaws (8% of patients who were upstaged by second TUR were excluded from the study after randomization, albeit accounted for in the cystectomy rates), with probable overestimation of the benefits of second TUR.[43] Nevertheless, there are ample data in this study to show the decreased recurrence and progression rates with a second TUR.

TREATMENT OPTIONS

Intravesical Therapy

Over the past 2 decades, a multitude of published studies established the effectiveness of adjuvant intravesical therapy for treatment of NMIBC. Both mitomycin C and doxorubicin were shown to reduce the risk recurrence and rate of progression, with mitomycin C possibly being more effective.[44] Over the years, BCG was shown to be superior to intravesical chemotherapy and became the treatment of choice for conservative management of high-grade disease. There are several studies reporting a wide range of recurrence and progression rates most likely because of the significant heterogeneity in the studied population including additional risk factors, use of second TUR, and use of maintenance therapy.[45–54] In one of the early studies published more than 20 years ago on adjuvant BCG following TUR for HGT1 disease, Cookson and Sarosdy[55] reported 91% tumor-free rate with a median follow-up of nearly 5 years with a progression rate of only 7%. Several randomized trials clearly documented the improvement in long-term tumor progression-free and disease-specific survival rates compared with TURBT alone. However, it became clear early on that patients who fail to achieve a complete response after the initial course of BCG were at significant risk of progression and death.[56] Short-term follow-up does not adequately document the continuous risk of recurrence and progression compared with cystectomy series in which most recurrences occur within 3 years.[57]

Cookson and colleagues[2] reported the results of 15 years of follow-up of high-risk patients (CIS, T1) randomized to TUR alone or combined with intravesical BCG. Of the 86 patients enrolled, 44% had stage T1 tumors. Forty-six (53%) patients had progression and 31 (36%) eventually underwent cystectomy. The 10-year and 15-year disease-specific survival rates were 70% and 63%, respectively. At 15 years, 34% of patients overall were dead of bladder cancer, underscoring the high-risk nature of this group of patients. These results support the use of initial aggressive local therapy in patients with high-risk superficial bladder cancer. Numerous studies have published long-term results of using adjuvant BCG for HGT1 disease (**Table 1**).[45–53,58–68] Only a few studies have reported results beyond 5 years.[48,49,51,53,54]

Although adjuvant intravesical BCG therapy after TUR for HGT1 bladder cancer is evidently effective, the study by Shahin and colleagues[53] showed that it may only delay the time to recurrence and cystectomy, and that BCG does not affect cancer-specific survival (CSS) in the long term. However, this study did not include maintenance therapy. In addition, a meta-analysis validated the benefit of adjuvant BCG on progression. This study, involving 24 trials and 4863 patients (including patients with Ta disease and CIS), showed a relative risk reduction of 27% for progression in patients receiving adjuvant BCG. However, this benefit was only seen in patients who received maintenance BCG therapy and overall there was no difference in treatment effect for CSS.[69]

Predictors of Progression

Some experts advocate an initial conservative approach to HGT1 disease, with deferred cystectomy on progression. The problem with this approach is that patients allowed to progress are inherently at a disadvantage, as shown by the death rates, despite cystectomy, which range from 16% to 34%.[2,53,54] This uncertainty has led some to investigate predictors of progression. In a review including more than 1000 patients with HGT1 disease treated with adjuvant BCG, Herr and colleagues[70] reported progression rates ranging from 13% to 48% with a median follow-up of 5 years. This wide range suggests the concept of risk stratification in patients with HGT1 disease.

Alkhateeb and colleagues[71] examined the prognostic significance of prior tumor resection in cases of HGT1 bladder cancer by comparing 95 primary with 96 nonprimary T1 tumors with similar clinicopathologic characteristics treated with BCG. The progression rate for the primary versus the nonprimary group was 24.2% versus 39.6%, respectively ([HR 2.07], P = .03). This difference remained significant on multivariate Cox regression analysis; however, there was no difference between the groups in regards to recurrence or disease-specific mortality. Kakiashvili and colleagues[72] examined clinicopathologic features of 136 patients from two university centers to find predictors of recurrence and progression, and found CIS as the only independent predictor for recurrence in multivariate analysis (P = .011). The investigators found no independent predictors of progression in 30% of the patients, many of which occurred beyond 3 years, again highlighting the significant and unpredictable risk in this patient

Table 1
Select series reporting long-term results with BCG for HGT1 bladder cancer

Study	No. Patients	Median Follow-up (mo)	Recurrence (%)	Progression (%)	DOD (%)
Pansadoro et al,[45] 1995	50	42	16	12	2
Baniel et al,[46] 1998	78	56	28	8	0
Lebret et al,[47] 1998	35	45	23	17	6
Hurle et al,[48] 1999	51	85	37	18	14
Patard et al,[49] 2001	50	65	52	22	14
Kulkarni and Gupta,[50] 2002	69	45	46	12	6
Pansadoro et al,[51] 2002	81	76	33	15	6
Peyromaure et al,[52] 2003	57	56	42	23	12
Shahin et al,[53] 2003	92	64	70	33	23
Margel et al,[54] 2007	78	107	35	18	16

Abbreviation: DOD, dead of disease.

population.[72] Orsola and colleagues[73] recently reported on risk factors for finding disease following BCG therapy in HGT1 disease. Tumor size and CIS were associated with finding positive disease at 3 months following initial TURBT and adjuvant BCG therapy. Other studies have corroborated the finding that the presence of CIS is associated with an increased risk of progression and death caused by disease.[19,74] The EORTC has recognized associated CIS as the most significant factor associated with risk of recurrence and progression at 5 years after BCG therapy.[75] It is therefore imperative that pathologists report associated CIS as a separate finding in the presence of HGT1 disease so patients can be counseled appropriately regarding their risk profile.

In addition, patients who have tumor recurrence and are treated with a second course of BCG are at significant risk of progression and death. In a study of 214 patients with high-risk disease who recurred with a T1 tumor, there was a 71% cumulative incidence of progression to muscle-invasive disease in those treated with a second course of BCG, with nearly half of these patients dying of disease compared with 28% of those who underwent cystectomy (31% dead of disease).[76] Thus a HGT1 recurrence following adjuvant BCG therapy portends a poor prognosis and there is ample evidence that supports early cystectomy for this extremely high-risk patient population. Response rates to repeat BCG therapy for HGT1 disease is poor and delaying definitive therapy has a profound effect on the ultimate outcome.

Some others studies have documented a higher risk of progression with tumor morphology with solid tumors having more than twice the risk of progression and death from bladder cancer as papillary tumors. Other factors such as tumor size and aberrant histology,[77] in addition to the number of T1 lesions (multifocality), have been associated with higher progression rates.[21,78] LVI is an important pathologic finding in cystectomy specimens and has also been shown to have prognostic significance in HGT1 lesions.[78,79]

Chemoradiation

The data relating to radiation therapy (RT) in the treatment of HGT1 bladder cancer are limited. There are some data suggesting that concurrent chemotherapy with RT can be effective in high-grade urothelial carcinoma. Results from Erlangen, Germany, on 84 patients with HGT1 tumors using a trimodality bladder-sparing approach with concurrent chemotherapy and radiation showed a 10-year progression-free rate of 71% and a 10-year disease-specific survival rate of 71%.[80] More than 80% of the survivors had an intact bladder and 70% were 'delighted' or 'pleased' with their urinary function. In contrast with these promising results, a randomized trial comparing RT with conservative therapy (observation or intravesical therapy with mitomycin C [MMC] or BCG) for HGT1 disease showed no difference in progression-free survival or RFS (29% in the control vs 31% in the RT arm ($P = .65$).[81] There are few reports of the effectiveness of trimodality therapy as a second-line treatment of bladder preservation in patients with recurrent HGT1 disease following BCG therapy. The Radiation Therapy Oncology Group (RTOG) opened a clinical trial (RTOG 0926, Douglas Dahl, principal investigator) to explore the efficacy of chemoradiation in patients with HGT1 disease. To be eligible for this trial, all patients must undergo a restaging TURBT with muscularis propria present in the specimen and no evidence of muscle-invasive disease. The primary objective is avoiding cystectomy without compromising survival.

RADICAL CYSTECTOMY

Most cystectomy series for HGT1 tumors include patients with high-risk disease who have failed prior intravesical therapy. Because cystectomy generally represents the most aggressive and ultimate treatment of HGT1 disease, any comparison with more conservative treatment is hampered at the start by significant selection bias. Because of the substantial understaging of disease, it is important to scrutinize these series to distinguish those reporting on clinical versus pathologic T1 disease. Given the significant clinical understaging of HGT1 disease, series without restaging TURBT cannot be directly compared with those who were adequately staged. Nevertheless, the outcome from early cystectomy for HGT1 disease is generally excellent, with recurrence and disease-specific survival curves generally flattening after 2 to 3 years. In addition, the number of patients with clinical (c) T1 disease who harbor occult lymph node metastasis is important in series that include an extended pelvic lymph node dissection. In one study of 66 patients with cT1 disease, 27% of the cases were upstaged and 12% of those patients who had concomitant CIS had pathologic nodal involvement. Patients with cT1 tumors with CIS had a significantly worse CSS. Cancer-specific mortality for the cohort of patients with cT1 disease was 22% but those who had pathologic T1 disease had 10-year CSS of 92%.[5] If cystectomy is performed when the tumor is still confined to the lamina propria, most patients are cured. If treatment is delayed until muscle invasion is clinically evident, cure rates decrease significantly.

Early Versus Delayed Cystectomy

Timing of cystectomy is of paramount importance and affects pathologic stage and outcome. There is continued debate on whether patients presenting with high-risk features can be first treated with intravesical therapy or should undergo immediate cystectomy. Notwithstanding the limitations of nonrandomized comparisons, numerous studies have shown an unfavorable effect on outcome for patients who undergo delayed cystectomy. Herr and Sogani[82] examined the long-term outcome of 307 patients with high-risk NMIBC initially treated with TURBT and BCG, of whom 29% ultimately underwent cystectomy during a 15-year to 20-year follow-up period. Of the 90 patients who underwent cystectomy, 49% survived. Only 18% of the patients survived when cystectomy was performed for muscle-invasive disease after 2 years of follow-up, compared with 41% when cystectomy was performed before 2 years. Multivariate analysis revealed improved survival in those who underwent earlier rather than delayed cystectomy for relapse.[82]

Although there are no randomized trials comparing early cystectomy with conservative management with intravesical therapy, Denzinger and colleagues[83] compared the long-term outcome in patients with HGT1 disease treated with early versus deferred cystectomy for recurrent or progressive disease after initial conservative management. They compared patients who had at least 2 of the known risk factors for progression (multifocality, tumor size, and CIS) during initial TURBT. All the patients were offered up-front cystectomy and 51% opted for early cystectomy, with the other 49% undergoing deferred cystectomy for recurrence of progressive disease. Similar to all other studies, there was a 30% upstaging seen in the cystectomy specimen. The 10-year CSS was 78% in the early cystectomy cohort compared with 51% in the deferred cystectomy group ($P<.01$). The presence of CIS was correlated with a lower CSS in the deferred cystectomy group. The study had selection bias because the patients who underwent deferred cystectomy had failed conservative management and therefore presumably were at higher risk than those who underwent immediate cystectomy. Nevertheless, the patients in the 2 groups were well matched and had similar initial risk factors. Because there will probably never be a randomized trial comparing immediate cystectomy with intravesical therapy, this study provides more convincing evidence that patients with HGT1 disease who have more aggressive treatment early in the course of the disease have improved outcomes.

Other investigators have published similar results. Hautmann and colleagues[84] reported on a series of 274 patients with cT1 disease, of whom 175 were treated with immediate cystectomy compared with 99 who underwent delayed cystectomy for recurrence following intravesical treatment. The patients who underwent immediate cystectomy did not have a restaging TUR. The reported CSS was 78% for the immediate cystectomy group compared with 65% in the deferred group. The survival disadvantage in the deferred group was calculated at 17%. However, in a large series of 523 patients from Memorial Sloan Kettering with HGT1 disease who had undergone restaging TUR, Dalbagni and colleagues[85] did not find any difference in survival between the immediate versus deferred cystectomy group. Of the 523 patients, 417 were deemed true HGT1, of whom 84 underwent immediate cystectomy. Of the 333 patients who were initially managed conservatively, 59 eventually undergoing cystectomy. The need for deferred cystectomy was higher in those who were found to have T1 disease on restaging TUR, again highlighting the high-risk nature of this group of patients and stratifying patients who would benefit most from early radical cystectomy. This series differs from the other series in that treatment approach was highly tailored and all patients underwent restaging TUR.

Results from Radical Cystectomy for HGT1 Disease

When counseling patients regarding treatment options, it is important to discuss long-term results from cystectomy performed for HGT1 disease. There are several series from high-volume centers reporting excellent outcomes for up-front radical cystectomy, for clinical T1 (**Table 2**),[5,8,13,83,86–91] or pathologic T1 disease (**Table 3**).[92–96] Gupta and colleagues[88] reported outcomes on 167 patients with HGT1 disease who underwent radical cystectomy at 3 academic centers in the United States. Median follow-up was short at just less than 3 years. Nevertheless, the CSS was 81.5%. However, 17.5% of patients had lymph node metastases, although there was 50% understaging with 27.5% having extravesical disease. The only factor predicting disease recurrence (HR = 2.13) and mortality (HR = 2.75) was concomitant presence of CIS before cystectomy. In a larger multicenter study of 1136 patients who underwent radical cystectomy for clinical HGT1 disease, half were upstaged to muscle-invasive disease, one-third had

Table 2
Outcomes of radical cystectomy for HGT1 urothelial carcinoma of the bladder

Immediate or Early Radical Cystectomy for Clinical HGT1 Tumor							
Study	N	Median Follow-up	Prior BCG Therapy (%)	Upstaging (%)	LN+ (%)	Recurrence (%)	DSS (%)
Amling et al,[86] 1969–1990	166	120	—	—	7	—	76
Thalmann et al,[87] 1980–99	29	47	0	41	14	21	69
Gupta et al,[88] 1984–2003	167	34	44	50	18	29	82
Weisner et al,[89] 1989–2002	188	—	—	34	16	—	—
Bianco et al,[5] 1990–2000	66	48	27	27	9	78	78
Lambert et al,[8] 1990–2005	104	—	44	40	—	48	93
Masood and Mufti,[90] 1992–2002	30	57	30	27	—	—	88
Dutta et al,[13] 1995–99	78	—	37	40	12	—	78
Denzinger et al,[83] 1995–2005	54	61	0	26	—	—	78
Fritsche et al,[91] 2010 (multicenter)	113	48	—	51	16	—	65

Abbreviations: DSS, disease-specific survival; LN+, lymph node positive.

non–organ-confined disease, and 16% had positive lymph nodes. With a median follow-up of 48 months, 36% died of metastatic bladder cancer.[91] The investigators concluded that patients with high risk of progression may benefit from early cystectomy. However, substantial understaging and high incidence of extravesical disease argues for better clinical staging (through updated imaging, restaging TUR) to identify patients who would be candidates for neoadjuvant chemotherapy to improve survival rates.

In an analysis from the Surveillance Epidemiology and End Results (SEER) database from 2004 to 2007, Canter and colleagues[97] stratified patients who underwent radical cystectomy within 1 year of diagnosis of HGT1 bladder cancer. Of the nearly 8500 patients who were registered in the database as having HGT1 disease, less than 5% underwent radical cystectomy. As expected, these patients were significantly younger. However, CSS was not different between patients who underwent cystectomy versus nonsurgical management up to 3 years from diagnosis, although patients who did not undergo cystectomy had a significantly higher death rate from other causes. Only about one-third of the patients who progressed to muscle-invasive disease achieved a durable cure. However, interpretation of SEER-based studies on HGT1 disease are limited given the short-term follow-up, the lack of information on use of BCG therapy, and the information on patients who underwent delayed cystectomy beyond 1 year after initial diagnosis of HGT1 disease. The Canadian Bladder Cancer Network series involving 306 patients from 8 different Canadian centers with 3-year follow-up, revealed a 5-year and 10-year disease-specific survival of 77% and 67%, respectively, 29% of the patients were upstaged to extravesical disease, and 26% had positive lymph nodes.[98]

At our institution, there has always been a selective, but aggressive, approach to management of patients with high-grade T1 disease. In the large cohort of patients who underwent radical cystectomy at University of Southern California with long-term follow-up, 34% of the patients with clinical T1 bladder cancer were pathologically understaged, with only half having organ-confined disease and 14% having lymph node metastasis.[93]

Table 3
Results from large cystectomy cohorts reporting on pT1 disease

Study	N	Median Follow-up	LN+ (%)	RFS
Pagano et al,[92] 1979–1987	74	60	—	71
Stein et al,[93] 1971–1997	208	120	7	80 (5 y)
Madersbacher et al,[94] 1985–2000	77	45	3	76 (5 y)
Hautman et al,[95] 1986–2009	127	38	4	71 (10 y)
Shariat et al,[96] 1984–2003 (multiinstitutional)	114	39	—	89 (20 y)

As expected, those who were upstaged at cystectomy had significantly worse RFS than those who remained at T1 or less on final pathology at cystectomy.[99] These results, published in 2001, predated routine use of restaging TUR. Most published results of outcomes following cystectomy focus on clinical T1 disease and have a heterogeneous group of patients many of whom have extravesical and lymph node–positive (LN+) disease. Many of these series do not include restaging TUR and have significant clinical understaging, and therefore do not reflect the outcome of pathologic disease. In our updated cohort of more than 1600 patients undergoing radical cystectomy for urothelial carcinoma of the bladder, we found 222 patients with no prior history of muscle-invasive disease who underwent radical cystectomy for high-grade disease (≤cT1N0M0) and had pathologic T1 disease at cystectomy. Median follow-up of this cohort was 14.3 years, thereby allowing adequate analysis of the long-term outcome of patients with pT1 disease. In this cohort, 24 patients (11%) had LVI and 13 patients (6%) had positive lymph nodes. RFS at 5 and 10 years was 81% and 74%, respectively. In the patients with LN+ disease, the RFS at 5 years was 46%. In a multivariable analysis including age, p53 status, grade, CIS, multifocality, gender, prior intravesical therapy, lymph node status, and LVI, lymph node status and LVI were the only factors significantly associated with RFS (LN+, $P = .0002$; LVI, $P = .0071$) (**Fig. 1**, Daneshmand, 2012, unpublished data).

Indications for Immediate Cystectomy in HGT1

After more than 20 years of retrospective studies, it is still not possible to reliably predict the outcome of patients who present with high-grade T1 disease. These patients do not have superficial disease and such a designation should be reserved for patients with Ta or CIS disease only. Patients with HGT1 disease have invasive disease

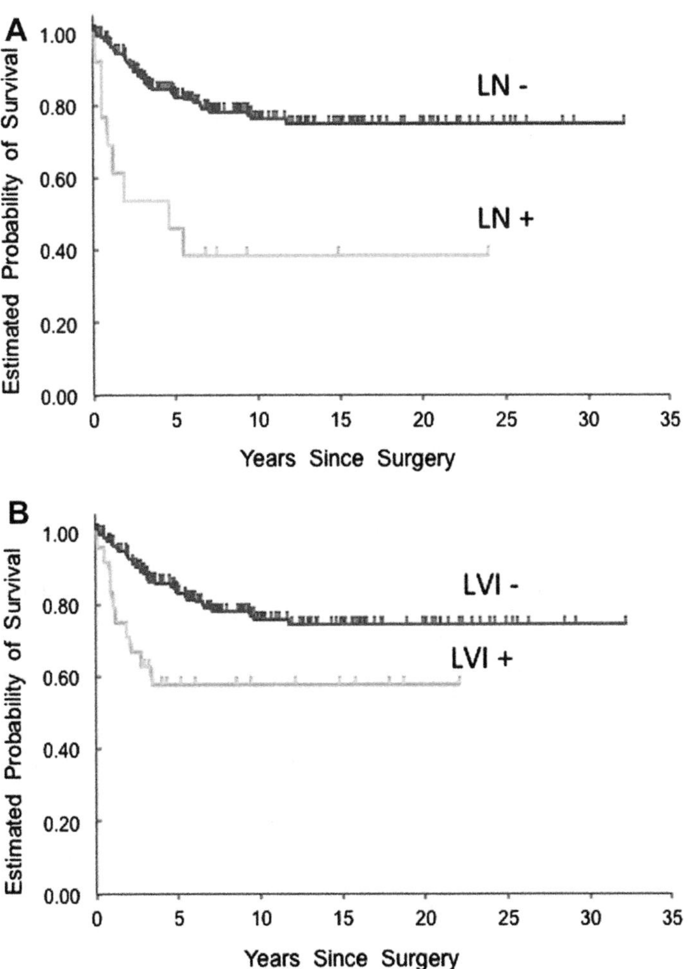

Fig. 1. Factors significantly associated with RFS in patients with pathologic T1 at cystectomy. LN−, lymph node negative.

that can progress to metastases and death. Owing to the vast difference in treatment strategy, there will probably never be a randomized study of radical cystectomy versus conservative treatment with cystectomy at progression. At this point, clinicians therefore have to rely on the wealth of retrospective data that can be used to guide optimal treatment strategies based on all available clinicopathologic data. In a review article on treatment strategy for newly diagnosed HGT1 disease, Kulkarni and colleagues[68] presented a treatment algorithm for newly diagnosed HGT1 tumors and summarized the available data on risk factors for progression of the disease to use in recommending immediate or early cystectomy. Presence of concomitant CIS, tumor multifocality, hydronephrosis, tumor size (greater than 3 cm), stage T1b, and presence of residual T1 deem patients high risk. They suggested that patients with 2 or more risk factors of HGT1 disease at diagnosis should be advised to undergo immediate cystectomy. In cases of conservative management, presence of tumor at first surveillance cystoscopy following BCG, recurrent T1 disease, or prostatic urethral involvement during follow-up should trigger the decision to proceed with cystectomy. The international consensus panel has also recognized stratification of HGT1 tumors into low-risk and high-risk groups.[100] Others have also recommended management based on risk stratification including age and comorbidity status.[101]

The question remains whether patients with significant risk factors should still undergo restaging TUR to identify those at risk for extravesical disease or lymph node metastasis. Better approaches are necessary to identify the subset of patients with non–organ-confined disease who would benefit from neoadjuvant chemotherapy. The incidence of nodal involvement in patients treated with radical cystectomy for HGT1 bladder cancer is reportedly 12% to 15%.[5,89,102,103] Clinical staging should be based on all available information, including bimanual examination in addition to cross-sectional imaging, not just TURBT stage, which may not give a clear picture of the aggressive nature of the disease. Patients who have clinical evidence of extravesical disease on imaging or have hydronephrosis are at higher risk of upstaging and should be considered for neoadjuvant chemotherapy before cystectomy.[104]

In the era of restaging TUR, the indications for immediate cystectomy following initial TURBT for HGT1 tumors should be patients with 1 or more of the following:

- No evidence of extravesical disease on cross-sectional imaging performed at most 8 weeks before cystectomy, in whom restaging TUR will not change management
- Endoscopically unresectable disease
- Patient preference
- Poorly functioning bladder in a patient who will not tolerate intravesical therapy
- Multiple poor prognostic factors in a patient in whom restaging TUR will not change management (ie, potentially identify eligibility for neoadjuvant therapy)
- HGT1 tumor in a diverticulum, which precludes obtaining adequate muscularis propria

As previously mentioned, the pathologic stage at repeat TUR is a critical prognostic factor. In the cases upstaged to T2 disease, the decision is straightforward and these patients should proceed immediately to cystectomy. If restaging TUR reveals residual T1 disease, strong consideration should be given to cystectomy. The 5-year progression rate in this high-risk group of patients is 76% in the series reported by Herr and colleagues.[105] Patients who have no residual disease on restaging TUR have a better prognosis and can be managed conservatively with induction and maintenance BCG treatment.[106,107]

The risks of both conservative (intravesical therapy) and aggressive (up-front radical cystectomy) treatment should be discussed with the patients. There is ample evidence that immediate cystectomy offers the best chance for cure, particularly in the presence of adverse features.[7] There are several advantages for undergoing immediate or early radical cystectomy for HGT1 disease. It not only offers accurate pathologic staging but also identifies and potentially cures the subset of patients who have LN+ disease. Even with restaging TUR, a proportion of patients are still upstaged to muscle-invasive and/or LN+ disease.[39] Cystectomy also offers definitive treatment obviating multiple intravesical therapies, surveillance cystoscopies, and biopsies. The morbidity and inconvenience of repeated treatment and evaluation during conservative management should not be underestimated. In addition, as mentioned previously, the risk of progression with conservative management is continuous and lifelong, whereas most recurrences following cystectomy occur within 3 years.[57] Also, delaying cystectomy is associated with worse outcomes. The longer ineffective treatments are used for high-grade disease, the higher the risk of progression and metastases. Wiesner and colleagues[89] noted that the number of TURs performed for NMIBC (86% T1) was significantly associated with upstaging and lymph node metastases.

DISCUSSION

Radical cystectomy with thorough lymph node dissection provides accurate staging information, simplifies follow-up, and most patients are considered cured after 3 years. However, radical cystectomy is associated with significant morbidity, including effects on urinary continence, sexual function, and gastrointestinal function. Early cystectomy performed for HGT1 disease allows nerve-sparing approaches and most patients are candidates for orthotopic reconstruction, which has excellent results at high-volume centers.[108,109] Reports of nerve-sparing cystectomy have shown good functional outcomes.[110,111] In a series of 21 male patients undergoing nerve-sparing cystectomy, 79% were potent postoperatively, 58% with spontaneous complete tumescence.[111]

The crux of the issue is balancing quality of life with effective cancer management. To that end, Kulkarni and colleagues[112] attempted to shed light on this dilemma by estimating quality-adjusted life expectancy (QALE). They used a decision analytical Markov model comparing immediate cystectomy with orthotopic neobladder with initial BCG with delayed cystectomy for refractory or progressive disease. For a sexually potent, 60-year-old, healthy male patient, the average life expectancy predicted by the model was almost 8 months longer with immediate cystectomy than with conservative management, whereas the QALE was 4.2 months longer with cystectomy. After age 70 years, the conservative treatment became the preferred approach. However, when considering QALE, this change in preferred treatment appeared at age 65 years. Additional comorbidities decreased the benefit of immediate cystectomy.

SUMMARY

HGT1 disease represents a heterogeneous group of tumors with variable clinical course. Current accepted treatment options include conservative management with induction and maintenance BCG therapy versus radical cystectomy with pelvic lymph node dissection. Clinical decisions should be made on risk of progression and patients with high-risk features including aberrant pathology, concomitant CIS, deep lamina propria invasion, LVI, involvement of prostatic urethra, large or multifocal tumors, and persistent HGT1 disease on restaging TUR should be strongly considered for immediate cystectomy. Up to 70% of patients with HGT1 disease may be able to retain their bladders with appropriate conservative management. If cancer cure is the goal, immediate radical cystectomy can provide a CSS of greater than 90% in properly staged patients. Those who are initially treated with conservative management but have high-grade disease recurrence at 3-month follow-up should also be advised to undergo cystectomy. Delay in definitive treatment with cystectomy in the high-risk patient is associated with significantly increased risk of progression and death caused by disease. Patients undergoing conservative treatment of HGT1 disease should undergo a 6-week course of induction BCG followed by maintenance BCG for the following 1 to 3 years with vigilant lifelong surveillance. At this point, investigational molecular markers have not substantially improved prognostication and their use needs further validation. Even radical cystectomy for pathologic T1 disease does not guarantee cure, indicating that a subset of HGT1 tumors have aggressive biologic behavior that requires identification and adjuvant therapy.

REFERENCES

1. van Rhijn BW, Burger M, Lotan Y, et al. Recurrence and progression of disease in non-muscle-invasive bladder cancer: from epidemiology to treatment strategy. Eur Urol 2009;56:430–42.
2. Cookson MS, Herr HW, Zhang ZF, et al. The treated natural history of high risk superficial bladder cancer: 15-year outcome. J Urol 1997;158:62–7.
3. Heney NM, Ahmed S, Flanagan MJ, et al. Superficial bladder cancer: progression and recurrence. J Urol 1983;130:1083–6.
4. Herr HW, Schwalb DM, Zhang ZF, et al. Intravesical bacillus Calmette-Guerin therapy prevents tumor progression and death from superficial bladder cancer: ten-year follow-up of a prospective randomized trial. J Clin Oncol 1995;13:1404–8.
5. Bianco FJ Jr, Justa D, Grignon DJ, et al. Management of clinical T1 bladder transitional cell carcinoma by radical cystectomy. Urol Oncol 2004;22:290–4.
6. Esrig D, Freeman JA, Stein JP, et al. Early cystectomy for clinical stage T1 transitional cell carcinoma of the bladder. Semin Urol Oncol 1997;15:154–60.
7. Skinner EC. The best treatment for high-grade T1 bladder cancer is cystectomy. Urol Oncol 2007;25:523–5.
8. Lambert EH, Pierorazio PM, Olsson CA, et al. The increasing use of intravesical therapies for stage T1 bladder cancer coincides with decreasing survival after cystectomy. BJU Int 2007;100:33–6.
9. Luciani LG, Neulander E, Murphy WM, et al. Risk of continued intravesical therapy and delayed cystectomy in BCG-refractory superficial bladder cancer: an investigational approach. Urology 2001;58:376–9.

10. O'Donnell MA, Lilli K, Leopold C. Interim results from a national multicenter phase II trial of combination bacillus Calmette-Guerin plus interferon alfa-2b for superficial bladder cancer. J Urol 2004;172:888–93.
11. Van Der Meijden A, Sylvester R, Collette L, et al. The role and impact of pathology review on stage and grade assessment of stages Ta and T1 bladder tumors: a combined analysis of 5 European Organization for Research and Treatment of Cancer trials. J Urol 2000;164:1533–7.
12. Mark JR, Gelpi-Hammerschmidt F, Trabulsi EJ, et al. Blue light cystoscopy for detection and treatment of non-muscle invasive bladder cancer. Can J Urol 2012;19:6227–31.
13. Dutta SC, Smith JA Jr, Shappell SB, et al. Clinical under staging of high risk nonmuscle invasive urothelial carcinoma treated with radical cystectomy. J Urol 2001;166:490–3.
14. Herr HW. The value of a second transurethral resection in evaluating patients with bladder tumors. J Urol 1999;162:74–6.
15. Jancke G, Rosell J, Jahnson S. Residual tumour in the marginal resection after a complete transurethral resection is associated with local recurrence in Ta/T1 urinary bladder cancer. Scand J Urol Nephrol 2012;46:343–7.
16. Orsola A, Trias I, Raventos CX, et al. Initial high-grade T1 urothelial cell carcinoma: feasibility and prognostic significance of lamina propria invasion microstaging (T1a/b/c) in BCG-treated and BCG-non-treated patients. Eur Urol 2005;48:231–8 [discussion: 238].
17. Platz CE, Cohen MB, Jones MP, et al. Is microstaging of early invasive cancer of the urinary bladder possible or useful? Mod Pathol 1996;9: 1035–9.
18. Holmang S, Hedelin H, Anderstrom C, et al. The importance of the depth of invasion in stage T1 bladder carcinoma: a prospective cohort study. J Urol 1997;157:800–3 [discussion: 804].
19. Smits G, Schaafsma E, Kiemeney L, et al. Microstaging of pT1 transitional cell carcinoma of the bladder: identification of subgroups with distinct risks of progression. Urology 1998;52:1009–13 [discussion: 1013–4].
20. Younes M, Sussman J, True LD. The usefulness of the level of the muscularis mucosae in the staging of invasive transitional cell carcinoma of the urinary bladder. Cancer 1990;66:543–8.
21. Angulo JC, Lopez JI, Grignon DJ, et al. Muscularis mucosa differentiates two populations with different prognosis in stage T1 bladder cancer. Urology 1995;45:47–53.
22. van Rhijn BW, van der Kwast TH, Alkhateeb SS, et al. A new and highly prognostic system to discern T1 bladder cancer substage. Eur Urol 2012;61:378–84.
23. Bertz S, Denzinger S, Otto W, et al. Substaging by estimating the size of invasive tumour can improve risk stratification in pT1 urothelial bladder cancer-evaluation of a large hospital-based single-centre series. Histopathology 2011;59:722–32.
24. Tilki D, Shariat SF, Lotan Y, et al. Lymphovascular invasion is independently associated with bladder cancer recurrence and survival in patients with final stage T1 disease and negative lymph nodes after radical cystectomy. BJU Int 2012. [Epub ahead of print].
25. Shariat SF, Svatek RS, Tilki D, et al. International validation of the prognostic value of lymphovascular invasion in patients treated with radical cystectomy. BJU Int 2010;105:1402–12.
26. Segal R, Yafi FA, Brimo F, et al. Prognostic factors and outcome in patients with T1 high-grade bladder cancer: can we identify patients for early cystectomy? BJU Int 2012;109:1026–30.
27. van Rhijn BW, Liu L, Vis AN, et al. Prognostic value of molecular markers, sub-stage and European Organisation for the Research and Treatment of Cancer risk scores in primary T1 bladder cancer. BJU Int 2012;110:1169–76.
28. Acikalin D, Oner U, Can C, et al. Predictive value of maspin and Ki-67 expression in transurethral resection specimens in patients with T1 bladder cancer. Tumori 2012;98:344–50.
29. Quek ML, Sanderson K, Daneshmand S, et al. New molecular markers for bladder cancer detection. Curr Opin Urol 2004;14:259–64.
30. Esrig D, Elmajian D, Groshen S, et al. Accumulation of nuclear p53 and tumor progression in bladder cancer. N Engl J Med 1994;331:1259–64.
31. Kim SI, Kwon SM, Kim YS, et al. Association of cyclooxygenase-2 expression with prognosis of stage T1 grade 3 bladder cancer. Urology 2002; 60:816–21.
32. Lopez-Knowles E, Hernandez S, Kogevinas M, et al. The p53 pathway and outcome among patients with T1G3 bladder tumors. Clin Cancer Res 2006;12:6029–36.
33. Shariat SF, Zippe C, Ludecke G, et al. Nomograms including nuclear matrix protein 22 for prediction of disease recurrence and progression in patients with Ta, T1 or CIS transitional cell carcinoma of the bladder. J Urol 2005;173:1518–25.
34. deVere White RW, Deitch AD, Daneshmand S, et al. The prognostic significance of S-phase analysis in stage Ta/T1 bladder cancer. A Southwest Oncology Group Study. Eur Urol 2000;37:595–600.
35. Jakse G, Algaba F, Malmstrom PU, et al. A second-look TUR in T1 transitional cell carcinoma: why? Eur Urol 2004;45:539–46 [discussion: 546].

36. Miladi M, Peyromaure M, Zerbib M, et al. The value of a second transurethral resection in evaluating patients with bladder tumours. Eur Urol 2003;43: 241–5.
37. Schwaibold HE, Sivalingam S, May F, et al. The value of a second transurethral resection for T1 bladder cancer. BJU Int 2006;97:1199–201.
38. Soloway MS, Lee CT, Steinberg GD, et al. Difficult decisions in urologic oncology: management of high-grade T1 transitional cell carcinoma of the bladder. Urol Oncol 2007;25:338–40.
39. Dalbagni G, Herr HW, Reuter VE. Impact of a second transurethral resection on the staging of T1 bladder cancer. Urology 2002;60:822–4 [discussion: 824–5].
40. Herr HW, Donat SM, Dalbagni G. Can restaging transurethral resection of T1 bladder cancer select patients for immediate cystectomy? J Urol 2007; 177:75–9 [discussion: 79].
41. Herr HW. Restaging transurethral resection of high risk superficial bladder cancer improves the initial response to bacillus Calmette-Guerin therapy. J Urol 2005;174:2134–7.
42. Divrik RT, Sahin AF, Yildirim U, et al. Impact of routine second transurethral resection on the long-term outcome of patients with newly diagnosed pT1 urothelial carcinoma with respect to recurrence, progression rate, and disease-specific survival: a prospective randomised clinical trial. Eur Urol 2010;58:185–90.
43. Novara G, Ficarra V. Does routine second transurethral resection affect the long-term outcome of patients with T1 bladder cancer? Why a flawed randomized controlled trial cannot address the issue. Eur Urol 2010;58:193–4.
44. Jauhiainen K, Alfthan O. Instillation of mitomycin C and doxorubicin in the prevention of recurrent superficial (Ta-T1) bladder cancer. Br J Urol 1987;60:54–9.
45. Pansadoro V, Emiliozzi P, Defidio L, et al. Bacillus Calmette-Guerin in the treatment of stage T1 grade 3 transitional cell carcinoma of the bladder: long-term results. J Urol 1995;154:2054–8.
46. Baniel J, Grauss D, Engelstein D, et al. Intravesical bacillus Calmette-Guerin treatment for stage T1 grade 3 transitional cell carcinoma of the bladder. Urology 1998;52:785–9.
47. Lebret T, Gaudez F, Herve JM, et al. Low-dose BCG instillations in the treatment of stage T1 grade 3 bladder tumours: recurrence, progression and success. Eur Urol 1998;34:67–72.
48. Hurle R, Losa A, Manzetti A, et al. Intravesical bacille Calmette-Guerin in stage T1 grade 3 bladder cancer therapy: a 7-year follow-up. Urology 1999; 54:258–63.
49. Patard J, Moudouni S, Saint F, et al. Tumor progression and survival in patients with T1G3 bladder tumors: multicentric retrospective study comparing 94 patients treated during 17 years. Urology 2001; 58:551–6.
50. Kulkarni JN, Gupta R. Recurrence and progression in stage T1G3 bladder tumour with intravesical bacille Calmette-Guerin (Danish 1331 strain). BJU Int 2002;90:554–7.
51. Pansadoro V, Emiliozzi P, de Paula F, et al. Long-term follow-up of G3T1 transitional cell carcinoma of the bladder treated with intravesical bacille Calmette-Guerin: 18-year experience. Urology 2002;59:227–31.
52. Peyromaure M, Guerin F, Amsellem-Ouazana D, et al. Intravesical bacillus Calmette-Guerin therapy for stage T1 grade 3 transitional cell carcinoma of the bladder: recurrence, progression and survival in a study of 57 patients. J Urol 2003;169:2110–2.
53. Shahin O, Thalmann GN, Rentsch C, et al. A retrospective analysis of 153 patients treated with or without intravesical bacillus Calmette-Guerin for primary stage T1 grade 3 bladder cancer: recurrence, progression and survival. J Urol 2003;169:96–100 [discussion: 100].
54. Margel D, Tal R, Golan S, et al. Long-term follow-up of patients with stage T1 high-grade transitional cell carcinoma managed by Bacille Calmette-Guerin immunotherapy. Urology 2007;69:78–82.
55. Cookson MS, Sarosdy MF. Management of stage T1 superficial bladder cancer with intravesical bacillus Calmette-Guerin therapy. J Urol 1992; 148:797–801.
56. Eure GR, Cundiff MR, Schellhammer PF. Bacillus Calmette-Guerin therapy for high risk stage T1 superficial bladder cancer. J Urol 1992;147:376–9.
57. Mitra AP, Quinn DI, Dorff TB, et al. Factors influencing post-recurrence survival in bladder cancer following radical cystectomy. BJU Int 2012;109: 846–54.
58. Lamm DL, Blumenstein BA, Crissman JD, et al. Maintenance bacillus Calmette-Guerin immunotherapy for recurrent TA, T1 and carcinoma in situ transitional cell carcinoma of the bladder: a randomized Southwest Oncology Group study. J Urol 2000;163:1124–9.
59. Zhang GK, Uke ET, Sharer WC, et al. Reassessment of conservative management for stage T1N0M0 transitional cell carcinoma of the bladder. J Urol 1996;155:1907–9.
60. Herr HW. Tumour progression and survival in patients with T1G3 bladder tumours: 15-year outcome. Br J Urol 1997;80:762–5.
61. Gohji K, Nomi M, Okamoto M, et al. Conservative therapy for stage T1b, grade 3 transitional cell carcinoma of the bladder. Urology 1999;53:308–13.
62. Brake M, Loertzer H, Horsch R, et al. Recurrence and progression of stage T1, grade 3 transitional

cell carcinoma of the bladder following intravesical immunotherapy with bacillus Calmette-Guerin. J Urol 2000;163:1697–701.
63. Iori F, Di Seri M, De Nunzio C, et al. Long-term maintenance bacille Calmette-Guerin therapy in high-grade superficial bladder cancer. Urology 2002;59:414–8.
64. Griffiths TR, Charlton M, Neal DE, et al. Treatment of carcinoma in situ with intravesical bacillus Calmette-Guerin without maintenance. J Urol 2002;167:2408–12.
65. Hara I, Miyake H, Takechi Y, et al. Clinical outcome of conservative therapy for stage T1, grade 3 transitional cell carcinoma of the bladder. Int J Urol 2003;10:19–24.
66. McHugh LA, Griffiths TR. T1G3 transitional cell carcinoma of the bladder: recurrence, progression and survival. BJU Int 2004;94:193.
67. Peyromaure M, Zerbib M. T1G3 transitional cell carcinoma of the bladder: recurrence, progression and survival. BJU Int 2004;93:60–3.
68. Kulkarni GS, Hakenberg OW, Gschwend JE, et al. An updated critical analysis of the treatment strategy for newly diagnosed high-grade T1 (previously T1G3) bladder cancer. Eur Urol 2010;57:60–70.
69. Sylvester RJ, van der MA, Lamm DL. Intravesical bacillus Calmette-Guerin reduces the risk of progression in patients with superficial bladder cancer: a meta-analysis of the published results of randomized clinical trials. J Urol 2002;168: 1964–70.
70. Herr HW, Jakse G, Sheinfeld J. The T1 bladder tumor. Semin Urol 1990;8:254–61.
71. Alkhateeb SS, Van Rhijn BW, Finelli A, et al. Nonprimary pT1 nonmuscle invasive bladder cancer treated with bacillus Calmette-Guerin is associated with higher risk of progression compared to primary T1 tumors. J Urol 2010;184:81–6.
72. Kakiashvili DM, van Rhijn BW, Trottier G, et al. Long-term follow-up of T1 high-grade bladder cancer after intravesical bacille Calmette-Guerin treatment. BJU Int 2011;107:540–6.
73. Orsola A, Cecchini L, Raventos CX, et al. Risk factors for positive findings in patients with high-grade T1 bladder cancer treated with transurethral resection of bladder tumour (TUR) and bacille Calmette-Guerin therapy and the decision for a repeat TUR. BJU Int 2010;105:202–7.
74. Zieger K, Olsen PR, Wolf H, et al. Long term follow-up of superficial invasive bladder carcinoma with or without concomitant epithelial atypia–recurrence and progression. Scand J Urol Nephrol 2002;36: 52–9.
75. Sylvester RJ, van der Meijden AP, Oosterlinck W, et al. Predicting recurrence and progression in individual patients with stage Ta T1 bladder cancer using EORTC risk tables: a combined analysis of 2596 patients from seven EORTC trials. Eur Urol 2006;49:466–77. [discussion: 475–7].
76. Raj GV, Herr H, Serio AM, et al. Treatment paradigm shift may improve survival of patients with high risk superficial bladder cancer. J Urol 2007; 177:1283–6 [discussion: 1286].
77. Kamat AM, Dinney CP, Gee JR, et al. Micropapillary bladder cancer: a review of the University of Texas M. D. Anderson Cancer Center experience with 100 consecutive patients. Cancer 2007;110: 62–7.
78. Andius P, Johansson SL, Holmang S. Prognostic factors in stage T1 bladder cancer: tumor pattern (solid or papillary) and vascular invasion more important than depth of invasion. Urology 2007; 70:758–62.
79. Lopez JI, Angulo JC. The prognostic significance of vascular invasion in stage T1 bladder cancer. Histopathology 1995;27:27–33.
80. Weiss C, Wolze C, Engehausen DG, et al. Radiochemotherapy after transurethral resection for high-risk T1 bladder cancer: an alternative to intravesical therapy or early cystectomy? J Clin Oncol 2006;24:2318–24.
81. Harland SJ, Kynaston H, Grigor K, et al. A randomized trial of radical radiotherapy for the management of pT1G3 NXM0 transitional cell carcinoma of the bladder. J Urol 2007;178:807–13 [discussion: 813].
82. Herr HW, Sogani PC. Does early cystectomy improve the survival of patients with high risk superficial bladder tumors? J Urol 2001;166: 1296–9.
83. Denzinger S, Fritsche HM, Otto W, et al. Early versus deferred cystectomy for initial high-risk pT1G3 urothelial carcinoma of the bladder: do risk factors define feasibility of bladder-sparing approach? Eur Urol 2008;53:146–52.
84. Hautmann RE, Volkmer BG, Gust K. Quantification of the survival benefit of early versus deferred cystectomy in high-risk non-muscle invasive bladder cancer (T1 G3). World J Urol 2009;27:347–51.
85. Dalbagni G, Vora K, Kaag M, et al. Clinical outcome in a contemporary series of restaged patients with clinical T1 bladder cancer. Eur Urol 2009;56:903–10.
86. Amling CL, Thrasher JB, Frazier HA, et al. Radical cystectomy for stages Ta, Tis and T1 transitional cell carcinoma of the bladder. J Urol 1994;151: 31–5 [discussion: 35–6].
87. Thalmann GN, Markwalder R, Shahin O, et al. Primary T1G3 bladder cancer: organ preserving approach or immediate cystectomy? J Urol 2004; 172:70–5.
88. Gupta A, Lotan Y, Bastian PJ, et al. Outcomes of patients with clinical T1 grade 3 urothelial cell

bladder carcinoma treated with radical cystectomy. Urology 2008;71:302–7.
89. Wiesner C, Pfitzenmaier J, Faldum A, et al. Lymph node metastases in non-muscle invasive bladder cancer are correlated with the number of transurethral resections and tumour upstaging at radical cystectomy. BJU Int 2005;95:301–5.
90. Masood S, Mufti GR. Outcomes of patients with clinical T1 grade 3 urothelial cell bladder carcinoma treated with radical cystectomy. Urology 2008;72:952 [author reply: 952].
91. Fritsche HM, Burger M, Svatek RS, et al. Characteristics and outcomes of patients with clinical T1 grade 3 urothelial carcinoma treated with radical cystectomy: results from an international cohort. Eur Urol 2010;57:300–9.
92. Pagano F, Bassi P, Galetti TP, et al. Results of contemporary radical cystectomy for invasive bladder cancer: a clinicopathological study with an emphasis on the inadequacy of the tumor, nodes and metastases classification. J Urol 1991; 145:45–50.
93. Stein JP, Lieskovsky G, Cote R, et al. Radical cystectomy in the treatment of invasive bladder cancer: long-term results in 1,054 patients. J Clin Oncol 2001;19:666–75.
94. Madersbacher S, Hochreiter W, Burkhard F, et al. Radical cystectomy for bladder cancer today–a homogeneous series without neoadjuvant therapy. J Clin Oncol 2003;21:690–6.
95. Hautmann RE, de Petriconi RC, Pfeiffer C, et al. Radical cystectomy for urothelial carcinoma of the bladder without neoadjuvant or adjuvant therapy: long-term results in 1100 patients. Eur Urol 2012; 61:1039–47.
96. Shariat SF, Karakiewicz PI, Palapattu GS, et al. Outcomes of radical cystectomy for transitional cell carcinoma of the bladder: a contemporary series from the Bladder Cancer Research Consortium. J Urol 2006;176:2414–22 [discussion: 2422].
97. Canter D, Egleston B, Wong YN, et al. Use of radical cystectomy as initial therapy for the treatment of high-grade T1 urothelial carcinoma of the bladder: A SEER database analysis. Urol Oncol 2011. [Epub ahead of print].
98. Chalasani V, Kassouf W, Chin JL, et al. Radical cystectomy for the treatment of T1 bladder cancer: the Canadian Bladder Cancer Network experience. Can Urol Assoc J 2011;5:83–7.
99. Stein JP, Penson DF. Invasive T1 bladder cancer: indications and rationale for radical cystectomy. BJU Int 2008;102:270–5.
100. Nieder AM, Brausi M, Lamm D, et al. Management of stage T1 tumors of the bladder: International Consensus Panel. Urology 2005;66:108–25.
101. Bostrom PJ, Alkhateeb S, van Rhijn BW, et al. Optimal timing of radical cystectomy in T1 high-grade bladder cancer. Expert Rev Anticancer Ther 2010;10:1891–902.
102. Solsona E, Iborra I, Rubio J, et al. The optimum timing of radical cystectomy for patients with recurrent high-risk superficial bladder tumour. BJU Int 2004;94:1258–62.
103. Nieder AM, Simon MA, Kim SS, et al. Radical cystectomy after bacillus Calmette-Guerin for high-risk Ta, T1, and carcinoma in situ: defining the risk of initial bladder preservation. Urology 2006; 67:737–41.
104. Ahmadi H, Mitra AP, Abdelsayed GA, et al. Principal component analysis based pre-cystectomy model to predict pathological stage in patients with clinical organ-confined bladder cancer. BJU Int 2012. [Epub ahead of print].
105. Herr HW, Donat SM. A re-staging transurethral resection predicts early progression of superficial bladder cancer. BJU Int 2006;97:1194–8.
106. Brauers A, Buettner R, Jakse G. Second resection and prognosis of primary high risk superficial bladder cancer: is cystectomy often too early? J Urol 2001;165:808–10.
107. Brausi M, Witjes JA, Lamm D, et al. A review of current guidelines and best practice recommendations for the management of nonmuscle invasive bladder cancer by the International Bladder Cancer Group. J Urol 2011;186:2158–67.
108. Hautmann RE, Abol-Enein H, Hafez K, et al. Urinary diversion. Urology 2007;69:17–49.
109. Ahmadi H, Skinner EC, Simma-Chiang V, et al. Urinary functional outcome following radical cystoprostatectomy and ileal neobladder reconstruction in male patients. J Urol 2012. [Epub ahead of print].
110. Puppo P, Introini C, Bertolotto F, et al. Potency preserving cystectomy with intrafascial prostatectomy for high risk superficial bladder cancer. J Urol 2008;179:1727–32 [discussion: 1732].
111. Hekal IA, El-Bahnasawy MS, Mosbah A, et al. Recoverability of erectile function in post-radical cystectomy patients: subjective and objective evaluations. Eur Urol 2009;55:275–83.
112. Kulkarni GS, Finelli A, Fleshner NE, et al. Optimal management of high-risk T1G3 bladder cancer: a decision analysis. PLoS Med 2007;4: e284.

The Conundrum of Prostatic Urethral Involvement

Johann P. Ingimarsson, MD, John D. Seigne, MB*

KEYWORDS

• Non-muscle invasive bladder cancer • Prostatic urethra • Stromal involvement • Urothelial cancer

KEY POINTS

- The presence and depth of urothelial cancer involvement in the prostatic urethra can significantly affect the management of a patient with non-muscle invasive bladder cancer.
- Bladder tumor multifocality, carcinoma in situ, and tumor of the trigone and bladder neck have been associated with prostatic involvement.
- Transurethral resection loop biopsy of the precollicular area between 5 and 7 o'clock will identify most prostatic urethral involvement.
- Superficial and subendothelial tumors can be treated with bacillus Calmette-Guérin (BCG) instillation and close follow-up, and ductal involvement with BCG or cystoprostatectomy; however, stromal involvement warrants cystoprostatectomy.

INTRODUCTION

Urothelial carcinoma is a multifocal disease of the urothelium that can develop anywhere in the urinary tract, including the prostatic urethra. The lining of the prostatic urethra and the prostatic ducts have the same transitional cell urothelium as the bladder; therefore, it is not surprising that a patient who develops non-muscle invasive bladder cancer (NMIBC) can develop urothelial carcinoma in the prostatic urethra or ducts, either as an extension from the primary process or as a de novo entity.

Knowledge of urothelial cancer of the prostate is pertinent to the management on NMIBC for 3 reasons: the presence and depth of prostate urothelial cancer will affect prognosis[1]; its presence in the prostatic urethra may suggest understaging of the primary tumor in the bladder[2]; and NMIBC managed conservatively can recur in the prostatic urethra.[3]

This article offers an overview of urothelial cancer in the setting of NMIBC, and its incidence, diagnosis, and management.

DEFINITIONS, CLASSIFICATIONS, AND STAGING

The prostate contains glands that consist of ducts and terminal acini that are in continuity with the transitional urothelium of the prostatic urethra and bladder. The ducts and acini are surrounded by the stroma, consisting of connective tissues and smooth muscle cells. The urothelium and the stroma are separated only by a thin basement membrane. The differences in anatomic and functional structure of the prostate, as well as the absence of muscularis propria, alter the natural history, staging, and management of urothelial cancer that occurs in this area. Involvement of prostatic urethra, ducts, acini, and stroma have all been described in patients with non-muscle invasive bladder transitional cell carcinoma.[1,4,5] These entities each have distinctly different clinical significance and prognosis.[1]

Conceptually urothelial cancer of the prostatic urethra can be confusing, so it is important to

The authors are employees of the above institutions and have no other affiliations or conflict of interest to disclose.
Section of Urology, Department of surgery, Dartmouth Hitchcock Medical Center, Norris Cotton Cancer Center, Geisel School of Medicine, One Medical Center Drive, Lebanon, NH 03756, USA
* Corresponding author.
E-mail address: john.d.seigne@hitchcock.org

Urol Clin N Am 40 (2013) 249–259
http://dx.doi.org/10.1016/j.ucl.2013.01.010
0094-0143/13/$ – see front matter

establish classifications and definitions before further discussion on diagnosis and management. A significant contributor to this problem is the different anatomic structure of the prostate and the fact that prostatic urothelial cancer can arise primarily in the prostate or as a direct extension of a primary bladder tumor.

As a result, prostatic urothelial cancer is included in two separate staging systems: first, a staging system for primary urothelial cancer arising in the prostate, and second, a staging system for primary urothelial cancer of the bladder that extends into the prostate. **Table 1** illustrates the similarities and differences between the staging systems for these 2 anatomic sites.

It should be noted that the American Joint Cancer Committee staging system was only changed in 2010 to reflect these differences. Before the 2010 revision, any involvement of the prostate in a patient with bladder cancer was classified as stage T4a bladder cancer, regardless of depth of invasion.[6] This classification was justly criticized, as convincing survival data suggest that primary prostatic urothelial cancer, as opposed to bladder cancer directly invading the prostate, carries a different prognosis, as does involvement of the prostatic urethra with urothelial cancer of different depths of invasion.[1,7–12] Examining the first question, Pagano and colleagues[10] compared survival in patients with contiguous spread of bladder cancer to the prostate with those with a noncontiguous urothelial cancer arising within the prostate. Only 7% of the patients with a contiguous tumor were alive at 5 years compared with 46% of patients with a noncontiguous tumor. Examining the second question of prostatic stromal involvement in comparison with lesser degrees of tumor invasion, Esrig and colleagues[7] investigated 143 men who underwent cystectomy and were found to have prostatic involvement; 5-year overall survival rates with and without stromal invasion were 36% and 71%, respectively. In addition, men without stromal invasion had a prognosis no worse than men without any prostatic involvement at all. Similarly, Solsona and colleagues[8] found patients with prostatic stromal involvement to have a hazard ratio of 2.89 for cancer-specific mortality in comparison with those without stromal involvement. Herr and Donat[3] investigated patients with NMIBC who had been treated with intravesical bacillus Calmette-Guérin (BCG) and had late recurrences

Table 1
American Joint Cancer Committee staging system, seventh (2010) version

Urothelial Cancer of the Bladder	Urothelial Cancer of the Prostate
TX: Primary tumor cannot be assessed	
T0: No evidence of a primary tumor	
Ta: Noninvasive papillary carcinoma	
Tis: Noninvasive flat carcinoma (flat carcinoma in situ, or carcinoma in situ)	Tis pu: Carcinoma in situ, involvement of prostatic urethra
	Tis pd: Carcinoma in situ, involvement of prostatic ducts
T1: Tumor invades subepithelial connective tissue	T1: Tumor invades urethral subepithelial connective tissue
T2: The tumor invades muscularis propria T2a: Tumor invades the inner half of muscularis propria T2b: Tumor invades the outer half of muscularis propria	
T3: Tumor invades perivesicle tissue T3a: Microscopically T3b: Macroscopically	
T4: Tumor invades any of the following: prostatic stroma, seminal vesicles uterus, vagina, pelvic wall, abdominal wall T4a: Tumor invades prostatic stroma, uterus, vagina T4b: Tumor invades pelvic wall or abdominal wall	T2: Tumor invades prostatic stroma, corpus spongiosum, periurethral muscle T3: Tumor invades beyond prostatic capsule, corpus cavernosum, bladder neck T4: Tumor invades adjacent organs

Data from Edge SB, Byrd DR, Compton CC, et al, editors. AJCC cancer staging manual. 7th edition. New York: Springer; 2010.

in the prostate. Prognosis was highly dependent on depth of invasion, whereby survival rate was 82% in patients with prostatic urethral or ductal involvement, compared with 48% with those with stromal involvement.[3] Examining the question of lesser degrees of prostatic involvement, Barocas and colleagues[1] investigated 3-year overall survival among 162 cystoprostatectomy patients with prostatic involvement. Three-year survival was 59% if the prostatic urethral involvement was carcinoma in situ (Tis pu), 52% if there was ductal involvement, and only 17% if there was stromal involvement.

INCIDENCE

When discussing the incidence of urothelial cancer involving the prostate it should be realized that isolated primary prostatic urothelial cancer is rare; instead this tumor is almost always associated with the presence of, or history of, urothelial cancer of the bladder.[13] There is a moderate amount of data available on the incidence of urothelial cancer arising within the prostate in patients with bladder cancer, with reported overall incidence rates of 6% to 48%, with a 7% to 17% incidence of prostatic stromal involvement.[14] Most of these data come from the cystoprostatectomy literature, which is heavily focused on muscle invasive bladder cancer and only includes NMIBC that has failed more conservative therapy. Therefore, much of the information is not directly applicable to the patient with newly diagnosed NMIBC.

The incidence figures for NMIBC-associated prostatic involvement also vary depending on the method by which the prostatic urethra is assessed (visual inspection, cold-cup biopsy, resectoscope biopsy, or pathologic analysis of the cystoprostatectomy specimen) and the timing and indications for the sample collection (diagnosis, investigation of isolated positive cytology, following intravesical therapy, or at the time of cystectomy).

In regard of the different sampling methodologies, the incidence of prostatic involvement reported following cold-cup biopsy is 24% to 27%. In these series Tis constitutes 69% to 100% of prostate pathology, and only 1 case of stromal invasion has been found.[15,16] However, with cold-cup biopsy there is clearly a high frequency of inadequate sampling of the ducts and stroma. Most studies use a resectoscope to sample the prostate. Studies using a resectoscope loop biopsy have found a 6% to 36% rate of prostatic involvement with urothelial cancer.[4,5,17,18] Many of these studies were designed to monitor outcomes of intravesical therapy whereby stromal and sometimes ductal involvement were exclusion criteria; therefore, establishing the true incidence of ductal involvement can be difficult. In a series of 49 patients undergoing transurethral resection (TUR) for a bladder tumor and with biopsy of their prostatic urethra, Schellhammer and colleagues[5] reported that 18 (37%) had prostatic involvement. Of these patients, 13 had identifiable ducts in the specimen and 7 of 13 (56%) harbored ductal urothelial cancer. Cystectomy data, although heavily focused on muscle invasive bladder cancer, have been reported in a few series that allow for subanalysis of NMIBC. In a cystectomy series of 192 patients, Nixon and colleagues[19] found 42 men with Tis, or T1, bladder disease, 8 (19%) of whom had prostatic involvement. Similarly, in series by Liedberg and colleagues[20] and Mazzucchelli and colleagues,[21] 5 of 19 men (26%) and 26 of 70 men (37%), respectively, with NMIBC were found to have prostatic involvement. Although these studies reported the overall rates of prostatic stromal involvement, this was not specified for the subset with NMIBC.

To sum up, the incidence rates of prostatic urethral involvement at initial diagnosis range from 6% to 37% and are dependent on sampling method and patient risk. The frequency of recurrence of urothelial cancer in the prostate following therapy for NMIBC ranges from 8% to 48%, and is explored in more detail in the next section.[3,19,22–25]

RISK FACTORS FOR PROSTATIC URETHRAL INVOLVEMENT

If diagnosed, prostatic involvement may drastically affect both prognosis[1] and management of NMIBC. However, in most cases identification and diagnosis requires transurethral biopsy or resection of the prostatic urethra. As tissue biopsy of the prostate is not without potential morbidity, a moderate amount of work has gone into trying to identify which patients might benefit from sampling of the prostate. Numerous factors have been evaluated.

Much information can be gained from the cystectomy literature. Nixon and colleagues[19] looked at 192 prostatectomy samples, of which 30 (15%) had prostatic urethral involvement. Patients with tumor multifocality and bladder carcinoma in situ (CIS) had rates of prostatic involvement of 34% and 31%, respectively. In a study by Mazzucchelli and colleagues,[21] 94 out of 248 (38%) cystoprostatectomy specimens had prostatic urethral involvement. Trigonal or bladder neck tumor location, pT and pN stage, and previous history of recurrence were significant risk factors. Based on their data, a formula was constructed that uses number of tumor foci in bladder, history of prior recurrence, and location of bladder tumor, which was able to predict with 61% sensitivity and 78% specificity whether there was a concomitant prostatic involvement. Other series have found numerous other factors associated with prostatic urethral involvement, including multifocal CIS, trigonal CIS, periurethral tissue invasion, ureter invasion, vascular invasion, history of bladder tumor recurrence, and history of prior bladder intillations.[1,20,22,26,27]

In the transurethral literature it has been reported that macroscopic tumor in the urethra correctly identifies prostatic urethral involvement with a sensitivity of 83% and a specificity of 95%.[19] However, Mungan and colleagues[4] reported a series with an overall prostatic urethral involvement rate of 6.2% whereby macroscopic involvement was seen in 3.5% of cases. In the other 2.7% the urethra appeared normal. The same study found that on univariate analysis, stage, grade, and multifocality of the bladder tumors correlated with prostatic involvement, not macroscopic appearance of the prostatic urethra. On multivariate analysis, only bladder tumor multifocality significantly correlated with prostatic involvement. In this study the risk of developing prostatic involvement in the presence of multiple bladder tumors was 16 times higher than the risk conferred by stage or grade.

Cystoscopic inspection, therefore, has a high specificity in correctly identifying a macroscopic tumor but a low sensitivity in correctly identifying the presence of tumor when the urethra appears normal, especially in a high-risk patient. The risk factors that correlate best with the presence of prostatic urethral carcinoma include the presence of multifocal bladder tumors, CIS, and tumors located on the trigone or bladder neck.

The European Association of Urology (EAU) 2011 guidelines on NMIBC recommend biopsy of the prostatic urethra for cases of bladder-neck tumor, when bladder CIS is present or suspected, when there is positive cytology without evidence of tumor in the bladder, or when abnormalities of the prostatic urethra are visible.[28] The National Comprehensive Care Network (NCCN) recommends considering a TUR biopsy of the prostatic urethra if the bladder tumor is sessile, or there is suspicion of high-grade bladder tumor or bladder CIS.[29]

Finally, whereas bladder tumor parameters can predict the presence of a prostatic urethral cancer, at least one study has investigated the converse, that is, the presence of prostatic urethral involvement as a risk factor for understaging of the primary bladder tumor. Huguet and colleagues[2] evaluated 62 patients with Tis, T1, or Ta bladder cancer that had failed TUR and BCG and eventually went onto cystoprostatectomy. In their series, initial prostatic involvement was the only significant risk factor of upstaging of the bladder tumor to muscle or stromal invasive disease, with a hazard ratio of 12.2 (95% confidence interval 2.2–65.5).

DIAGNOSTIC METHOD

There are numerous reports of the different methods used to diagnose prostatic urothelial cancer. Most describe cold-cut biopsy or TUR, although fine-needle aspiration and transrectal ultrasound-guided biopsy have been used.[22]

As mentioned in the previous section, the finding of a cystoscopically visible papillary lesion in the prostatic urethra on initial inspection has a high sensitivity and specificity for the presence of urothelial cancer.[19] However, one should be cautious in patients with a prior history of intravesical BCG treatment. A study by Orihuela and colleagues[23] reported that 48% of biopsies of suspicious lesions were negative. The patient with a normal-appearing urethra, in the absence of risk factors (multiple bladder tumors, CIS, tumor at the bladder neck, and so forth), has a relatively low absolute risk of the presence of tumor (~6%); however, approximately 43% of prostatic urethral tumors are not visually apparent.[4]

Several studies have examined the sensitivity and specificity as well as the most appropriate technique with which to perform a prostatic urethral biopsy with the resectoscope loop. Donat and colleagues[30] performed a prospective TUR loop biopsy on 246 male patients who subsequently underwent cystoprostatectomy, and found the sensitivity and specificity for Tis to be 53% and 77%, for T1 57% and 89%, and for stromal invasion 56% and 93%. Liedberg and colleagues[20] reported a similar 66% sensitivity and 89% specificity for any prostatic urothelial cancer in their 175-patient cystoprostatectomy series.

Various investigators have studied how extensively and where the prostatic urethra ought to be sampled. Hillyard and colleagues[17] initially described cold-cup biopsies and TUR biopsies of the lateral lobes. Taylor and colleagues,[31] in a long-term follow-up of the same series, described additionally taking TUR resections proximal to the verumontanum. Liedberg and colleagues[20] described transurethral loop biopsies from the bladder neck to the verumontanum, obtained at the 4- and 8-o'clock positions. This approach is supported by Sakamoto and colleagues[32] who, based on pathologic evaluation of cystoprostatectomy specimens, found that firstly, 93% of urothelial cancer involving the prostatic urethra is superficial enough to be identified with a superficial resection and secondly, that 84% are located at the 5- and 7-o'clock positions. In their series, only 1 patient had deep stromal involvement without a superficial tumor being identified. Given that most of the tumors are detected superficially in the prostate, a complete TUR of the prostate is not indicated. Parenthetically, should a TUR of the prostate be indicated for lower urinary tract symptoms at the time of a bladder tumor resection, a recent meta-analysis suggests that this is quiet safe, with a low risk of tumor implantation in the prostate resection bed.[33]

Accordingly, the technique most used to sample the prostatic urethra is a TUR at the 5- and 7-o'clock positions just proximal to the verumontanum, as this allows the surgeon to obtain a specimen of adequate depth and size to allow for pathologic assessment of mucosa, ducts, and stroma. This procedure is in agreement with the 2011 EAU guideline, which suggests that the biopsy should be taken "from abnormal areas and from the precollicular area (between 5 and 7 o'clock position) using a resection loop."[28]

MANAGEMENT

The management of NMIBC with prostatic urethral involvement falls into 3 categories: Group 1, noninvasive papillary tumors and CIS of the prostatic urethra (pTa/T1 and pTis pu); Group 2, CIS involving the prostatic ducts (pTIS pd); and Group 3, prostatic stromal involvement (pT2–pT4). This section also discusses management of the urethra in patients undergoing cystectomy who have known preoperative prostatic urethral involvement.

Group 1: Noninvasive Papillary Tumors and CIS of the Prostatic Urethra (pTa/T1 and pTis pu)

There is mounting evidence that Tis pu and T1 can be managed with TUR and/or intravesical instillation. In the study by Donat and colleagues[30] discussed previously, a TUR (biopsy) was performed on 246 men with bladder cancers who subsequently underwent a cystoprostatectomy. Of those diagnosed with prostatic urothelial cancer by TUR, 45% had no urothelial cancer identified on whole-mount examination of the prostate. These findings suggest that TUR alone will be curative in a proportion of patients.

Chemotherapeutic agents such as mitomycin C, adriamycin, epirubicin, and BCG have been used for intravesical therapy in the conservative management of superficial tumors involving the prostatic urethra. Of these BCG has been most extensively investigated, and multiple small case series have reported complete response rates in the range of 48% to 87%.[5,17,18,23,24] Intravesical chemotherapy has been reported to be somewhat less effective than BCG, with a complete response rate of 37% in a study by Solsona and colleagues[25] that used mitomycin C or adriamycin. In another small retrospective review of 19 patients, epirubicin was noted to have a response rate of 29% compared with 58% for BCG.[34]

As the intravesical agents only make contact with the prostatic urothelium briefly during instillation and voiding, there is controversy as to the extent of penetration of intravesical therapy into the prostate. LaFontaine and colleagues[35] examined cystoprostatectomy specimens, and found that 75% of men with prior history of BCG bladder instillations had developed granulomatous prostatitis compared with 11% of men without prior BCG treatment. A similar finding by Oates and colleagues[36] of granulomatous response in 100% of prostates biopsied after BCG treatment supports the notion that BCG penetrates deeply. However, as a caveat, granulomatosis inflammation can be seen in the prostate of patients who have not undergone BCG therapy, and a transurethral biopsy of the prostate has itself been shown to cause granulomatous prostatitis on occasion.[23]

Some investigators have argued for TUR resections before BCG therapy to allow better penetration of the instillation into the prostate.[17] Although BCG without TUR has been reported with a 78% initial complete response rate,[18] most reported series use TUR with BCG. The outcomes of reported series evaluating BCG are shown in **Table 2**. **Table 2**a shows studies on Tis pu and Ta only while **Table 2**c shows data that include Tis pd, as these series are larger and with long follow-up.

EAU and NCCN guidelines, and a World Health Organization/Societé Internationale d'Urologie (WHO/SIU) consensus, all state that Tis pu and T1 can be treated with BCG and that TUR can increase BCG contact with the prostate.[28,29,37,38]

Limited data exist on how to manage prostatic recurrence of urothelial cancer after BCG treatment, as most series are reporting fewer than 5 recurrences.[23] TUR, another course of BCG, and cystoprostatectomy have all been described. Both NCCN and WHO/SIU recommend cystoprostatectomy for recurrent disease.[29,38]

Table 2
Summary of the results of studies examining the efficacy of bacillus Calmette-Guérin (BCG) in patients with prostatic involvement

Authors,[Ref.] Year	Complete Response (%)	Late Recurrence (%)	Progression	Transitioned to Cystectomy	Transitioned to Systemic Chemotherapy or Irradiation	Mean Follow-Up (mo)	Comment
(a) Ta and Tis pu Disease							
Orihuela et al,[23] 1989	13/15 (87)	1/13 (8)	1/15	1/15[a]		?	Tis pu + Ta Recurrence responded to TUR
Ovesen et al,[16] 1993	10/10 (100)	2/10 (20)				26	Tis pu
Palou et al,[18] 1996	14/18 (78)	5/14 (36)	3/18	3/18		31	Tis pu
Canda et al,[34] 2004	7/12 (58)	2/12 (17)	3/12	1/12[a]	4/12[a]	64	Tis pu + Ta Recurrence responded to second round of BCG
(b) Tis pd Disease							
Palou Redorta et al,[39] 2006	5/10 (50)	1/5	2/10	2/10	1/10		Tis pd
(c) Ta, Tis pu, and Tis pd Disease							
Bretton et al,[24] 1989	13/23 (56)		10/23	8/10	2/10	42	Tis pu + Tis pd + Ta
Taylor et al,[31] 2007	18/28 (64)	10/18	15/28	8/28		89	Tis pu + Tis pd + Ta

[a] These patients were nonresponders to intravesical BCG therapy.

Group 2: CIS Involving the Prostatic Ducts (pTis pd)

Treatment when there is acinar or ductal involvement is more controversial. There are essentially two options, TUR followed by BCG with surveillance cystoscopies or immediate cystoprostatectomy. The argument for BCG is the potential to avoid cystoprostatectomy and the associated morbidities with the need for urinary diversion. Most studies have very few patients, and head-to-head comparison has not been attempted. Studies from Bretton and colleagues[24] and Taylor and colleagues[31] used TUR and BCG for patients with prostatic urethral involvement. Their data included Tis du disease.[5] These studies showed reasonable complete response rates (see **Table 2**c), but long-term outcomes for patients with ductal involvement are not specifically stated. Palou Redorta and colleagues[39] report a BCG treatment series wherein all the patients had Tis pd (see **Table 2**b). Half of the 10 patients responded to therapy and 1 of 5 responders developed recurrence, thus only 40% were free of disease.

Some studies among patients who have undergone cystoprostatectomy show little or no difference in survival between patients with urethral tumors (Tis pu/Ta) and Tis pd patients.[1,40] However, Wishnow and Ro[41] report a series wherein 11% of patients with ductal disease went on to develop metastasis (although this number is small compared with the 100% of patients with stromal involvement). These investigators argue that because there is only a thin layer of connective tissue preventing ductal disease from becoming stromal disease, cystoprostatectomy with either adjuvant or neoadjuvant chemotherapy should be offered.

The EAU guidelines and WHO/SIU recommendations conclude that the data are insufficient to provide clear recommendations and, as there is no conclusive result regarding conservative therapy, a cystoprostatectomy should be considered in these patients.[28,38] The NCCN guidelines consider both BCG with surveillance cystoscopies or immediate cystoprostatectomy as options.

Group 3: Prostatic Stromal Involvement (pT2–pT4)

Bladder cancer with concomitant prostatic stromal invasion technically is considered as a bladder cancer of a higher stage, T4a, and as such should not be considered as NMIBC. It should be treated with systemic neoadjuvant chemotherapy followed by cystoprostatectomy and urethrectomy according to most investigators and guidelines,[28,29,38] and thus is not discussed further here.

Evaluation of the Prostatic Urethra at the Time of Routine Cystoscopic Follow-Up of NMIBC

Studies looking at the follow-up of patients with NMIBC undergoing intravesical therapy (regardless of initial prostatic involvement) have identified prostatic involvement in 8% to 48% of cases.[3,19,22–25] Herr and Donat[3] followed 186 men with NMIBC for 15 years, and found prostatic recurrence in 72 patients (39%) after a median follow-up of 28 months. Of these, 27 patients (15%) developed stromal invasion. Similarly, Solsona and colleagues[25] followed 242 men with NMIBC with cold-cup prostatic urethral biopsies, of whom 32 had recurrence in the prostatic urethra. Despite additional TUR and intravesical therapy, 20 eventually re-recurred, with 13 progressing to bladder muscle or prostatic stromal invasion or distant metastasis, necessitating cystoprostatectomy, radiation, or chemotherapy. Schwalb and colleagues[42] demonstrated that the prostatic urethra is the third most common site of recurrence at 16%, behind the bladder (64%) and ureter (20%), in patients who develop a positive urine cytology after having a complete response to BCG. Therefore, these investigators have recommended frequent random biopsies of the prostatic urethra at the time of routine cystoscopic follow-up, especially in the presence of bladder CIS or unexplained positive urine cytology.[25,30,43] The aforementioned studies used 3- to 6-month intervals, but the optimal frequency of prostatic urethra biopsies has not been examined. The NCCN guideline recommends TUR biopsy of the prostatic urethra if cytology is positive, and when cystoscopy and imaging studies are negative, whereas the EAU and WHO/SIU do not address this issue specifically.

Management of the Urethra in a Patient with Prostatic Involvement Undergoing Cystoprostatectomy

Although most men with NMIBC can initially be treated with conservative therapy, there is a subpopulation of patients with refractory disease for whom cystoprostatectomy is indicated. Among the decisions that need to be made in choosing the best surgery for the patient is whether the urethra should be left in place. Urothelial cancer can recur in the urethra after cystectomy, contemporary series reporting a rate of 3.7% to 8.1%.[44–47] Historically its prognosis has been poor, with median survival reported at 28 months, whereas more recent series report 63% 5-year cancer-specific survival.[46,48] In past decades it has been advised to perform urethrectomy at the time of surgery.[49] However, urethrectomy carries with it morbidity, including adverse effects on sexual functions,[50,51] arguing for urethral sparing. Therefore, selectively performing urethrectomy on those men with a higher risk of urethral recurrence would prevent overtreatment with its associated morbidity. Reported risk factors include bladder CIS, upper tract urothelial carcinoma, tumor at the bladder neck, and involvement of the prostatic urethra.[47] The most consistent risk factor reported in studies is prostatic involvement, with 37% to 71% of those with urothelial carcinoma involving the prostate developing urethral recurrence after cystoprostatectomy.[52,53] Of importance is that the depth of invasion affects the risk of recurrence. Urethral involvement (T1 or Tis pu) carries little risk of recurrence, ductal involvement (Tis pd) 10% to 25% risk, and stromal involvement 30% to 67% risk.[52,53]

There is evidence suggesting that patients undergoing cutaneous diversion have a higher rate of urethral recurrence than those having an orthotopic neobladder.[46] A study by Freeman and colleagues[47] found 3% recurrence in patients with neobladders compared with 11% in patients with cutaneous diversion. Here again, prostatic involvement affected recurrence rates. Of men with urothelial cancer in the prostate, 5% of those who had a neobladder developed recurrence, as opposed to 24% of those who had cutaneous diversion.

One could conclude that this argues for preoperative TUR biopsy of the prostatic urethra before surgery. However, comparative studies have shown that intraoperative frozen section at the time of cystoprostatectomy is more accurate than TUR in predicting urethral recurrence. Lebret and colleagues[54] reported a series of 118 cystoprostatectomy patients. Of these, 9 patients had positive TUR biopsies of the prostate, but negative urethral frozen-section margin. At 10 years of follow-up, none had recurred in the prostatic urethra. Cho and colleagues[44] found an 18-fold increase in risk of recurrence if urethral margins were positive.

EAU guidelines recommend urethrectomy if there are positive margins at the level of the urethra or any positive bladder margins, or if tumor extensively invades the prostate. Prophylactic urethrectomy is not justified.[55] The WHO/SIU conclude that urothelial carcinoma of the prostate diagnosed by TUR in not an absolute indication for prophylactic urethrectomy. Furthermore, a negative frozen-section of the prostatic urethra is accurate in identifying patients at very low risk of developing a second primary or urethral tumor recurrence. However, a positive frozen-section should be considered a contraindication to performing an orthotopic neobladder.[38,56]

SUMMARY

- In a male patient with NMIBC, urothelial cancer of the prostatic urethra can occur simultaneously or metachronously.
- The incidence is 6% to 37%, based on patient risk and diagnostic method.
- Tumor multifocality, CIS, and tumor involvement of the trigone and bladder neck have been associated with a higher risk of concomitant prostate involvement.
- Transurethral resection loop biopsy of the precollicular area between 5 and 7 o'clock will identify most prostatic urethral involvement.
- The presence of prostatic urothelial cancer may suggest understaging of an associated primary bladder tumor.
- The presence and depth of invasion of the prostatic urethra affects the prognosis and management.
  - Noninvasive papillary tumors and CIS of the prostatic urethra (T1 and Tis pu) carries the best prognosis, and can be treated with TUR and intravesical BCG and close follow-up.
  - Ductal urothelial carcinoma (Tis pd) has intermediate prognosis, and there is inconsistency between studies. Although TUR and intravesical BCG treatment has been described and is considered an option in the NCCN guidelines, cystoprostatectomy is commonly recommended.
  - Prostate stromal urothelial carcinoma (T4a) has the worst prognosis, and is treated with neoadjuvant therapy followed by cystoprostatectomy and urethrectomy.
- NMIBC managed conservatively can recur in the prostatic urethra at fairly high rates (8%–48%), often with stromal involvement. Some investigators recommend routine prostatic urethral biopsies.
- In patients undergoing cystoprostatectomy for bladder cancer with known prostatic involvement, a neobladder is an acceptable form of urinary diversion as long as a frozen section of the tip of the prostate is negative; in all other circumstances a urethrectomy should be performed.
- **Table 3** summarizes the recommendations from the various relevant guidelines.

Table 3
Summary of relevant guidelines/consensus

	EAU	NCCN	WHO/SIU
Indications for prostate biopsy for UCP	Bladder neck tumor, CIS present or suspected, positive cytology without evidence of tumor in the bladder, visible abnormalities of the prostatic urethra	Sessile bladder tumors, high grade cytology, suspicion of bladder CIS	—
Mode of diagnosis	TUR of precollicular area between 5 and 7 o'clock	TUR	—
Management of Tis pu and T1	TUR + intravesical BCG	TUR + intravesical BCG	TUR + intravesical BCG
Management of Tis pd	Cystoprostatectomy	TUR + intravesical BCG Or Cystoprostatectomy	Cystoprostatectomy
Management of T4 (stromal involvement)	Cystoprostatectomy	Cystoprostatectomy	Cystoprostatectomy
Follow-up biopsies of the prostate after BCG	—	Cytology is positive and cystoscopy and imaging studies are negative	—
Management of urethra at the time of cystoprostatectomy	Urethrectomy if: Positive margins at the level of the urethra, any positive bladder margins, tumor extensively invades the prostate	—	Urothelial carcinoma on TUR is not an absolute indication for prophylactic urethrectomy Negative frozen section accurate in identifying very low risk of urethra recurrence Positive frozen section is a contraindication for an orthotopic neobladder

Abbreviations: BCG, bacillus Calmette-Guérin; CIS, carcinoma in situ; EAU, European Association of Urology; NCCN, National Comprehensive Care Network; SIU, Societé Internationale d'Urologie; TUR, transurethral resection; UCP, urothelial carcinoma of the prostate; WHO, World Health Organization.
Data from Refs.[28,29,38,55,56]

REFERENCES

1. Barocas D, Patel S, Chang S, et al. Outcomes of patients undergoing radical cystoprostatectomy for bladder cancer with prostatic involvement on final pathology. BJU Int 2009;104(8):1091–7.
2. Huguet J, Crego M, Sabaté S, et al. Cystectomy in patients with high risk superficial bladder tumors who fail intravesical BCG therapy: pre-cystectomy prostate involvement as a prognostic factor. Eur Urol 2005;48(1):53–9.
3. Herr H, Donat S. Prostatic tumor relapse in patients with superficial bladder tumors: 15-year outcome. J Urol 1999;161(6):1854–7.
4. Mungan M, Canda A, Tuzel E, et al. Risk factors for mucosal prostatic urethral involvement in superficial transitional cell carcinoma of the bladder. Eur Urol 2005;48(5):760–3.
5. Schellhammer P, Ladaga L, Moriarty R. Intravesical bacillus Calmette-Guérin for the treatment of superficial transitional cell carcinoma of the prostatic urethra in association with carcinoma of the bladder. J Urol 1995;153(1):53–6.

6. Greene F, Page D, Fleming I, et al, editors. AJCC cancer staging manual. 6th edition. NewYork: Springer; 2002.
7. Esrig D, Freeman J, Elmajian D, et al. Transitional cell carcinoma involving the prostate with a proposed staging classification for stromal invasion. J Urol 1996;156(3):1071–6.
8. Solsona E, Iborra I, Dumont R, et al. Risk groups in patients with bladder cancer treated with radical cystectomy: statistical and clinical model improving homogeneity. J Urol 2005;174(4 Pt 1): 1226–30.
9. Shen S, Lerner S, Muezzinoglu B, et al. Prostatic involvement by transitional cell carcinoma in patients with bladder cancer and its prognostic significance. Hum Pathol 2006;37(6):726–34.
10. Pagano F, Bassi P, Ferrante G, et al. Is stage pT4a (D1) reliable in assessing transitional cell carcinoma involvement of the prostate in patients with a concurrent bladder cancer? A necessary distinction for contiguous or noncontiguous involvement. J Urol 1996;155(1):244–7.
11. Cheville J, Dundore P, Bostwick D, et al. Transitional cell carcinoma of the prostate: clinicopathologic study of 50 cases. Cancer 1998;82(4):703–7.
12. Ayyathurai R, Gomez P, Luongo T, et al. Prostatic involvement by urothelial carcinoma of the bladder: clinicopathological features and outcome after radical cystectomy. BJU Int 2007;100(5):1021–5.
13. Seemayer T, Knaack J, Thelmo W, et al. Further observations on carcinoma in situ of the urinary bladder: silent but extensive intraprostatic involvement. Cancer 1975;36(2):514–20.
14. Walsh DL, Chang SS. Dilemmas in the treatment of urothelial cancers of the prostate. Urol Oncol 2009; 27(4):352–7.
15. Rikken C, van Helsdingen P, Kazzaz B. Are biopsies from the prostatic urethra useful in patients with superficial bladder carcinoma? Br J Urol 1987; 59(2):145–7.
16. Ovesen H, Poulsen A, Steven K. Intravesical Bacillus Calmette-Guérin with the Danish strain for treatment of carcinoma in situ of the bladder. Br J Urol 1993; 75(5 Pt 2):744–8.
17. Hillyard R Jr, Ladaga L, Schellhammer P. Superficial transitional cell carcinoma of the bladder associated with mucosal involvement of the prostatic urethra: results of treatment with intravesical bacillus Calmette-Guérin. J Urol 1998;139(2):290–3.
18. Palou J, Xavier B, Laguna P, et al. In situ transitional cell carcinoma involvement of prostatic urethra: bacillus Calmette-Guérin therapy without previous transurethral resection of the prostate. Urology 1996;47(4):482–4.
19. Nixon R, Chang S, Lafleur B, et al. Carcinoma in situ and tumor multifocality predict the risk of prostatic urethral involvement at radical cystectomy in men with transitional cell carcinoma of the bladder. J Urol 2002;167(2 Pt 1):502–5.
20. Liedberg F, Anderson H, Bläckberg M, et al. Prospective study of transitional cell carcinoma in the prostatic urethra and prostate in the cystoprostatectomy specimen. Incidence, characteristics and preoperative detection. Scand J Urol Nephrol 2007;41(4):290–6.
21. Mazzucchelli R, Barbisan F, Santinelli A, et al. Prediction of prostatic involvement by urothelial carcinoma in radical cystoprostatectomy for bladder cancer. Urology 2009;74(2):385–90.
22. Wood D Jr, Montie J, Pontes J, et al. Identification of transitional cell carcinoma of the prostate in bladder cancer patients: a prospective study. J Urol 1989; 142(1):83–5.
23. Orihuela E, Herr H, Whitmore W Jr. Conservative treatment of superficial transitional cell carcinoma of prostatic urethra with intravesical BCG. Urology 1989;34(5):231–7.
24. Bretton P, Herr H, Whitmore W Jr, et al. Intravesical bacillus Calmette-Guérin therapy for in situ transitional cell carcinoma involving the prostatic urethra. J Urol 1989;141(4):853–6.
25. Solsona E, Iborra I, Ricós J, et al. Recurrence of superficial bladder tumors in prostatic urethra. Eur Urol 1991;19(2):89–92.
26. Honda N, Yamada Y, Okada M, et al. Clinical study of transitional cell carcinoma of the prostate associated with bladder transitional cell carcinoma. Int J Urol 2002;9(1):71–2.
27. Tabibi A, Simforoosh N, Parvin M, et al. Predictive factors for prostatic involvement by transitional cell carcinoma of the bladder. Urol J 2011;8(1): 43–7.
28. Babjuk M, Oosterlinck W, Sylvester R, et al. EAU guideline son non-muscle-invasive urothelial carcinoma of the bladder, the 2011 update. Eur Urol 2011;59(6):997–1008.
29. NCCN clinical practice guidelines in oncology. Bladder cancer. Version 1.2013. 2012. Available at: http://www.nccn.org.
30. Donat S, Wei D, McGuire M, et al. The efficacy of transurethral biopsy for predicting the long-term clinical impact of prostatic invasive bladder cancer. J Urol 2001;165(5):1580–4.
31. Taylor J, Davis J, Schellhammer P. Long-term follow-up of intravesical bacillus Calmette-Guérin treatment for superficial transitional-cell carcinoma of the bladder involving the prostatic urethra. Clin Genitourin Cancer 2007;5(6):386–9.
32. Sakamoto N, Tsuneyoshi M, Naito S, et al. An adequate sampling of the prostate to identify prostatic involvement by urothelial carcinoma in bladder cancer patients. J Urol 1993;149:318–21.
33. Picozzi S, Ricci C, Gaeta M, et al. Is it oncologically safe performing simultaneous transurethral resection

of the bladder and prostate? A meta-analysis on 1,234 patients. Int Urol Nephrol 2012;44(5):1325–33.
34. Canda A, Tuzel E, Mungan M, et al. Conservative management of mucosal prostatic urethral involvement in patients with superficial transitional cell carcinoma of the bladder. Eur Urol 2004;45(4):465–9.
35. LaFontaine P, Middleman B, Graham S Jr, et al. Incidence of granulomatous prostatitis and acid-fast bacilli after intravesical BCG therapy. Urology 1997;49(3):363–6.
36. Oates R, Stilmant M, Freedlund M, et al. Granulomatous prostatitis following bacillus Calmette-Guérin immunotherapy of bladder cancer. J Urol 1988; 140(7):751–4.
37. Edge SB, Byrd DR, Compton CC, et al, editors. AJCC cancer staging manual. 7th edition. New York: Springer; 2010.
38. Palou J, Baniel J, Klotz L, et al. Urothelial carcinoma of the prostate. Urology 2007;69(Suppl 1):50–61.
39. Palou Redorta J, Schatteman P, Huguet Pérez J, et al. Intravesical instillations with bacillus Calmette-Guérin for the treatment of carcinoma in situ involving prostatic ducts. Eur Urol 2006;49(5):834–8.
40. Njinou Ngninkeu B, Lorge F, Moulin P, et al. Transitional cell carcinoma involving the prostate: a clinicopathological retrospective study of 76 cases. J Urol 2003;169(1):149–52.
41. Wishnow KI, Ro JY. Importance of early treatment of transitional cell carcinoma of prostatic ducts. Urology 1988;32(1):11–2.
42. Schwalb M, Herr H, Sogani P, et al. Positive urinary cytology following a complete response to intravesical bacillus Calmette-Guérin therapy: pattern of recurrence. J Urol 1994;152(2 Pt 1):382–7.
43. Montie J, Wood D Jr, Mendendorp S, et al. The significance and management of transitional cell carcinoma of the prostate. Semin Urol 1990;8(4): 262–8.
44. Cho K, Seo J, Park S, et al. The risk factor for urethral recurrence after radical cystectomy in patients with transitional cell carcinoma of the bladder. Urol Int 2009;82(3):306–11.
45. Stein J, Clark P, Miranda G, et al. Urethral tumor recurrence following cystectomy and urinary diversion: clinical and pathological characteristics in 768 male patients. J Urol 2005;173(4):1163–8.
46. Boorjian S, Kim S, Weight C, et al. Risk factors and outcomes of urethral recurrence following radical cystectomy. Eur Urol 2011;60(6):1266–72.
47. Freeman J, Tarter T, Esrig D, et al. Urethral recurrence in patients with orthotopic ileal neobladders. J Urol 1996;156:1615–9.
48. Clark P, Stein J, Groshen S, et al. The management of urethral transitional cell carcinoma after radical cystectomy for invasive bladder cancer. J Urol 2004;172(4 Pt 1):1324–47.
49. Schellhammer P, Whitmore W Jr. Transitional cell carcinoma of the urethra in men having cystectomy for bladder cancer. J Urol 1976;115(1):56–60.
50. Kitamura T, Moriyama N, Shibamoto K, et al. Urethrectomy is harmful for preserving potency after radical cystectomy. Urol Int 1987;42(5):375–9.
51. Tomić R, Sjödin J. Sexual function in men after radical cystectomy with or without urethrectomy. Scand J Urol Nephrol 1992;26(2):127–9.
52. Hardeman S, Soloway M. Urethral recurrence following radical cystectomy. J Urol 1990;144(3): 666–9.
53. Levinson A, Johnson D, Wishnow K. Indications for urethrectomy in an era of continent urinary diversion. J Urol 1990;144(1):73–5.
54. Lebret T, Hervé J, Barré P, et al. Urethral recurrence of transitional cell carcinoma of the bladder. Predictive value of preoperative latero-montanal biopsies and urethral frozen sections during prostatocystectomy. Eur Urol 1998;33(2):170–4.
55. Stenzl A, Cowan N, De Santis M, et al. Treatment of muscle-invasive and metastatic bladder cancer: update of the EAU guidelines. Eur Urol 2011;59(6): 1009–18.
56. World Health Organization (WHO) Consensus Conference on Bladder Cancer, Hautmann R, Abol-Enein H, Hafez K, et al. Urinary diversion. Urology 2007;69(Suppl 1):17–49.

The Costs of Non-Muscle Invasive Bladder Cancer

Andrew C. James, MD[a,*], John L. Gore, MD, MS[a,b]

KEYWORDS

• Bladder cancer • Cost-effectiveness • Quality of care

KEY POINTS

- Bladder cancer is the costliest cancer to treat in the United States on a per capita basis. Diagnosis, treatment, and continued surveillance all contribute to the economic burden of non-muscle invasive bladder cancer (NMIBC).
- Novel urinary markers are being investigated to replace cystoscopy and cytology in hopes of diminishing the burden associated with surveillance in NMIBC. Although showing promise, they currently lack the sensitivity and specificity to replace cystoscopy and cytology. In addition, the use of newer endoscopic methods such as fluorescence and narrow-band cystoscopy have yet to show superiority in detecting clinically meaningful lesions compared with traditional white-light cystoscopy.
- Characterization of the risk of recurrence and progression of patients with NMIBC can optimize surveillance strategies and lower expenditures associated with surveillance.
- The indirect costs of NMIBC include decreased productivity, reduced physical and social functioning, and a lowered health-related quality of life.
- Improved adherence to evidence-based practices such as recommendations for mitomycin C instillation, repeat resection of high-grade NMIBC, and induction bacille Calmette-Guérin would decrease the burden of NMIBC.
- Urologist-led quality collaboratives would likely improve on compliance with evidence-based recommendations and further optimize surveillance strategies in patients with NMIBC.

INTRODUCTION

Bladder cancer is one of the most common cancer diagnoses in the United States, with an estimated 68,810 new cases in 2010, accounting for 7% of all cancers and 3% of cancer deaths.[1] Approximately 70% of bladder cancers do not invade the underlying muscle at diagnosis[2]; this type of malignancy is broadly referred to as non-muscle invasive bladder cancer (NMIBC). Among NMIBCs, disorders can range from low-grade, superficial disease that often behaves in an indolent fashion to more aggressive high-grade lesions such as carcinoma in situ (CIS) and lesions invading the underlying lamina propria. These high-risk, high-grade lesions have the potential to progress to muscle-invasive disease that is typically not amenable to the bladder-sparing treatments often used for NMIBC.

Treatment of bladder cancer is costly, in both direct and indirect terms. Of all cancers, bladder cancer is the ninth most costly in the United States in terms of overall expenditures,[3] and has the greatest lifetime treatment cost per patient diagnosed, surpassing colorectal, breast, prostate, and lung cancers.[4] Among the 5 commonest cancers in

Funding sources: Dr Gore, National Cancer Institute, National Institutes of Health.
Conflict of interest: Dr James, none; Dr Gore, previously served as advisor to ENDO Pharmaceuticals, Inc.
[a] Department of Urology, University of Washington, 1959 Northeast Pacific Street, Box 356510, Seattle, WA 98195, USA; [b] Department of Surgery, Fred Hutchinson Cancer Research Center, University of Washington, 1100 Fairview Avenue North, Seattle, WA 98109, USA
* Corresponding author.
E-mail address: acjames@u.washington.edu

Urol Clin N Am 40 (2013) 261–269
http://dx.doi.org/10.1016/j.ucl.2013.01.004

elderly patients, review of Medicare data expenditures also found bladder cancer to be the costliest.[5] Of patients diagnosed with low-grade NMIBC, approximately 50% recur and 5% progress to muscle-invasive disease.[2] These recurrences necessitate multiple endoscopic resections and intravesical treatments combined with lifelong surveillance. Beyond the direct costs, NMIBC treatment also results in indirect costs such as lost productivity or the heightened psychological burden of a cancer diagnosis.

PATHOLOGY/STAGING

NMIBC is defined by the stage classification of the cancer according to American Joint Committee on Cancer (AJCC) specifications.[6] Cancer grade is an important component of risk stratification within NMIBC. The World Health Organization (WHO) recently adopted the term urothelial cell carcinoma (UCC) to replace the traditional term transitional cell carcinoma.[7] UCC was formerly graded from 1 to 3, with grade 1 lesions representing well-differentiated UCC and grade 3 lesions representing poorly differentiated UCC. However, as per WHO recommendation, this has been replaced by dichotomous histologic grading with UCC lesions now categorized as either high grade or low grade. This grading decreases some of the histologic discrepancy and interpathologist variability that was often present with grade 2 tumors with the earlier classification. Papillary urothelial neoplasm of low malignant potential (PUNLMP) and papillomas are two additional noninvasive bladder lesions that are rarely aggressive. PUNLMPs progress in fewer than 3% of cases; however, because of the possibility of local recurrence and the low probability of progression, many advocate maintenance of surveillance.[8] Papillomas do not progress and do not require long-term follow-up.[9]

The bladder wall comprises 3 histologic layers. The inner urothelium is approximately 7 cell layers thick. Just deep to this, the lamina propria is a layer of blood vessels and lymphatics. The outermost muscularis propria predominantly functions to give the bladder its contracting ability. Stage classification Ta tumors are papillary tumors that do not extend deep to the urothelium. CIS (stage classification Tis) refers to a flat, high-grade lesion confined to the urothelium. Stage classification T1 tumors invade the lamina propria but do not extend into the underlying muscularis propria. This article focuses on the costs associated with management of lesions confined to the urothelium or lamina propria (ie, stage classification Ta, Tis, and T1), which are collectively referred to as NMIBC.

RISK FACTORS AND DEMOGRAPHICS

Tobacco smoking is the greatest known external risk factor for the development of bladder cancer. The relative risk among smokers for the development of bladder cancer is 2.8 in men and 2.7 in women compared with nonsmokers.[10] This risk increases in proportion to a patient's duration of tobacco use and with the amount of tobacco exposure over time. Other environmental exposures also increase the risk for the development of UCC. Certain occupations with frequent contact with petroleum products, stains, and dyes have an increased risk for bladder cancer.[11] Such individuals include mechanics, leather workers, miners, and hairdressers.

Men outnumber women in bladder cancer diagnoses at a ratio of 3:1.[12] Although bladder cancer is more common in men, women often present with late-stage UCC, likely as a result of misinterpretation of presentation with hematuria. The incidence of bladder cancer increases with age; most diagnoses occur during the eighth decade of life. UCC is more prevalent in the white population, with white men and women having a 3-fold increase in the risk of developing bladder cancer compared with African Americans.[13]

DIRECT ECONOMIC BURDEN

The economic burden of diagnosis, treatment, and surveillance of NMIBC is substantial. Bladder cancer care in the United States in 2010 cost an estimated $3.98 billion.[3] Lifetime per capita costs have been estimated between $96,000 and $187,000 in 2001 US dollars, or more than $230,000 in 2010 US dollars.[4] Modeling patients whose course follows the best possible bladder cancer outcomes (patients with NMIBC with projected recurrences at the mean NMIBC rate), Avritcher and colleagues[14] found that the lifetime cost of treatment of patients in a best-case scenario was $120,684. Management of recurrences accounted for approximately 60% of this lifetime cost. If all patients newly diagnosed with NMIBC in the last year received recommended surveillance care with no recurrences (a perfect case scenario), the cost to the health care system for the management of this cohort for 5 years would exceed $150 million.[15]

Several factors contribute to the cost of NMIBC. Most patients present with either gross or microscopic hematuria, and initial evaluation for hematuria consists of cystoscopy and cross-sectional imaging. Urine cytology is often performed to evaluate for CIS that may be difficult to visualize cystoscopically or to better define the anticipated grade of identified bladder lesions. In instances of chronic kidney disease or contrast allergy, the expense of the initial evaluation is often compounded by the need to evaluate the upper urinary tract endoscopically, typically by performing retrograde pyelography or ureteroscopy under a general anesthetic.

If tumor or a suspicious lesion is visualized on initial cystoscopic examination, on radiographic examination, or if the urine cytology is suspicious for malignant cells, the initial tumor resection or biopsy of suspicious areas is usually done under general anesthesia. Intravesical instillation of mitomycin C is commonly indicated to reduce the risk of recurrence of bladder tumors, especially if the tumor seems to be low grade and noninvasive. For those diagnosed with NMIBC, the treatment and follow-up vary depending on the stage and grade of tumor. A repeat resection within 6 weeks is recommended for patients with high-grade T1 NMIBC disease because of a 64% risk of understaging when muscularis propria is absent from the initial resection and a 40% overall risk of understaging.[16,17] Because management of upstaged NMIBC is different and cancer-specific outcomes suffer for mismanaged patients, repeat resection is not a candidate target for cost savings.

Following initial resection, among patients with high-grade NMIBC, intravesical bacille Calmette-Guérin (BCG) is typically indicated as first-line treatment. BCG is an attenuated mycobacterium that induces an immune response. Recommendations from the National Comprehensive Cancer Network (NCCN) advocate a 6-week induction course of BCG for those with high-grade Ta or T1 bladder cancer as well as those with CIS, followed by up to 3 years of maintenance therapy for multiple installations at varying time intervals,[18] based on high-level evidence.[19] Kilbridge and Kantoff[20] used a cost model to show that use of BCG in a 65-year-old man with high-grade NMIBC costs approximately $4820 per year of life saved (2010 US dollars), a remarkable cost-effectiveness figure.

For patients with low-grade NMIBC, treatment and surveillance are less vigilant. Patients are often managed conservatively with surgical treatment of recurrences, without consideration of induction intravesical immunotherapy or chemotherapy. However, patients should receive a single instillation of intravesical chemotherapy concordant with resections, based on high-level evidence. Randomized trials and meta-analyses show that intravesical administration of mitomycin C given immediately after resection of a bladder tumor decreases tumor recurrence by approximately 35%.[21,22]

For high-risk NMIBC refractory to treatment with BCG, salvage intravesical chemotherapy may help patients avoid major extirpative surgery, which is costly both in terms of expenditure and in the induced quality-of-life burden to the patient. Intravesical valrubicin has a single indication for its use as a salvage agent in high-risk NMIBC failing BCG. However, the cost-effectiveness of valrubicin for this indication may be marginally superior to that of radical cystectomy. Valrubicin showed durable benefit in 28% of patients with BCG-refractory NMIBC, and costs 6 times more than an induction course of BCG.[23] Cost-effectiveness models that incorporate the disutility of cystectomy with urinary diversion may better account for the benefit of salvage valrubicin.

Prediction algorithms have attempted to better classify patients' risks of recurrence and progression of bladder cancer to optimize surveillance strategies. The American Urological Association (AUA) categorizes patients into low-risk and high-risk groups based on grade and volume of cancer.[24] Low-risk patients have low-volume, low-grade NMIBC. Intermediate-risk patients have higher volume low-grade NMIBC. The AUA categorizes all patients with high-grade NMIBC as high risk. The NCCN describes a similar risk stratification classification, but the NCCN categorizes all patients with low-grade NMIBC as low risk, independently of tumor volume.[25] Intermediate-risk patients have high-grade stage classification Ta bladder cancer. High-risk patients with NMIBC have stage classification T1 and Tis tumors. The remainder of this article refers to the NCCN risk stratification and guidelines.

Patients with intermediate-risk or high-risk NMIBC require quarterly cystoscopies for the first 2 years after diagnosis with upper urinary tract evaluation every 1 to 2 years with cross-sectional imaging. Surveillance cystoscopy may be performed at increasing intervals if patients are recurrence free after 2 years. However, these patients are typically committed to a lifetime of upper tract surveillance. Although recommendations vary regarding surveillance for low-risk NMIBC, the presence of tumor at the initial 3-month cystoscopic evaluation is a prognostic marker for recurrent disease.[26,27] NCCN guidelines recommend initial cystoscopy 3 months after resection, with subsequent cystoscopies at increasing intervals if the initial cystoscopy is negative for recurrence.[18]

Long-term surveillance of NMIBC contributes substantially to the cost burden of the disease. Compared with muscle-invasive bladder cancer, in which costs are disproportionately driven by initial diagnosis and treatment, complications of these therapies and subsequent care, including end-of-life care, treatment complications account for only 4% of overall NMIBC costs.[14] Because NMIBC surveillance mandates frequent invasive procedures and periodic cross-sectional imaging, these components of care dominate determinants of NMIBC costs. Changes in surveillance and treatment strategies have previously mirrored changes in physician reimbursement. In an effort to decrease the cost of hospital-based procedures, in 2005, Medicare adopted changes in reimbursements for office-based endoscopic procedures,[28] which led to a large increase in office-based procedures and increased the cost of NMIBC surveillance and treatment.

To mitigate the costs associated with cystoscopic surveillance, to address concerns about patient noncompliance because of procedural discomfort, and to overcome the low sensitivity of cytology, other novel urinary markers have been examined that could obviate cystoscopy. Cytology has a median sensitivity of 69% for the detection of high-risk tumors within the bladder, 78% sensitivity for detection of CIS, but lower sensitivity for upper tract lesions within the ureter and renal pelvis.[29] Thus, a negative cytology does not preclude cystoscopy, particularly in the setting of low-grade NMIBC or upper urinary tract tumors.

Commercial urinary markers for bladder tumor antigens (BTA stat and BTA trak) have superior sensitivity for low-grade tumors (48% vs 13% for cytology), but limited sensitivity overall, failing to detect 47% of tumors identified cystoscopically.[30] In addition, these tests had low specificity and frequent false-positive results in the setting of urinary tract infections. ImmunoCyt tests for markers of exfoliated UCCs. Similar to BTA stat and BTA trak, ImmunoCyt has improved sensitivity for low-grade NMIBC compared with cytology, but has low specificity. ImmunoCyt seems to be particularly confounded in patients with cystitis or benign prostatic hyperplasia.[31,32] Urinary testing for NMP22 has sensitivity of 59%, 90%, and 70% for low-grade NMIBC, high-risk NMIBC, and CIS, respectively. Reduced sensitivity in cases of infection, bladder calculi, and prior urinary tract instrumentation curtail its usefulness in the evaluation and surveillance of NMIBC.[33,34]

Fluorescence in situ hybridization (FISH) detects aneuploidy in chromosomes 3, 7, and 17, as well as loss of the 9p21 locus of the P16 tumor suppressor gene.[35] Sensitivity is limited in low-grade NMIBC, but increases in the detection of high-grade NMIBC.[36] FISH urinary testing does have some usefulness in patients undergoing treatment with intravesical BCG, a setting in which cytology has limited usefulness, and may be of benefit in certain patients undergoing intravesical treatment who have ambiguous cytology results.[37] Kamat and colleagues[38] reported that high false-positive rates incurred with FISH tripled the cost associated with each additional cancer diagnosis compared with cystoscopy alone. To date, urinary markers have yet to be identified with adequate sensitivity or specificity to obviate cystoscopy and cytology and the potential cost reductions that could produce.

Novel endoscopic techniques have been developed to improve on detection of bladder cancer. Narrow-band imaging cystoscopy and fluorescence cystoscopy after intravesical instillation of 5-aminolevulinic acid or hexaminolevulinate have been shown to increase tumor detection rates compared with traditional white-light cystoscopy.[39,40] Better detection was associated with decreased recurrence rates at 3-month surveillance, presumably because of complete treatment of all identified lesions at initial resection. Cauberg and colleagues[39] showed significantly decreased recurrence rates from 30.5% with conventional cystoscopy to 15.0% with narrow-band imaging cystoscopy 3 months after initial resection. A large multicenter study identified a 9% absolute reduction in the recurrence of bladder tumors using fluorescence cystoscopy.[40] However, these novel cystoscopic techniques are costly, and the proportion of lesions detected through fluorescence and narrow-band cystoscopy that are clinically important is unknown.

Management and surveillance of NMIBC remains costly. Unlike cancers that may be followed with serum laboratory tests or dedicated physical examinations, NMIBC requires expensive invasive procedures. Risk stratification can direct the intensity of surveillance required; patients with low-risk NMIBC can probably be followed less vigilantly than those with intermediate-risk or high-risk NMIBC. However, the investigation of other biomarkers for bladder cancer recurrence has not produced a test that has replaced the need for cystoscopy. Augmentation of conventional cystoscopy with new technologies has not shown convincing cost-effectiveness.

INDIRECT ECONOMIC BURDEN

Although the diagnosis, treatment, and surveillance of NMIBC consume substantial health care resources, there are indirect costs as well. Few studies have quantified the indirect costs of NMIBC treatment. The loss of work related to bladder cancer care can exert a major burden on patients. Patients with NMIBC undergo initial diagnostic evaluation, definitive biopsy in the operating room, a possible repeat resection depending on the initial pathology, induction intravesical BCG, surveillance visits with cystoscopy every 3 months, the possibility of maintenance intravesical therapy, and additional time off depending on their threshold for recovery after each procedure. Among those who return to work is the probability of diminished productivity.

The socioeconomic profile of the average patient with bladder cancer suggests that loss of work could disproportionately affect those with NMIBC. Given primary risk factors of tobacco use and chemical exposure, professions associated with a bladder cancer diagnosis tend to be blue collar.[11] In contrast, because bladder cancer disproportionately affects older men and women, many patients with NMIBC are of retirement age and unaffected by work concerns. However, among younger patients yet to retire, the time from work required for NMIBC care could adversely affect their personal financial situation.

More awareness is being given to the psychological burden of bladder cancer and its treatment. Several health-related quality-of-life instruments have been validated for use in assessment of patient with bladder cancer, comprising questions pertinent to NMIBC and muscle-invasive bladder cancer care. The Bladder Cancer Index measures urinary, sexual, and bowel function and shows reliability among patients with muscle-invasive bladder cancer undergoing cystectomy and among patients with NMIBC.[41,42] The Functional Assessment of Cancer Therapy Bladder Cancer (FACT-BL) similarly can be applied to patients with both muscle-invasive cancer and NMIBC but includes more generic quality-of-life questions.[43] The European Organization for Research and Treatment of Cancer (EORTC) likewise produced an instrument for quality-of-life assessment in NMIBC, the EORTC QLQ-BLS24.[44] The 24-item questionnaire is specific to patients with NMIBC and has questions devoted to the impact of intravesical therapy and cystoscopic procedures.

Applying these and generic quality-of-life questionnaires, several investigators have evaluated the outcomes of NMIBC survivors. Compared with age-matched and sex-matched controls, the mental health of patients undergoing resection was lower after the initial resection but eventually returned to normal on repeat resection.[45] Physical functioning, social functioning, and emotional quality of life were also lower among patients with NMIBC than among controls. Intravesical treatment with BCG also affects generic quality of life, irrespective of the cancer outcome, with increased psychological distress among BCG recipients.[46] Among bladder cancer–specific domains, a cross section of patients with NMIBC showed superior urinary, sexual, and bowel function compared with patients with muscle-invasive bladder cancer following radical cystectomy.[42] Patients who had received intravesical therapy had worse urinary function scores than patients with NMIBC who were naive to intravesical agents. Using FACT-BL, Allareddy and colleagues[47] showed similar disease-specific quality-of-life scores between patients with NMIBC and those having radical cystectomy, which may be a function of the generic nature of many FACT-BL items. Few studies have longitudinally evaluated patients with NMIBC to quantify whether resections, cystoscopies, or intravesical treatment courses have a cumulative impact on generic or bladder cancer–specific quality of life.

OPPORTUNITIES FOR IMPROVEMENT

The cost of health care in the United States currently accounts for approximately 17% of gross domestic product (GDP) and will increase to approximately 25% of the GDP by 2025. The expensive modalities of diagnosis, treatment, and surveillance of bladder cancer are potential targets for health care savings.[48] Diagnosis, predicated on imaging and cystoscopy, is unlikely to change. The domain of bladder cancer treatment could realize better cost-effectiveness. Despite level I evidence supporting instillation of chemotherapy after bladder tumor resection for prevention of cancer recurrence,[22] review of practice patterns from population-based cohorts suggests that this may rarely occur in real-world practice.[49,50] If accurate, this would be associated with marked harm to patients with NMIBC and to the health care system. Lee and colleagues[51] estimated that 1025 quality-adjusted life years are lost in the United States every 2 years because of underuse of intravesical mitomycin C, which amounts to 8.1 quality-adjusted life days per patient. Because underuse of mitomycin C would be associated with an excess of more than 7800 recurrent NMIBC cases, better compliance could save more than $30 million. Because a recurrence extends the need for frequent surveillance care, this study may underestimate the economic burden of underuse of postresection intravesical chemotherapy. The reduction in recurrences would also, almost certainly, reduce the psychological impact of NMIBC care.

Surveillance care represents a domain of bladder cancer care delivery with an opportunity to obtain better health care value. NMIBC surveillance guidelines are based on expert opinion. Studies of population-based practice patterns show robust variation in adherence to these guidelines. Analyses using Surveillance, Epidemiology, and End Results (SEER) cancer registry data linked with Medicare claims (SEER-Medicare) have indicated that adherence to recommended NMIBC surveillance protocols may be very poor.[50,52] Fewer than 40% of patients comply with a relaxed definition of recommended care.[50,52] Applying more stringent criteria, almost no patients with high-risk NMIBC receive all recommended components of NMIBC care including repeat resection, induction BCG, and vigilant cystoscopic surveillance with cytology. The treating urologist affects patient compliance. Chamie and colleagues[50] found that 45% of the variance in compliance with NMIBC care is attributable to the treating clinician.

This appearance of noncompliance with guideline-recommended care may be a reflection of the lack of evidence underlying surveillance schedules. Hollenbeck and colleagues[53] critically evaluated the intensity of NMIBC surveillance using SEER-Medicare. The investigators found no difference in need for radical cystectomy or in survival outcomes for patients with high-intensity surveillance compared with patients with low-intensity surveillance. The investigators classified intensity by terciles of observed practice patterns, in which high-intensity care may still be noncompliant. To address this, a follow-up study stratified patients by the number of cystoscopic examinations and again found no difference in deaths from bladder cancer.[54] Current recommendations based on expert opinion may overestimate the needed burden of surveillance and tailored surveillance strategies could potentially lessen both the monetary and emotional costs associated with NMIBC follow-up. New technologies could guide surveillance schedules. Mutations in fibroblast growth factor receptor 3 (FGFR3) are common and have shown an association with less aggressive behavior than wild-type FGFR3 NMIBC tumors.[55,56] Pending further studies, FGFR3 could be used to indicate patients in whom more relaxed surveillance strategies could be adopted. Decision analysis models comparing standard surveillance protocols with modified protocols informed by FGFR3 showed impressive cost savings with the modified schedule halving the expected costs for a standard protocol.[57] Other urinary biomarkers may similarly inform better risk stratification that could direct surveillance care.

In addition to the improvements in surveillance, more conservative treatment strategies might decrease operative resection of low-risk lesions. Low-grade tumors have a smaller chance of progressing to muscle-invasive bladder cancer than high-grade lesions. Because the likelihood of progression is low, expectant management is an option for small lesions. Pruthi and colleagues[58] examined 22 patients with a history of low-grade NMIBC who underwent expectant management of their small papillary bladder tumors. At mean follow-up of 25 months, 17 had minimal growth and 5 had moderate growth of their tumors. Two patients required repeat resection because of tumor growth and worrisome cytology, both of whom showed grade or stage progression. Thus, expectant management is safe for patients with a known history of low-grade NMIBC who present with small-volume recurrences. Prospective studies may reinforce expectant management of small low-grade recurrences.

Because many of the quality detriments and clinical decisions that affect NMIBC costs are urologist driven, urologist-led quality improvement collaboratives have potential as a solution. For equivocal clinical situations, collaboratives can generate real-world comparative effectiveness estimates through transparent reporting of management outcomes and ascertainment of best practices. General surgical collaboratives have achieved remarkable cost savings for patients having bariatric and colorectal surgery with lower complication rates than regionally matched hospitals not participating in the collaboratives.[59–62] Urologic collaboratives are already in operation. The Urologic Surgery Quality Collaborative[63] used practice feedback reports to reduce the overuse of advanced staging imaging studies for patients newly diagnosed with low-risk prostate cancer.[64] A similar initiative could address the underuse of intravesical chemotherapy after bladder tumor resection.

SUMMARY

Bladder cancer is a costly health condition. Because NMIBC is the predominant new bladder cancer diagnosis, understanding the drivers of the high cost of NMIBC care would identify targets for cost reduction initiatives and quality-improvement efforts. These costs affect the health care system, but the patient-centered costs of lost work, decreased productivity, and incurred quality-of-life detriments are similarly substantial. Ensuring better compliance with NMIBC treatments that are known to reduce recurrence rates could also reduce both direct and indirect costs. One emerging avenue for addressing compliance and the quality of bladder cancer care is urologist participation in clinician-led quality collaboratives, in which transparent reporting and benchmarking could affect the underuse of adjunctive NMIBC therapies.

REFERENCES

1. Siegel R, Ward E, Brawley O, et al. Cancer statistics, 2011: the impact of eliminating socioeconomic and racial disparities on premature cancer deaths. CA Cancer J Clin 2011;61(4):212–36.
2. Jones JS, Larchian WA. Non-muscle-invasive bladder cancer (Ta, T1, and CIS). In: Wein AJ, Kavoussi LR, Novick AC, et al, editors. Campbell-Walsh urology. 10 edition. Philadelphia: Saunders; 2012. p. 2335–54.
3. Mariotto AB, Yabroff KR, Shao Y, et al. Projections of the cost of cancer care in the United States: 2010-2020. J Natl Cancer Inst 2011;103(2):117–28.
4. Botteman MF, Pashos CL, Redaelli A, et al. The health economics of bladder cancer: a comprehensive review of the published literature. Pharmacoeconomics 2003;21(18):1315–30.
5. Riley GF, Potosky AL, Lubitz JD, et al. Medicare payments from diagnosis to death for elderly cancer patients by stage at diagnosis. Med Care 1995; 33(8):828–41.
6. Edge SB, American Joint Committee on Cancer, American Cancer Society. AJCC cancer staging handbook: from the AJCC cancer staging manual. 7th edition. New York: Springer; 2010.
7. Eble JN, Sauter G, Epstein JI, et al. World Health Organization classification of tumours. Pathology and genetics of tumours of the urinary system and male genital organs. Lyon: IARC Press; 2004.
8. Epstein JI, Amin MB, Reuter VR, et al. The World Health Organization/International Society of Urological Pathology consensus classification of urothelial (transitional cell) neoplasms of the urinary bladder. Bladder Consensus Conference Committee. Am J Surg Pathol 1998;22(12):1435–48.
9. Donat SM. Evaluation and follow-up strategies for superficial bladder cancer. Urol Clin North Am 2003; 30(4):765–76.
10. Gandini S, Botteri E, Iodice S, et al. Tobacco smoking and cancer: a meta-analysis. Int J Cancer 2008;122(1):155–64.
11. Wood DP. Urothelial tumors of the bladder. In: Wein AJ, Kavoussi LR, Novick AC, et al, editors. Campbell-Walsh urology. 10 edition. Philadelphia: Saunders; 2012. p. 2309–34.
12. Jemal A, Siegel R, Ward E, et al. Cancer statistics, 2008. CA Cancer J Clin 2008;58(2):71–96.
13. Hayat MJ, Howlader N, Reichman ME, et al. Cancer statistics, trends, and multiple primary cancer analyses from the Surveillance, Epidemiology, and End Results (SEER) Program. Oncologist 2007;12(1): 20–37.
14. Avritscher EB, Cooksley CD, Grossman HB, et al. Clinical model of lifetime cost of treating bladder cancer and associated complications. Urology 2006;68(3): 549–53.
15. Han M, Schoenberg MP. The use of molecular diagnostics in bladder cancer. Urol Oncol 2000; 5(3):87–92.
16. Herr HW. The value of a second transurethral resection in evaluating patients with bladder tumors. J Urol 1999;162(1):74–6.
17. Dutta SC, Smith JA Jr, Shappell SB, et al. Clinical under staging of high risk nonmuscle invasive urothelial carcinoma treated with radical cystectomy. J Urol 2001;166(2):490–3.
18. Montie JE, Clark PE, Eisenberger MA, et al. Bladder cancer. J Natl Compr Canc Netw 2009;7(1):8–39.
19. Lamm DL, Blumenstein BA, Crissman JD, et al. Maintenance bacillus Calmette-Guerin immunotherapy for recurrent TA, T1 and carcinoma in situ transitional cell carcinoma of the bladder: a randomized Southwest Oncology Group Study. J Urol 2000; 163(4):1124–9.
20. Kilbridge KL, Kantoff P. Intravesical therapy for superficial bladder cancer: is it a wash? J Clin Oncol 1994;12(1):1–4.
21. Tolley DA, Parmar MK, Grigor KM, et al. The effect of intravesical mitomycin C on recurrence of newly diagnosed superficial bladder cancer: a further report with 7 years of follow up. J Urol 1996;155(4):1233–8.
22. Sylvester RJ, Oosterlinck W, van der Meijden AP. A single immediate postoperative instillation of chemotherapy decreases the risk of recurrence in patients with stage Ta T1 bladder cancer: a meta-analysis of published results of randomized clinical trials. J Urol 2004;171(6 Pt 1):2186–90 [quiz: 2435].
23. Marchetti A, Wang L, Magar R, et al. Management of patients with Bacilli Calmette-Guerin-refractory carcinoma in situ of the urinary bladder: cost implications of a clinical trial for valrubicin. Clin Ther 2000;22(4): 422–38.
24. Smith JA, Labasky RF, Montie JE, et al. Guideline for the management of nonmuscle invasive bladder cancer: (stages Ta, T1, and Tis): 2007 Update. 2007. Available at: http://www.auanet.org/content/guidelines-and-quality-care/clinical-guidelines/main-reports/bladcan07/chapter1.pdf. Accessed December 3, 2012.
25. Brausi M, Witjes JA, Lamm D, et al. A review of current guidelines and best practice recommendations for the management of nonmuscle invasive bladder cancer by the International Bladder Cancer Group. J Urol 2011;186(6):2158–67.
26. Holmang S, Johansson SL. Stage Ta-T1 bladder cancer: the relationship between findings at first followup cystoscopy and subsequent recurrence and progression. J Urol 2002;167(4):1634–7.
27. Mariappan P, Smith G. A surveillance schedule for G1Ta bladder cancer allowing efficient use of check cystoscopy and safe discharge at 5 years based on a 25-year prospective database. J Urol 2005;173(4): 1108–11.

28. Hemani ML, Makarov DV, Huang WC, et al. The effect of changes in Medicare reimbursement on the practice of office and hospital-based endoscopic surgery for bladder cancer. Cancer 2010; 116(5):1264–71.
29. Mowatt G, Zhu S, Kilonzo M, et al. Systematic review of the clinical effectiveness and cost-effectiveness of photodynamic diagnosis and urine biomarkers (FISH, ImmunoCyt, NMP22) and cytology for the detection and follow-up of bladder cancer. Health Technol Assess 2010;14(4):1–331, iii–iv.
30. Raitanen MP. The role of BTA stat test in follow-up of patients with bladder cancer: results from FinnBladder studies. World J Urol 2008;26(1):45–50.
31. Mian C, Pycha A, Wiener H, et al. Immunocyt: a new tool for detecting transitional cell cancer of the urinary tract. J Urol 1999;161(5):1486–9.
32. Olsson H, Zackrisson B. ImmunoCyt a useful method in the follow-up protocol for patients with urinary bladder carcinoma. Scand J Urol Nephrol 2001;35(4):280–2.
33. Nguyen CT, Jones JS. Defining the role of NMP22 in bladder cancer surveillance. World J Urol 2008; 26(1):51–8.
34. Lotan Y, Roehrborn CG. Sensitivity and specificity of commonly available bladder tumor markers versus cytology: results of a comprehensive literature review and meta-analyses. Urology 2003;61(1):109–18 [discussion: 118].
35. Halling KC, Kipp BR. Bladder cancer detection using FISH (UroVysion assay). Adv Anat Pathol 2008;15(5):279–86.
36. Moonen PM, Merkx GF, Peelen P, et al. UroVysion compared with cytology and quantitative cytology in the surveillance of non-muscle-invasive bladder cancer. Eur Urol 2007;51(5):1275–80 [discussion: 1280].
37. Savic S, Zlobec I, Thalmann GN, et al. The prognostic value of cytology and fluorescence in situ hybridization in the follow-up of nonmuscle-invasive bladder cancer after intravesical bacillus Calmette-Guerin therapy. Int J Cancer 2009; 124(12):2899–904.
38. Kamat AM, Karam JA, Grossman HB, et al. Prospective trial to identify optimal bladder cancer surveillance protocol: reducing costs while maximizing sensitivity. BJU Int 2011;108(7):1119–23.
39. Cauberg EC, Mamoulakis C, de la Rosette JJ, et al. Narrow band imaging-assisted transurethral resection for non-muscle invasive bladder cancer significantly reduces residual tumour rate. World J Urol 2011;29(4):503–9.
40. Stenzl A, Burger M, Fradet Y, et al. Hexaminolevulinate guided fluorescence cystoscopy reduces recurrence in patients with nonmuscle invasive bladder cancer. J Urol 2010;184(5):1907–13.
41. Gilbert SM, Dunn RL, Hollenbeck BK, et al. Development and validation of the Bladder Cancer Index: a comprehensive, disease specific measure of health related quality of life in patients with localized bladder cancer. J Urol 2010;183(5):1764–9.
42. Gilbert SM, Wood DP, Dunn RL, et al. Measuring health-related quality of life outcomes in bladder cancer patients using the Bladder Cancer Index (BCI). Cancer 2007;109(9):1756–62.
43. Cella DF. FACIT manual. Manual of the Functional Assessment of Chronic Illness Therapy (FACIT) scales version 4. Evanston (IL): Evanston Northwestern Healthcare and Northwestern University; 1997.
44. Sprangers MA, Cull A, Groenvold M, et al. The European Organization for Research and Treatment of Cancer approach to developing questionnaire modules: an update and overview. EORTC Quality of Life Study Group. Qual Life Res 1998; 7(4):291–300.
45. Yoshimura K, Utsunomiya N, Ichioka K, et al. Impact of superficial bladder cancer and transurethral resection on general health-related quality of life: an SF-36 survey. Urology 2005;65(2):290–4.
46. Mack D, Frick J. Quality of life in patients undergoing bacille Calmette-Guerin therapy for superficial bladder cancer. Br J Urol 1996;78(3):369–71.
47. Allareddy V, Kennedy J, West MM, et al. Quality of life in long-term survivors of bladder cancer. Cancer 2006;106(11):2355–62.
48. Hemani ML, Bennett CL. The excessive cost of early stage bladder cancer care: are providers really to blame? Cancer 2010;116(15):3530–2.
49. Madeb R, Golijanin D, Noyes K, et al. Treatment of nonmuscle invading bladder cancer: do physicians in the United States practice evidence based medicine? The use and economic implications of intravesical chemotherapy after transurethral resection of bladder tumors. Cancer 2009;115(12):2660–70.
50. Chamie K, Saigal CS, Lai J, et al. Compliance with guidelines for patients with bladder cancer: variation in the delivery of care. Cancer 2011;117(23): 5392–401.
51. Lee CT, Barocas D, Globe DR, et al. Economic and humanistic consequences of preventable bladder tumor recurrences in nonmuscle invasive bladder cancer cases. J Urol 2012;188(6):2114–9.
52. Schrag D, Hsieh LJ, Rabbani F, et al. Adherence to surveillance among patients with superficial bladder cancer. J Natl Cancer Inst 2003;95(8):588–97.
53. Hollenbeck BK, Ye Z, Dunn RL, et al. Provider treatment intensity and outcomes for patients with early-stage bladder cancer. J Natl Cancer Inst 2009; 101(8):571–80.
54. Hollingsworth JM, Zhang YS, Miller DC, et al. Identifying better practices for early-stage bladder cancer. Med Care 2011;49(12):1112–7.

55. Hernandez S, Lopez-Knowles E, Lloreta J, et al. Prospective study of FGFR3 mutations as a prognostic factor in nonmuscle invasive urothelial bladder carcinomas. J Clin Oncol 2006;24(22):3664–71.
56. van Oers JM, Zwarthoff EC, Rehman I, et al. FGFR3 mutations indicate better survival in invasive upper urinary tract and bladder tumours. Eur Urol 2009; 55(3):650–7.
57. van Kessel KE, Kompier LC, de Bekker-Grob EW, et al. FGFR3 mutation analysis on voided urine samples to reduce cystoscopies and cost in non-muscle invasive bladder cancer surveillance: a comparison of three different strategies. J Urol 2012. [Epub ahead of print].
58. Pruthi RS, Baldwin N, Bhalani V, et al. Conservative management of low risk superficial bladder tumors. J Urol 2008;179(1):87–90 [discussion: 90].
59. Birkmeyer NJ, Share D, Campbell DA Jr, et al. Partnering with payers to improve surgical quality: the Michigan plan. Surgery 2005;138(5):815–20.
60. Flum DR, Fisher N, Thompson J, et al. Washington State's approach to variability in surgical processes/outcomes: Surgical Clinical Outcomes Assessment Program (SCOAP). Surgery 2005;138(5):821–8.
61. Share DA, Campbell DA, Birkmeyer N, et al. How a regional collaborative of hospitals and physicians in Michigan cut costs and improved the quality of care. Health Aff (Millwood) 2011;30(4):636–45.
62. Kwon S, Florence M, Grigas P, et al. Creating a learning healthcare system in surgery: Washington State's Surgical Care and Outcomes Assessment Program (SCOAP) at 5 years. Surgery 2012;151(2): 146–52.
63. Miller DC, Murtagh DS, Suh RS, et al. Establishment of a urological surgery quality collaborative. J Urol 2010;184(6):2485–90.
64. Miller DC, Murtagh DS, Suh RS, et al. Regional collaboration to improve radiographic staging practices among men with early stage prostate cancer. J Urol 2011;186(3):844–9.

New Imaging Techniques for Non-Muscle Invasive Bladder Cancer: Ready for Primetime

Joseph A. Gillespie, MD, Michael A. O'Donnell, MD*

KEYWORDS

• Non-muscle invasive bladder cancer • Transurethral resection • White light cystoscopy
• Fluorescence cystoscopy • Narrow band imaging • Optical coherence tomography
• Confocal laser endomicroscopy

KEY POINTS

- Non-muscle invasive bladder cancer (NMIBC) is confined to the epithelium and lamina propria.
- Complete eradication and bladder preservation is the goal of transurethral resection (TUR).
- Technological limitations contribute to failure of TUR.
- Failure results in recurrence and progression.
- New imaging modalities that increase the urologist's ability to detect, stage, and treat NMIBC at TUR can have a significant impact in the treatment of NMIBC.

FLUORESCENCE CYSTOSCOPY

- Enhances tumor detection at initial resection for all stages and grades.
- Detection of carcinoma in situ is particularly enhanced with fluorescence cystoscopy (FC).
- Decreases rates of recurrence.

NARROW BAND IMAGING

- Shows similar efficacy in detection of tumors as FC.
- Does not require instillation of fluorophore in bladder before usage.

OPTICAL COHERENCE TOMOGRAPHY

- Provides real-time tumor grading during TUR.

CONFOCAL LASER ENDOMICROSCOPY

- Allows microscopic examination of urothelium in real-time for histopathologic analysis.

Bladder cancer remains one of the most difficult clinical conundrums for the practicing urologist. On the extremities of the disease, management of bladder cancer is simplified. The progressive nature of muscle-invasive disease dictates definitive management and the gold standard remains radical cystectomy. At the other extreme, the likelihood of a single, subcentimeter, superficial (Ta) low-grade tumor progressing to muscle invasion is less than 1%.[1] Adequate management

Disclosures: Dr Gillespie: None; Dr O'Donnell: Consultant: Viventia, Spectrum, Allergan, Endo Pharmaceuticals, Merck, Medical Enterprises.
Potential Conflict of Interest: Dr Gillespie: None; Dr O'Donnell: Scientific Advisory Board, Photocure.

Department of Urology, University of Iowa, 200 Hawkins Drive, 3 RCP, Iowa City, IA 52242-1089, USA
* Corresponding author.
E-mail address: michael-odonnell@uiowa.edu

Urol Clin N Am 40 (2013) 271–279
http://dx.doi.org/10.1016/j.ucl.2013.01.014

of such a lesion is eradication by transurethral resection (TUR) and a single instillation of intravesical chemotherapy at the time of resection. Recurrence and progression are monitored by quarterly cystoscopy for 1 year, decreasing in frequency thereafter if the patient remains free of tumor. Most patients, however, lie in between these 2 extremes. For these patients with non-muscle invasive bladder cancer (NMIBC), tumor recurrence and progression to muscle-invasive disease are a lifelong risk despite the multimodal application of chemotherapeutics, immune therapies, and repeated surgical resections.

Non-muscle invasive disease is confined to the epithelium (Ta) or the lamina propria (T1). A patient suspected of having bladder cancer undergoes evaluation with upper tract imaging, urine cytology, and cystoscopy.[2] The standard for evaluation of the lower urinary tract is white light cystoscopy (WLC), followed by TUR of any tumor that is discovered. Accurate assessment of histopathologic grade and depth of tumor invasion is required for the implementation of proper treatment. This implementation is accomplished by complete and accurate endoscopic resection at the time of TUR. For TUR to be successful, the tumor must be removed in its entirety, along with a sufficient margin of surrounding mucosae and the muscle directly beneath the tumor.[2]

WLC is, however, a technology fraught with deficiencies. Complete resection of papillary tumors is problematic and, as Brausi and colleagues[3] demonstrated, often leads to early recurrence. As a result, a single TUR is often insufficient for the task. A repeat TUR, performed within 2 to 6 weeks of the initial TUR, shows residual disease a significant portion of the time depending on stage, grade, and tumor multiplicity. For pathologically confirmed disease confined to the epithelium (pTa), residual tumor is seen between 6% and 37% of the time.[4,5] The rate is higher for disease that has been pathologically confirmed to invade into, but not through, the lamina propria (pT1) (33%–78%) and carcinoma in situ (CIS) (70%–80%)[5,6] and incomplete resection is not the only limitation. High-grade Ta or T1 tumors are understaged 10% of the time even when muscle is present in the original resection specimen and will be found to be muscle invasive at re-resection. To what degree deficiencies of surgical technique contribute to this phenomenon is unknown. It is doubtless a factor, but there are also significant technological limitations that contribute to a surgeon's inability to eradicate a bladder tumor completely at the time of resection.

Further evidence supporting this comes from the difficulty of finding and eradicating CIS as reported from trials that have recently explored the utility of random bladder biopsies. Despite the relative ease with which CIS is detected by bladder wash—fully 90% of patients with CIS are thought to have a positive cytology[2]—standard WLC fails to detect a lesion 50% of the time.[7] CIS is a flat, high-grade noninvasive lesion that, unlike Ta and T1 disease, has a high potential for progression when left untreated.[8] Classically described as a red "velvety" lesion, CIS is often multifocal and may be macroscopically invisible. Occult CIS is common when high-grade pTa or pT1 lesions have been identified and is present upward of 40% of the time.[8]

Of prognostic significance, CIS is, after tumor histopathologic grade, the second most important factor predicting progression to muscle invasive disease.[8] Its detection is therefore paramount for accurate risk stratification and the implementation of treatment. Random bladder biopsies are often performed for just such a reason, as a random survey of the bladder mucosae for occult CIS. One recent study demonstrated random biopsies to be positive for CIS 8% of the time.[9] Of clinical significance was the fact that, in a different study of random biopsying, random biopsies changed the indicated therapy 4.6% of the time.[10]

Finally, the economic impact of bladder cancer is immense. From diagnosis to death, bladder cancer is the most expensive cancer in the United States.[11] The inefficacy of cystoscopy for diagnosis and surveillance, in conjunction with the recurrent nature of the disease, is responsible for much of its financial burden. Technological advancements that can decrease recurrence have the potential to have a significant financial impact on health care costs if implemented properly.

FLUORESCENCE CYSTOSCOPY

The topical application of the protoporphyrin 5-aminolevulinic acid (5-ALA) was first performed in the early 1990s by a group of Munich urologists.[12] Before this, it had been shown that the intravenous injection of heme derivatives preferentially accrued in urothelial carcinomas.[13] Heme derivatives are photoactive substances that absorb light at one wavelength and emit at another. Initially, the practical implementation of photodynamic tumor detection using heme derivatives, in particular porphyrin II, was attempted, but ultimately abandoned because of the systemic effects of skin photosensitization due to the porphyrins. Of practical importance, however, was the exposition that a photosensitizer could be used to enhance cystoscopy and tumor detection.

The Munich group, along with several other pioneering groups,[14,15] showed that WLC could be effectively enhanced by the topical application of the protoporphyrin 5-ALA with minimal risk to the patient. Topical application managed to avoid the systemic complications associated with intravenous administration; however, the lipophilicity of 5-ALA still allowed for reasonably rapid local absorption over a period of several hours. These small proof-of-principle studies hinted, but were insufficiently powered to prove, that the instillation of 5-ALA before TUR could result in increased detection of all lesions and, in particular, 5-ALA had a distinct advantage in the enhanced detection of CIS. Subsequent randomized, prospective clinical trials would support these initial claims. 5-ALA has been consistently shown to enhance the detection of CIS greatly, with 33% to 36.7% more lesions detected.[16,17] An advantage was also seen with the detection of pTa lesions and pT1 lesions, but it is not as pronounced (7%–11% and 3.6%–13%, respectively).

Enhanced detection at initial resection should lead to an increase in the rate of complete resection and a decrease of residual tumors seen at re-resection. Filbeck and colleagues[18] demonstrated this in a randomized, prospective clinical trial. The WLC group had a 25.2% rate of residual tumor at 6 weeks, compared with 4.5% for the 5-ALA arm of the trial. On a stage-by-stage basis, the rate of residual tumor at 6 weeks for pTa was 17.8% and 3% for WLC and fluorescence cystoscopy (FC), respectively. pT1 had a greater rate of residual tumor for both, with the WLC arm having a rate of residual tumor of 36% and the FC arm having a rate of 11.8%. The difference was even greater when comparing residual CIS. In the WLC arm, CIS was found in 80% of patients at 6 weeks, whereas there was no residual CIS seen in the FC arm. This group also looked at the rate of recurrence in this trial and in a subsequent study with an 8-year follow-up.[19] The rate of overall recurrence for the WLC arm was 44% versus 16% for the FC arm. Further analysis based on risk stratification was also performed by this group. At 8 years there was a significant difference in recurrence-free survival (RFS) when comparing the FC arm to the WLC arm for all risk groups. The WLC group performed remarkably similarly regardless of risk stratification at 8 years (42%–45% for low, intermediate, and high risk stratification). The benefit of FC was greatest for low-risk patients (patients with solitary low-grade pTa or pT1 tumors), with 81% having no recurrence at 8 years. As tumor multiplicity and grade increased, however, the advantage narrowed but was still significant. The intermediate-risk group had the same grade and stage as the low-risk group, but presented with multiple tumors initially, which resulted in an RFS of 70% in the FC arm at 8 years. High-grade disease, including CIS, conferred additional risk of recurrence at 8 years. Nonetheless, 60% of patients remained recurrence-free in the high-risk group.

Further refinements have resulted in hexaminolevulinate (HAL)—Hexvix in Europe (Photocure ASA, Oslo, Norway) and Cysview in North America (Photocure USA, Princeton, NJ)—largely supplanting 5-ALA as the protoporphyrin of choice. HAL is a hexyl ester derivative of 5-ALA. It is significantly more potent than 5-ALA due to its increased lipophilicity and tissue solubility. This increased lipophilicity and tissue solubility allow for decreased instillation time and surgeon convenience for practical usage during TUR without any increase in its complications. Like 5-ALA, HAL absorbs blue light (wavelength 380–480) and emits red light (**Fig. 1**). Polarized light filters allow for visual enhancement of a tumor that appears red on a dark blue background.

Stenzl and colleagues[20] have shown similar results with HAL in an international randomized,

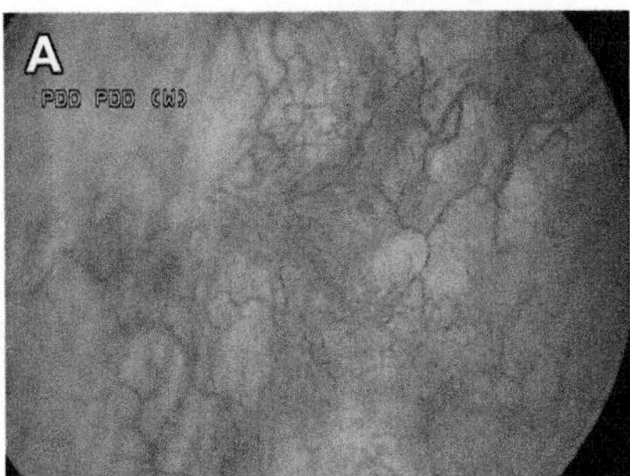

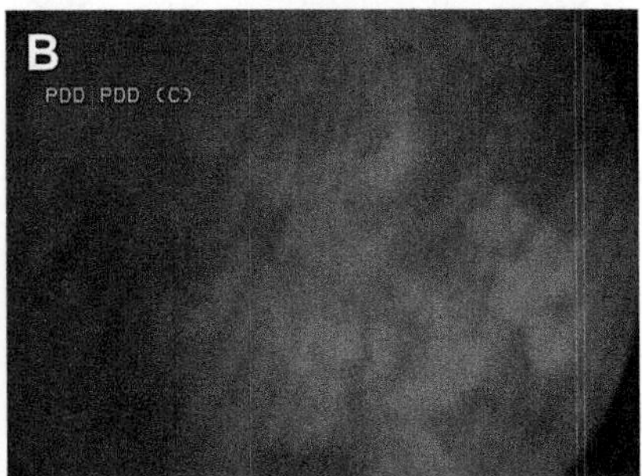

Fig. 1. (*A*) White light cystoscopy of a CIS lesion. Perception of lesion is limited to hypervascularity and subtle yellowish pigmentary discoloration of mucosae. (*B*) Fluorescent cystoscopy of the same lesion. The red enhancement of the tumor is not limited to identification but also extends the boundary of the lesion to be resected.

prospective trial that compared WLC-based and HAL-based FC. In this study there was a 32% increase in the detection of CIS in the fluorescence arm. Moreover, enhanced detection of tumors that were clinically relevant was also noted in this trial. The patients in the WLC arm underwent white light interrogation only, whereas the fluorescence arm group underwent an initial white light examination that was then followed by blue light interrogation. Tumors were mapped at both times and the results were recorded. In the fluorescence arm there was a 16% increase in the number of lesions detected. Of these lesions, 41% were high-grade Ta or T1 lesions that would not have been detected by WLC alone. This group also looked at rates of recurrence in a subsequent study.[21] The time to recurrence was significantly improved in the fluorescence arm when compared with the white light–only arm (16.4 months vs 9.4 months, respectively).

A further advantage that FC has over standard WLC is its ability to more accurately demarcate tumor from normal mucosae and aid in the complete resection of a tumor that is visible with both modalities. A single-center prospective, randomized trial by Geavlete and colleagues[22] found that 8.5% of tumors that had been resected under WLC had pathologically confirmed positive margins that could be visualized by FC (**Fig. 2**). This group also showed in a subsequent study that at the time of initial resection FC was superior in detecting multiple tumors when compared with WLC (35.2% vs 14.1%, respectively).[23] Furthermore, their analysis showed that HAL-based FC modified the risk stratification and the postoperative treatment regimen in several patients and aided a more accurate pathologic classification. Of particular note, patients who would had been declared "tumor free" by WLC, but the addition of HAL resulted in increased detection of bladder tumor. Stated another way, at initial TUR, there was a failure to find a tumor—the patient was "tumor-free"—7.7% of the time. In the FC arm, only 1.4% of patients were designated "tumor-free."

Not all studies to date have shown a uniform advantage of FC over WLC. Schumacher and colleagues,[16] in a randomized, multicenter, prospective trial, failed to show any advantage with respect to rates of recurrence for FC over WLC. An overall advantage for FC was seen in tumor detection and was consistent with other published trials—33% advantage in detecting CIS, 13% for pT1, and 6.7% for pTa—but no advantage was seen in rates of recurrence at 12 months in either low-risk or high-risk patients. One factor that could contribute to the difference seen in this trial is that it was a multicenter study. As a result, some of the surgeons who performed the TUR resections had limited experience with FC before their inclusion in the study.

Criticisms of HAL and 5-ALA are primarily twofold. One concern is its lack of specificity and high false-positive rate. The other concern is that neither influences disease progression and the number of individuals who progress to muscle-invasive disease is unchanged. Nonspecific uptake of heme derivatives does occur. This nonspecific uptake of heme derivatives is most notable in patients with a prior history of TUR and bacillus calmette-guerin (BCG) therapy. Inflammatory lesions, scars, and granulomas can all appear as red lesions on a blue background, the same as an FC-positive bladder tumor. Initial studies reported false-positive rates for FC as high as 51%.[24] However, the inability to diagnose strictly based on appearance is not unique to FC and false-positive biopsying occurs in even in the most experienced hands under WLC. Most recent large prospective, randomized trials have similar rates for false-positive biopsying (10%–15%) regardless

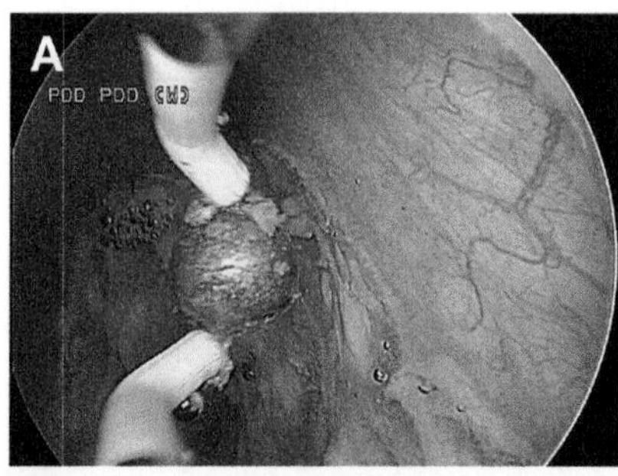

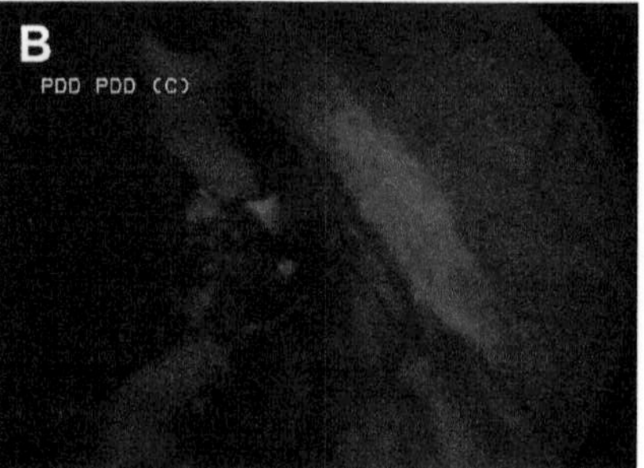

Fig. 2. (*A*) The bed of a papillary lesion that has been completely resected by WLC. Customarily, it is the authors' practice to extend the margin of the resected tumor to ensure complete resection of the tumor. (*B*) Reexamination of the tumor bed by fluorescent cystoscopy reveals a positive margin. Tumor resection margin was extended at the time of the resection accordingly.

of the modality directing the biopsy, with a slight increase of 1% or 2% for blue light–directed biopsies.[17,23]

With regard to progression, FC-based cystoscopy has not been conclusively shown to improve progression-free survival. Stenzl and colleagues[20] found no difference between the 2 arms, whereas others have shown a modest improvement of 1% or 2%, but these were not statistically significant.[16,23]

Several studies have looked into to the cost-effectiveness of fluorescence-based cystoscopy. Stenzl and colleagues[25] first looked into the cost-effectiveness of 5-ALA and found that the savings could be substantial if the difference in the rate of recurrence was 20%. The savings were largely due to avoided TURs. This savings covered the added expense of the supplemental equipment needed for FC by a factor of 3. Daniltchenko and colleagues[26] also found a significant cost-savings based primarily on the decrease in the total number of TURs that would need to be performed. Most convincingly, Zaak and colleagues[27] performed a cost analysis on a per-patient basis and analyzed patients who had undergone WLC and FC. They found a savings of about $250 per patient per year over a 7-year follow-up.

NARROW BAND IMAGING

The propensity of bladder cancers to be hypervascular is exploited in narrow band imaging (NBI). White light emanating from the lamp source is filtered into 2 discrete wavelengths—415 (blue) and 540 (green)—that have only superficial tissue penetration. Correspondingly, these are the peak absorptive ranges for hemoglobin. When combined with high-resolution magnifying endoscopy, the vascular architecture of a bladder lesion is accentuated and the disparity between malignant and benign is heightened. The technology was initially used for the characterization of colonic lesions[28,29] and was adapted to the cystoscope shortly thereafter.[28] Vascular structures appear dark brown (capillaries) and green (veins) on a pink-white background (normal mucosae) (**Fig. 3**). Unlike fluorescence cystoscopy, it does not require the instillation of a photoactive substance. Likewise, it avoids the added costs of the porphyrin and time associated with its instillation, and is more convenient to implement.

Initial studies have shown comparable efficacy to FC with regard to CIS, Ta, and T1 disease detection. Geavlete and colleagues,[30] in a single-center, prospective trial where patients were interrogated under WLC and then NBI, found a 33% difference in rates of detection for CIS in favor of NBI. pTa and pT1 also had increased rates of detection of 8.7% and 10.9%, respectively. This increased detection of tumors by NBI resulted in therapeutic augmentation in 10.6% of the patients where additional lesions were detected. Cauberg and colleagues[31] found a similar increase in total detection for NMIBC. Although their study tended to have low-grade disease and lower rates of CIS, 28 of 79 patients who were eventually diagnosed with NMIBC had additional lesions found by NBI. Conversely, WLC detected lesions that were not seen with NBI in only 3 of 78 patients. Of note, in this study the prevalence of CIS was 10.6%. NBI and WLC failed to detect CIS in 18% of the patients diagnosed with CIS and in these cases random biopsies were responsible for detection. Further studies that compare NBI with FC directly will be needed to determine which modality is superior for the detection of CIS.

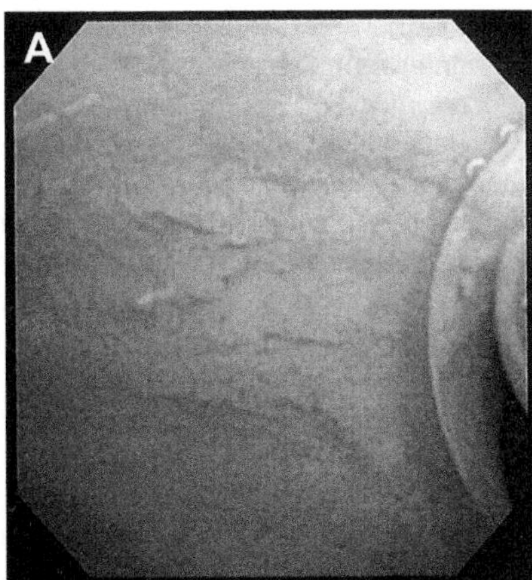

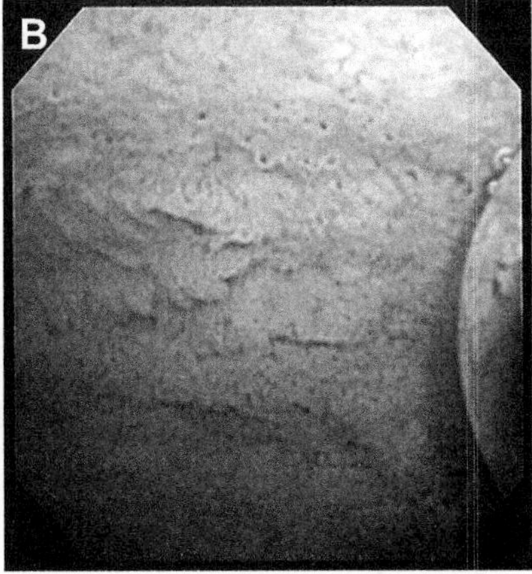

Fig. 3. (*A*) White light cystoscopy of a bladder tumor at the dome of the bladder (air bubble on the right side of the frame). (*B*) Enhanced contrast of tumor relative to WLC with brown tumor on green/white background.

Naselli and colleagues[32] analyzed NBI superiority to WLC during a second-look TUR in patients with high-grade NMIBC at 1 month. In this prospective observational study, patients underwent a second-look TUR under WLC first and then were interrogated for the first time by NBI. In all, 34% of patients had pathologically confirmed residual disease during the second-look TUR. Approximately one-third of these patients had lesions that were missed by the 2 TURs under WLC, but were detected by NBI. This same group also assessed rates of recurrence in a prospective, randomized trial.[33] NBI had 19.8% fewer recurrences at 1 year when compared with WLC. Similarly, Herr and Donat[34] found an RFS of 29 months versus 13 months for NBI and WLC, respectively, in patients with low-grade disease.

Early studies have shown high rates of false-positive biopsying, but this has not been borne out by later trials. This pattern is similar to what was observed in the early trials with HAL and 5-ALA. Herr and Donat[35] and Cauberg and colleagues[31] both reported a false-positive rate of biopsyof 36% and 31.6%, respectively, for NBI. Geavlete et al, in a recent prospective trial, had false-positive rates of 13.6% versus 11.5% for NBI and WLC, respectively.[30]

OPTICAL COHERENCE TOMOGRAPHY

Several new technologies allow for real-time, microscopic evaluation of the bladder mucosae. Optical coherence tomography (OCT) provides a cross-sectional image similar to an ultrasound, but uses near-infrared light instead of sound waves. Use of near-infrared light allows for increased resolution relative to high-frequency ultrasound. With a depth of penetration of 1 to 3 mm, the epithelia, lamina propria, and muscularis propria are readily identifiable. The corresponding layers have a different scatter and appearance. Tumors appear as disruptions in the tissue planes. A fiberoptic-based technology, OCT is adaptable to a rigid or flexible WLC and is used as an adjunct means of microscopic interrogation of the urothelium and underlying microarchitecture. Virtual tumor grading is performed by the surgeon in real-time during a TUR.

Early prospective studies have shown the significant limitations of early iterations of this technology. Karl and colleagues[36] were able to identify and stage all lesions correctly that were detected by WLC, but had an exceedingly high false-positive rate. Of 102 lesions identified by WLC and interrogated by OCT, 45 were suspected to be malignant by OCT. Malignancy was confirmed by biopsy on only 14 of these lesions. Encouragingly, there were no false negatives. Virtual histopathologic analysis was limited to tumor stage as the fidelity of the device did not allow for tumor grading. Device resolution in these early trials was 10 to 20 μm and depth of tissue penetration was limited to 2 mm. Recent advancements have increased resolution to submicrometer levels and are integrating Doppler and enhanced 3-dimensional imaging.[37] Furthermore, integrative software has been added to mitigate diagnostic subjectivity. Promising work has been performed by Ren and colleagues[38] in a transgenic mouse model for CIS. This group has additionally used OCT in conjunction with other imaging modalities (eg, WLC, NBI, and FC). The early results are promising for the combined use of OCT with both FC and NBI; however, further studies in humans will need to be performed as the applicability of the transgenic mouse model is not known.

CONFOCAL LASER ENDOMICROSCOPY

Confocal laser endomicroscopy (CLE) is another modality that, like OCT, is capable of examining the urothelium on a subcellular level. Fiberoptic advancements have allowed the conventionally bulky confocal laser microscope to be miniaturized and adapted to the working channels of endoscopes. Currently, it is approved for use within the respiratory and gastrointestinal tracts with promising results, particularly in identifying precancerous lesions in the esophagus.[39] Probes have been developed that accommodate both rigid and flexible cystoscopes. CLE does require administration of a fluorescent contrast agent, fluorescein, which has long been used by ophthalmologists and has an excellent safety profile when used optically and in the gastrointestinal tract. In the lower urinary tract, fluorescein is administered intravenously and/or intravesically. Fluorescein stains the extracellular matrix and penetrates the lamina propria regardless of whether it is administered intravenously or intravesically. It does not, however, allow visualization of nuclei or the muscularis propria. Wu and colleagues[40] compiled an atlas of upper and lower tract lesions and found a distinct profile for normal, inflammatory, and malignant lesions. The reproducibility and widespread applicability of CLE are currently unknown and further studies are needed.

DISCUSSION

Tumor multiplicity is the single greatest prognostic factor that influences cancer recurrence.[8] The enhanced ability to detect more tumors at initial resection and more accurately assess the boundary between normal mucosae and malignancy allows for a more complete resection at TUR and an increase in time to recurrence. Both NBI and FC have shown superiority with respect to WLC alone in tumor detection for all stages. The most pronounced advantage is with respect to the detection of CIS. Further trials will be needed to elucidate which method is superior.

NBI has the added advantage of not requiring instillation of contrast media. Not requiring instillation of contrast media avoids the costs of the contrast and associated disposables as well as the man-hours associated with its instillation. A similar advantage exists for OCT relative to CLE.

It should be reiterated that all the technologies mentioned in this article are meant to be used as an adjunct to WLC and are not meant to supplant WLC. As illustrated by Cauberg and colleagues,[31] NBI had a distinct advantage in CIS detection, but in approximately 4% of patients lesions were detected by WLC that were not seen by NBI. Furthermore, the addition of NBI or FC to WLC will not obviate random biopsies as persistent, occult CIS will not be eradicated by the universal adoption of either. The prevalence of occult CIS should decrease, but further studies are needed to define the advantage.

The addition of OCT or CLE has the potential to aid in enhancing the real-time accuracy of histopathologic analysis. This addition of OCT or CLE in turn could result in a decrease in pathologic specimens requiring processing and possibly even complication rates for TUR, but it will not likely influence rates of recurrence as the technologies currently exist. The field-of-view for both is limited. Furthermore, the lesion is still identified by WLC, or if used concurrently with NBI or FC, by those modalities. OCT and CLE are therefore dependent on those technologies for the identification of lesions. Universal interrogation of the bladder mucosae is not practicable by either OCT or CLE. Further limitations of OCT and CLE are the need for direct apposition of mucosae and device for use, proving untenable in certain areas of the bladder like the anterior bladder neck and posterior dome.

Progression and bladder preservation have not been conclusively shown to be affected by either FC or NBI. The greatest prognosticator of progression is tumor grade.[8] High-grade disease and, in particular, concomitant CIS carry a significant risk of progression.[41] Although FC and NBI greatly enhance the capability of WLC to detect CIS, and FC has been shown to more accurately demarcate tumor boundaries, the sensitivity of either modality is not absolute. Occult disease will persist in a minority of patients and progression can then occur. Larger trials are needed that compare NBI and FC and may be able to show an influence on progression.

REFERENCES

1. Babjuk M, Oosterlinck W, Sylvester R, et al, European Association of Urology (EAU). EAU guidelines on non-muscle-invasive urothelial carcinoma of the bladder, the 2011 update. Eur Urol 2011;59:997–1008.
2. Hall MC, Chang SS, Dalbagni G, et al. Guideline for the management of nonmuscle invasive bladder cancer (stages Ta, T1, and Tis): 2007 update. J Urol 2007;178:2314–30.
3. Brausi M, Collette L, Kurth K, et al. Variability in the recurrence rate at first follow-up cystoscopy after TUR in stage Ta T1 transitional cell carcinoma of the bladder: a combined analysis of seven EORTC studies. Eur Urol 2002;41:523–31.
4. Herr HW. The value of a second transurethral resection in evaluating patients with bladder tumors. J Urol 1999;162:74–6.
5. Schips L, Augustin H, Zigeuner RE, et al. Is repeated transurethral resection justified in patients with newly diagnosed superficial bladder cancer? Urology 2002;59:220–3.
6. Jakse G, Algaba F, Malmström PU, et al. A second-look TUR in T1 transitional cell carcinoma: why? Eur Urol 2004;45:539–46.
7. Fradet Y, Grossman HB, Gomella L, et al. A comparison of hexaminolevulinate fluorescence cystoscopy and white light cystoscopy for the detection of carcinoma in situ in patients with bladder cancer: a phase III, multicenter study. J Urol 2007; 178:68–73.
8. Sylvester RJ, van der Meijden A, Witjes JA, et al. High-grade Ta urothelial carcinoma and carcinoma in situ of the bladder. Urology 2005;66(6 Suppl 1): 90–107.
9. May F, Treiber U, Hartung R, et al. Significance of random bladder biopsies in superficial bladder cancer. Eur Urol 2003;44:47–50.
10. Librenjak D, Novakovic ZS, Situm M, et al. Biopsies of the normal-appearing urothelium in primary bladder cancer. Urol Ann 2010;2:71–5.
11. Botteman MF, Pashos CL, Redaelli A, et al. The health economics of bladder cancer: a comprehensive review of the published literature. Pharmacoeconomics 2003;21:1315–30.
12. Baumgartner R, Hofstetter A, Jocham D, et al. Photodynamic diagnosis in urology-first clinical experiences with a new method for detection of early stage cancer. Lasermedizin 1992;8:16–21.
13. Benson RC Jr, Farrow GM, Kinsey JH, et al. Detection and localization of in situ carcinoma of the bladder with hematoporphyrin derivative. Mayo Clin Proc 1982;57:548–55.

14. Kriegmair M, Baumgartner R, Kneuchel R, et al. Fluorescence photodetection of neloplastic urothelial lesions following intravesical instillation of 5-aminolevulinic acid. Urology 1994;44:836–41.
15. Jichlinski P, Forrer M, Mizeret J, et al. Clinical evaluation of a method for detecting superficial transitional cell carcinoma of the bladder by light-induced fluorescence of protoporphyrin IX following topical application of 5-aminolevulinic acid: preliminary results. Lasers Surg Med 1997;20:402–8.
16. Schumacher MC, Holmäng S, Davidsson T, et al. Transurethral resection of non–muscle-invasive bladder transitional cell cancers with or without 5-aminolevulinic acid under visible and fluorescent light: results of a prospective, randomised, multicentre study. Eur Urol 2010;57:293–9.
17. Stenzl A, Burger M, Fradet Y, et al. Hexaminolevulinate guided fluorescence cystoscopy reduces recurrence in patients with nonmuscle invasive bladder cancer. J Urol 2010;184:1907–14.
18. Filbeck T, Pichlmeier U, Knuechel R, et al. Clinically relevant improvement of recurrence-free survival with 5-aminolevulinic acid induced fluorescence diagnosis in patients with superficial bladder tumors. J Urol 2002;168:67–71.
19. Denzinger S, Burger M, Walter B, et al. Clinically relevant reduction in risk of recurrence of superficial bladder cancer using 5-aminolevulinic acid induced fluorescence diagnosis: 8 year results of prospective randomized study. Urology 2007;69:675–9.
20. Stenzl A, Penkoff H, Dajc-Sommerer E, et al. Detection and clinical outcome of urinary bladder cancer with 5-aminolevulinic acid-induced fluorescence cystoscopy. Cancer 2011;117:938–47.
21. Grossman HB, Stenzl A, Fradet Y, et al. Long-term decrease in bladder cancer recurrence with hexaminolevulinate enabled fluorescence cystoscopy. J Urol 2012;188:58–62.
22. Geavlete B, Jecu M, Multescu R, et al. HAL blue-light cystoscopy in high-risk nonmuscle-invasive bladder cancer–re-TURBT recurrence rates in a prospective, randomized study. Urology 2010;76:664–9.
23. Geavlete B, Multescu R, Georgescu D, et al. Treatment changes and long-term recurrence rates after hexaminolevulinate (HAL) fluorescence cystoscopy: does it really make a difference in patients with non-muscle-invasive bladder cancer (NMIBC)? BJU Int 2012;109:549–56.
24. De Dominicis C, Libertu M, Perugia G, et al. Role of 5-aminolevulinic acid in the diagnosis and treatment of superficial bladder cancer: improvement in diagnostic sensitivity. Urology 2001;57:1059–62.
25. Stenzl A, Hoeltl L, Bartsch G. Fluorescence assisted transurethral resection of bladder tumours: is it cost effective? Eur Urol 2001;39:31.
26. Daniltchenko DI, Riedl CR, Sachs MD, et al. Long-term benefit of 5-aminolevulinic acid fluorescence assisted transurethral resection of superficial bladder cancer: 5-year results of a prospective randomized study. J Urol 2005;174:2129–33.
27. Zaak D, Wieland WF, Stief CG, et al. Routine use of photodynamic diagnosis of bladder cancer: practical and economic issues. Eur Urol Suppl 2008;7: 536–41.
28. Machida H, Sano Y, Hamamoto Y, et al. Narrow-band imaging in the diagnosis of colorectal mucosal lesions: a pilot study. Endoscopy 2004;36: 1094–8.
29. Ohigashi T, Kozakai N, Mizuno R, et al. Endocytoscopy: novel endoscopic imaging technology for in-situ observation of bladder cancer cells. J Endourol 2006;20:698–701.
30. Geavlete B, Jecu M, Multescu R, et al. Narrow-band imaging cystoscopy in non-muscle-invasive bladder cancer: a prospective comparison to the standard approach. Ther Adv Urol 2012;4:211–7.
31. Cauberg EC, Kloen S, Visser M, et al. Narrow band imaging cystoscopy improves the detection of non-muscle-invasive bladder cancer. Urology 2010;76: 658–63.
32. Naselli A, Introini C, Bertolotto F, et al. Narrow band imaging for detecting residual/recurrent cancerous tissue during second transurethral resection of newly diagnosed non-muscle-invasive high-grade bladder cancer. BJU Int 2010;105:208–11.
33. Naselli A, Introini C, Timossi L, et al. A randomized prospective trial to assess the impact of transurethral resection in narrow band imaging modality on non-muscle-invasive bladder cancer recurrence. Eur Urol 2012;61:908–13.
34. Herr HW, Donat SM. Reduced bladder tumour recurrence rate associated with narrow-band imaging surveillance cystoscopy. BJU Int 2011;107: 396–8.
35. Herr H, Donat S. A comparison of white-light cystoscopy and narrow-band imaging cystoscopy to detect bladder tumour recurrences. BJU Int 2008; 102:1111–4.
36. Karl A, Stepp H, Willmann E, et al. Optical coherence tomography for bladder cancer—ready as a surrogate for optical biopsy? Results of a prospective mono-centre study. Eur J Med Res 2010;15: 131–4.
37. Yuan Z, Wang Z, Pan R, et al. High-resolution imaging diagnosis and staging of bladder cancer: comparison between optical coherence tomography and high-frequency ultrasound. J Biomed Opt 2008; 13:054007.
38. Ren H, Park KC, Pan R, et al. Early detection of carcinoma in situ of the bladder: a comparative study of white light cystoscopy, narrow band imaging, 5-ALA fluorescence cystoscopy and 3-dimensional optical coherence tomography. J Urol 2012;187:1063–70.

39. Wallace MB, Sharma P, Lightdale C, et al. Preliminary accuracy and interobserver agreement for the detection of intraepithelial neoplasia in Barrett's esophagus with probe-based confocal laser endomicroscopy. Gastrointest Endosc 2010;72:19–24.
40. Wu K, Liu JJ, Adams W, et al. Dynamic real-time microscopy of the urinary tract using confocal laser endomicroscopy. Urology 2011;78:225–31.
41. Babjuk M, Oosterlinck W, Sylvester R, et al. EAU guidelines on non-muscle invasive urothelial carcinoma of the bladder. Eur Urol 2008;54:303–14.

Diagnostically Challenging Cases: What are Atypia and Dysplasia?

Joseph Sanfrancesco, MD[a], J. Stephen Jones, MD[b], Donna E. Hansel, MD, PhD[a,b,c,d,*]

KEYWORDS

• Bladder • Urothelial carcinoma • Atypia • Dysplasia • Pathology

KEY POINTS

- *Atypia* and *dysplasia* are terms used to describe cellular abnormalities in the spectrum of reactive changes to neoplasia.
- Acute and chronic inflammation secondary to infectious, mechanical, or idiopathic causes can induce cytologic and architectural changes that can be interpreted by pathologists within the spectrum of atypia.
- Treatments, including systemic chemotherapy, intravesicular therapy, and radiotherapy, incite specific, often common, cellular changes that can microscopically be concerning for a neoplastic process.
- Despite improved investigation, the utility of immunohistochemistry as an ancillary tool in distinguishing benign processes from urothelial neoplasia remains unclear.

INTRODUCTION

The urothelial lining of the bladder presents diagnostic challenges, even under normal circumstances. A multitude of confounding factors, such as inflammation, reparative changes, distension state, and treatment effects, can hinder a diagnosis of early neoplasia. Thus, evaluation of biopsy and/or transurethral resection specimens requires pathologists to command a detailed understanding of the spectrum of histologic changes that can arise in the urinary bladder. Adding to the diagnostic challenge is that available ancillary studies, such as immunohistochemical (IHC) stains, are suboptimal in the diagnosis of bladder neoplasia. In light of these difficulties, pathologists have developed several diagnostic categories to address the histologic gray zones in bladder pathology. Despite what progress has been made, these categories are subjective and often do not correlate with outcomes.

WHAT ARE ATYPIA AND DYSPLASIA?

The definition of atypia has been a contentious topic within the field of pathology, not restricted to the genitourinary subspecialty. The lack of consensus on one of the most commonly used terms in pathology can be attributed to a variety of causes, such as the subjective nature of histologic evaluation, institutional bias, prior diagnosis, and preference of the evaluating pathologist.[1] Furthermore, some pathologists have used the terms, *atypia* and *dysplasia*, interchangeably, which can introduce problems in clinical management. It is implied that atypia represents a benign process in many instances whereas dysplasia describes a preneoplastic/neoplastic process,[1] although variation in defining these categories at the microscopic level often leads to confusion.

From a histologic perspective, atypia refers to a presence of 1 or more cellular or architectural features that deviate from that of an otherwise

[a] Pathology and Laboratory Medicine Institute, The Cleveland Clinic, 9500 Euclid Avenue, Cleveland, OH 44195, USA; [b] Glickman Urological and Kidney Institute, The Cleveland Clinic, 9500 Euclid Avenue, Cleveland, OH 44195, USA; [c] Taussig Cancer Institute, The Cleveland Clinic, 9500 Euclid Avenue, Cleveland, OH 44195, USA; [d] Genomic Medicine Institute, The Cleveland Clinic, 9500 Euclid Avenue, Cleveland, OH 44195, USA
* Corresponding author. Pathology and Laboratory Medicine Institute, 9500 Euclid Avenue, Desk L25, Cleveland, OH 44195.
E-mail address: hanseld@ccf.org

Urol Clin N Am 40 (2013) 281–293
http://dx.doi.org/10.1016/j.ucl.2013.01.006
0094-0143/13/$ – see front matter

normal-appearing cell or group of cells. Under normal conditions, urothelial cells contain oval nuclei, finely stippled chromatin, and minute to absent nucleoli as well as ample cytoplasm and distinct cell membranes (**Fig. 1**).[2] Even within the spectrum of normal, urothelial cells are permitted to have certain variations in cell size and cytoplasm, particularly in the most superficial layer of the urothelium (umbrella cell layer), which is in constant contact with the contents of the urinary space. These umbrella cells tend to be larger than cells in the intermediate and basal layers, with occasional binucleation and abundant eosinophilic cytoplasm. To further complicate matters for pathologists, bladder distension can lead to flattening of superficial (or umbrella) cells to a point where the layer can be difficult to identify microscopically.[3]

Despite the variety of appearances of normal urothelial cells, certain specific cellular features are evaluated when determining the presence of atypia. Abnormal nuclear features, including increased size (nucleomegaly), deviation from typical ovoid shape, coarse chromatin, and irregular nuclear membrane contour, are all contributory factors in classifying cells as atypical (**Fig. 2**).[4] In addition, the identification of an enlarged, prominent nucleolus or multiple nucleoli should raise concern.[1] Although eosinophilic (pink-appearing) cytoplasmic features are acceptable in the superficial urothelium, these cytoplasmic changes in other layers, as well as loss of cytoplasmic clearing, are also considered atypical features.[4]

Although atypia often refers specifically to cytologic (cellular) abnormalities, architectural changes can also guide pathologists to the appropriate diagnosis. Denudation of the urothelium can be associated with previous instrumentation, inflammation, or a neoplastic process (**Fig. 3**).[5] Conversely, thickening (hyperplasia) of the epithelium can result from a variety of causes, ranging from a benign proliferation to a reactive process secondary to inflammation, as well as being simply an artifact of tangential sectioning.[6] The presence of atypical cells in the background of varied epithelial thickness can pose a difficult diagnostic challenge. Assessment of histologic changes throughout the entire specimen, detailed clinical history, and cystoscopic findings are all necessary to ensure that correct diagnosis is made. As such, close communication with the treating urologist is critical for the appropriate diagnosis and management of a patient.[7]

DIAGNOSTIC CATEGORIES OF FLAT UROTHELIAL LESIONS

Reactive Urothelial Atypia

Reactive urothelial atypia remains one of the broadest categories used to describe abnormal-appearing urothelium but is generally considered at diagnosis to represent a benign process.[5] Reactive atypia is most often diagnosed in the setting of an acute and/or chronic inflammatory process that may arise in the setting of past instrumentation, infection, prior treatment, and other clinical scenarios that incite inflammation. The cytologic and architectural abnormalities that arise in these contexts are generally mild and uniform.[4] Increased nuclear size, vesicular-appearing chromatin, and pinpoint nucleoli are the most common features identified microscopically with reactive

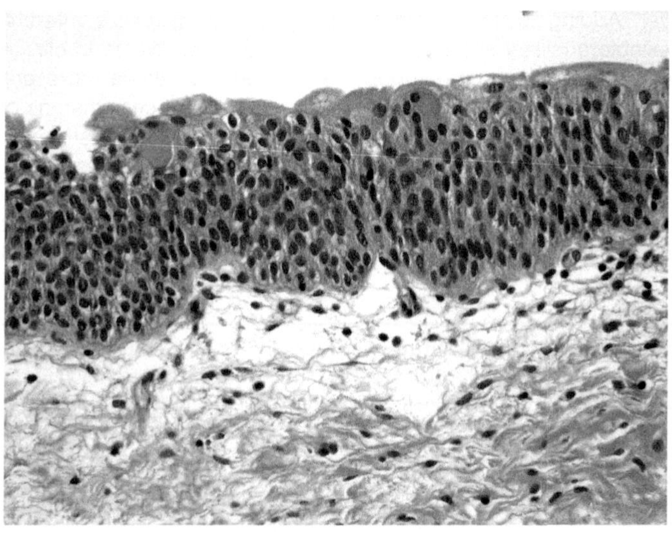

Fig. 1. Normal urothelium (hematoxylin-eosin, original magnification ×20).

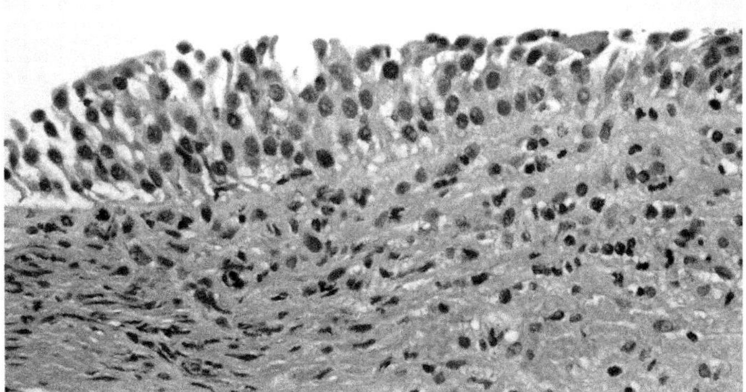

Fig. 2. Atypia demonstrates subtle changes from normal, which may include occasional hyperchromasia, disorganization, or increased nuclear/cellular variability (hematoxylin-eosin, original magnification ×20).

changes, which often occur in the presence of an inflammatory infiltrate within the urothelium (**Fig. 4**).[1] A key distinction for reactive atypia is uniformity of findings throughout the specimen. Pleomorphism (variation in nuclear size), hyperchromasia, and nuclear crowding are features that should raise concern for a probable preneoplastic or overt neoplastic process.[8]

Atypia of Unknown Significance

Atypia of unknown significance is a term introduced by an International Society of Urological Pathology consensus group in 1998[1] to classify histologic findings that meet various criteria for both reactive changes and dysplasia. Typically, this diagnosis is used in the setting of reactive nuclear and cytoplasmic changes with mild degrees of pleomorphism and/or hyperchromasia that are concerning for dysplasia. Additionally, this term has been used to describe histologic findings where the level of atypia is disproportionally greater than expected for the amount of inflammation. There is ongoing debate on whether this term is even an appropriate diagnosis.[4] The classification of histologic findings as atypia of unknown significance warrants clinical follow-up, ideally in the setting of resolved inflammation. Despite the inclination to monitor these patients prospectively, there is no evidence in the literature that has shown that this category of patients is predisposed to neoplastic progression, although further studies are needed to better clarify this entity.[8]

Urothelial Dysplasia

Urothelial dysplasia is considered to represent early preneoplastic/neoplastic change, with histologic features beyond those considered in the spectrum of benign or reactive urothelium.[9] In dysplasia, the thickness of the urothelium can be variable, but umbrella cells are usually present. Features of cellular crowding, multiple nucleoli,

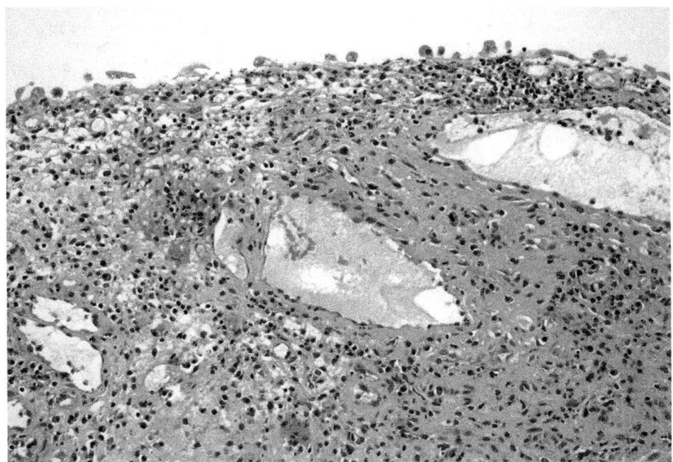

Fig. 3. Denudation may lead to a diagnosis of atypia (hematoxylin-eosin, original magnification ×10).

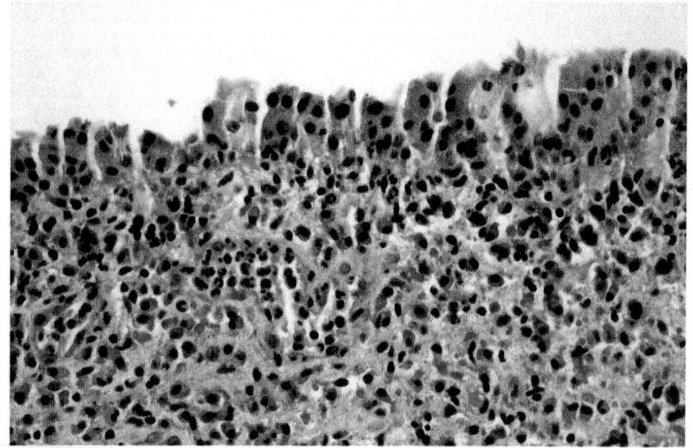

Fig. 4. Inflammation may complicate diagnostic accuracy, often leading to a diagnosis of atypia (hematoxylin-eosin, original magnification ×20).

and mild hyperchromasia are common in this diagnostic category (**Fig. 5**).[10] The diagnosis of dysplasia is used when some, but not all, of the criteria necessary for urothelial carcinoma in situ (CIS) are met. Currently, further subclassification of dysplasia as mild grade or moderate grade is no longer commonplace, whereas severe dysplasia is generally considered CIS.

Urothelial dysplasia can be further categorized into primary (de novo) and secondary dysplasia. Primary dysplasia is defined as dysplasia occurring in the absence of other histologic features of CIS and with no precedent history of urothelial neoplasia.[8] Because patients are usually asymptomatic and/or no gross lesion is visible on cystoscopy, true primary dysplasia is rarely seen by pathologists. Secondary dysplasia is classified as dysplasia identified in the setting of known neoplasia of the bladder, either current or prior. In either presentation, patients are currently undergoing screening to assess current symptoms or monitoring of a precedent high-grade lesion. Although both primary and secondary dysplasia are classified as true premalignant lesions, secondary dysplasia is more likely to progress to carcinoma.[8]

Carcinoma in Situ

Urothelial CIS is a neoplastic diagnosis, with malignant cells restricted within the urothelial lining of the bladder (noninvasive disease). In addition to the features of dysplasia, these cells demonstrate marked nuclear and cellular pleomorphism and

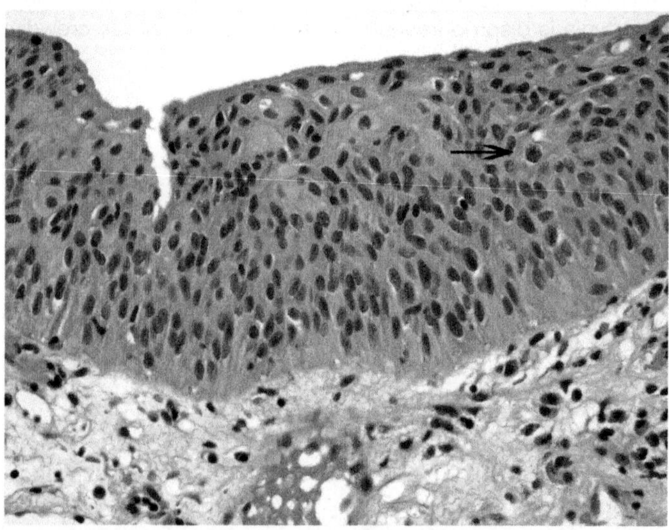

Fig. 5. Dysplasia is a subjective diagnosis. In this case, variable nuclear size, mild cellular disorganization, and occasional abnormal nuclear contours (*arrow*) support the diagnosis (hematoxylin-eosin, original magnification ×40).

hyperchromasia (**Fig. 6**).[9] CIS is commonly underdiagnosed when full-thickness cytologic atypia is absent or when umbrella cells are identified. Underdiagnosis of CIS may also occur in the setting of clinging CIS (single carcinoma cells are present in a background of otherwise denuded urothelium) and subtle involvement of von Brunn nests by CIS cells.[9]

INFLAMMATION AS A CONTRIBUTOR TO A DIAGNOSIS OF ATYPIA/DYSPLASIA

There are many inflammatory and infectious processes that incite reactive changes within the urinary bladder. Specifically, acute and chronic inflammation secondary to infectious, mechanical, or idiopathic causes can induce cytologic and architectural changes that can be interpreted by pathologists within the spectrum of atypia. The following categories represent a sampling of some of the common inflammatory processes that often lead to a diagnosis of atypia and/or dysplasia on bladder biopsy.

Acute and Chronic Cystitis

The most common cause of acute cystitis is infection, primarily, but not restricted to, gram-negative bacteria.[11] Additional causes of acute cystitis include prior instrumentation, trauma, and catheterization. In the acute setting, inflammatory-mediated cell responses lead to an influx of neutrophils, lymphocytes, and macrophages within the urothelium and lamina propria of the bladder. Edema and vascular congestion are also common.[12] Although reactive changes of the urothelium may not occur until the subacute or chronic inflammatory phase, pronounced inflammation can obscure underlying pathologic processes and make assessment difficult for pathologists, thus leading to a diagnosis of atypia. In the setting of chronic cystitis, a variety of changes can occur in the urothelium, including denudation, ulceration, or hyperplasia. In addition to difficulties in adequately visualizing the specimen microscopically secondary to copious amounts of granulation tissue and/or fibrosis, reactive atypia due to a persistent inflammatory process can raise suspicion for dysplasia in the bladder.[8]

Polypoid Cystitis

Polypoid cystitis, a common variant of cystitis in the bladder, remains a challenging inflammatory lesion for pathologists and urologists alike (**Fig. 7**).[13] On cystoscopy, the often exophytic growth pattern of polypoid cystitis may clinically resemble a papillary neoplasm. These lesions tend to appear in patients with a history of indwelling catheters, fistulas, chronic obstruction, or calculi. Microscopically, the lesion consists of large, bulbous outpouchings of the urothelial lining, with the lamina propria often edematous (**Fig. 8**).[13] Over time, ongoing inflammation may produce scarring of the lamina propria, leading to a more papillary-like appearance as well as inducing squamous metaplasia and reactive atypia.[14] In a 2008 study, 41 cases of polypoid cystitis previously misdiagnosed as papillary urothelial neoplasia were rereviewed.[13] Despite some mild atypia and mitotic figures in many of the cases, the cytologic features included uniform cell enlargement, similar vesicular chromatin patterns,

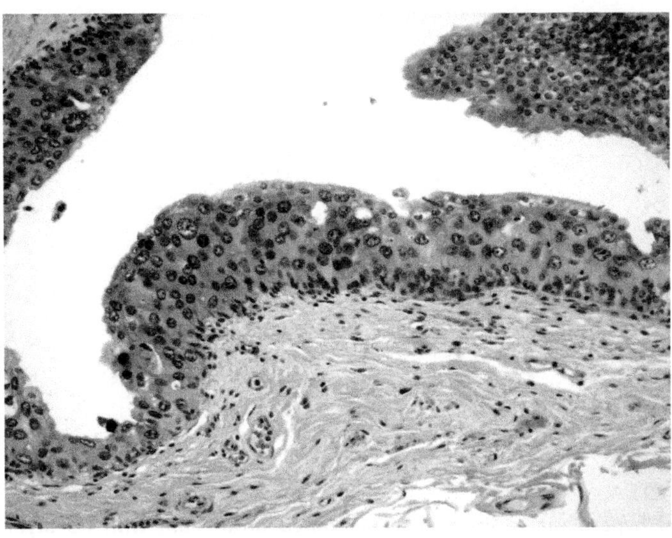

Fig. 6. CIS typically shows overt neoplastic features (hematoxylin-eosin, original magnification ×20).

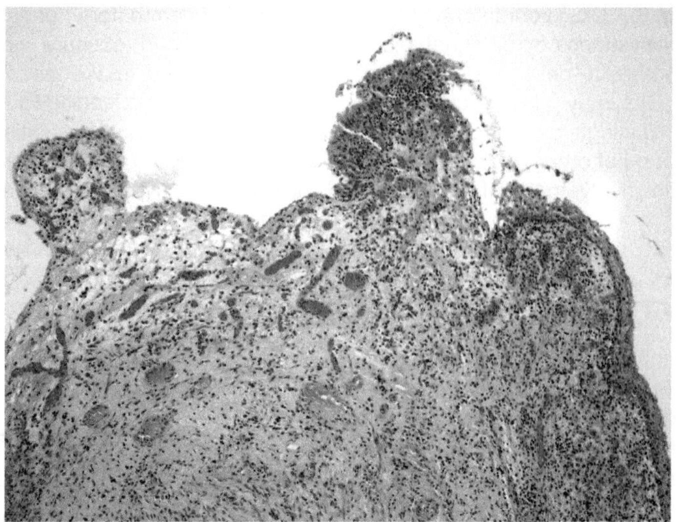

Fig. 7. Polypoid cystitis (hematoxylin-eosin, original magnification ×4).

and a single prominent nucleolus. Each of the 41 cases lacked definitive hyperchromasia and nuclear pleomorphism, which are key criteria in differentiating benign, reactive lesions from neoplasia.

Polyomavirus

BK and JC are double-stranded DNA viruses of the papovavirus family that can induce cytologic changes concerning for dysplasia.[15] These viruses live latently in the epithelium of the urinary tract and are asymptomatic. Use of systemic chemotherapeutic agents, primarily cyclophosphamide, as well as other clinical scenarios of immunodeficiency can lead to reactivation of these latent human polyoma viruses.[16] Atypical cellular features are usually first identified on urine cytology sampling where nuclear inclusions and/or chromatin irregularities are noted. Polyomavirus cellular changes often do not appear on histologic examination of biopsy specimens due to the virus' preference to infect the superficial cell layer, which can be lost in processing.[15] Efforts to use analysis of DNA content to differentiate virally infected cells from true neoplastic cells have historically been unsuccessful due to aneuploidy.[17] Correlation with clinical history, knowledge of patient immune status, and familiarity with common nuclear changes associated with reactivated viral infections are all crucial to avoid overdiagnosis of malignancy in this patient population.[16]

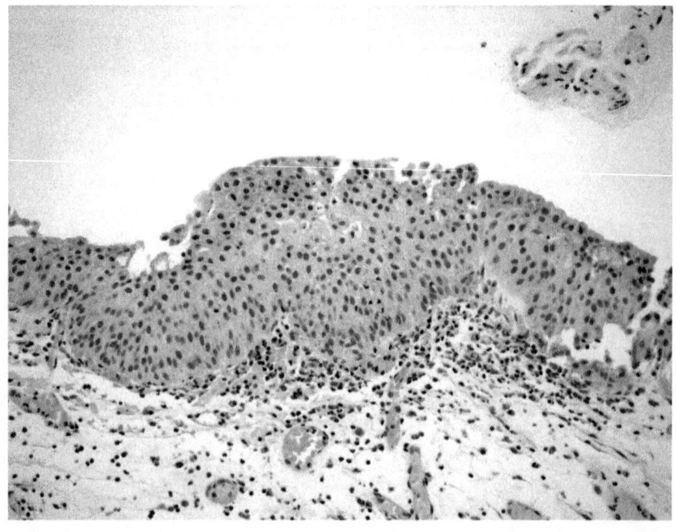

Fig. 8. Flat urothelial hyperplasia recognized as thickened urothelium with no atypia (hematoxylin-eosin, original magnification ×20).

HYPERPLASIA AS A CONTRIBUTOR TO A DIAGNOSIS OF ATYPIA/DYSPLASIA

The 2 most common types of hyperplasia identified in the urinary bladder are simple (flat) and papillary. Flat hyperplasia is defined as thickened, but cytologically normal, urothelium, usually greater than 7 cell layers in thickness (see **Fig. 8**).[1] Flat hyperplasia has occasionally been associated with the presence of mild atypia, but an evaluating pathologist should have a low threshold for addressing this in the diagnosis. Difficulty in definitively determining the presence of flat hyperplasia may be secondary to tangential sectioning of the tissue during processing.[6] Flat urothelial hyperplasia usually occurs in the clinical setting of inflammation or lithiasis (bladder stones) but has also been identified adjacent to papillary-type neoplasms.[9]

Papillary urothelial hyperplasia appears histologically as undulating epithelial thickening devoid of significant cellular atypia (**Fig. 9**). These papillary fronds may contain small, dilated vessels that appear as rudimentary vascular cores but lack the branching or more complex architecture that place this into a papillary neoplastic category.[18] Similar to flat hyperplasia, mild cytologic changes in the background of inflammation and instrumentation are permitted. Any indication that the atypical features are disproportional, given the clinical setting, should guide pathologists to consider a preneoplastic process and thus a diagnosis of papillary hyperplasia with dysplasia.[19] Taylor and colleagues[18] examined 16 cases of papillary hyperplasia and were unable to definitively determine if papillary hyperplasia, with no evidence of atypia, would progress to neoplasia without intervention. Furthermore, the investigators postulated that diagnosing papillary hyperplasia in a patient with a history of urothelial neoplasia likely represented a recurrence. Conversely, papillary hyperplasia with atypical features, dysplasia, or focal CIS may predispose patients to increased risk for disease progression.[19]

METAPLASTIC PROCESSES AND THEIR RELATIONSHIP TO BLADDER ATYPIA AND NEOPLASIA

Metaplasia is defined as a change (often reversible) from one differentiated cell type to another.[20] In cases of the urothelium, metaplasia often occurs in the setting of an inflammatory process or after instrumentation. Although metaplasia, by definition, is not a neoplastic process, atypia in these metaplastic cells can raise concern for less common malignancies of the bladder, such as adenocarcinoma or squamous cell carcinoma.

Squamous Metaplasia

Squamous metaplasia of the bladder involves replacement of urothelium by squamous epithelium and may be either nonkeratinizing or keratinizing. In some instances, nonkeratinizing squamous metaplasia is normal, such as in the trigone of the bladder in women.[21] Chronic inflammatory processes, often seen in patients with spinal cord injury or persistent in-dwelling catheters, may increase the likelihood of developing squamous metaplasia, which can present as leukoplakia on cystoscopy. Although keratinizing squamous metaplasia is traditionally associated with cystitis, bladder stones, and schistosomiasis, it may also be associated with concurrent or subsequent

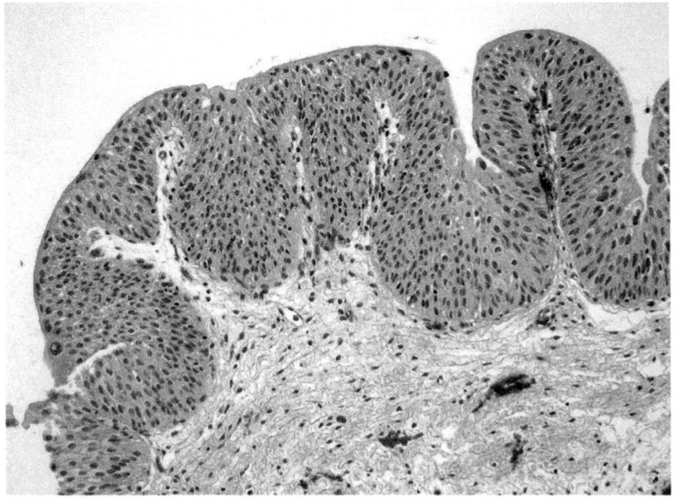

Fig. 9. Papillary hyperplasia shows upward tenting of vessels, suggesting a possible early papillary lesion in some instances (hematoxylin-eosin, original magnification ×20).

malignancy and thus should be regarded with higher suspicion and additional clinical follow-up (**Fig. 10**).[22]

Cystitis Cystica et Glandularis

Cystitis cystica et glandularis (CCEG) is a benign process defined as cystic changes within von Brunn nests (cystitis cystica) that develop metaplastic changes of the cellular lining to columnar or cuboidal epithelium (**Fig. 11**).[23] Similar to other metaplastic processes, CCEG is attributed to chronic inflammation/irritation and favors but is not restricted to the trigone of the bladder. CCEG is further subdivided into usual and intestinal types, although in practice this subcategorization is often not frequently used.

Intestinal Metaplasia

Intestinal metaplasia (IM) is a proliferation of epithelium in the urinary bladder characterized by gland-like structures lined with mucin-secreting cells (**Fig. 12**).[24] These mucin-secreting cells resemble goblet cells, which are found in the colonic mucosa of the lower gastrointestinal tract.[23] In a study by Corica and colleagues,[24] 53 cases of IM in the bladder were evaluated with long-term follow-up (mean >12 years among the 2 case groups[24]). The investigators determined that the presence of IM was not a strong risk factor for the development of overt malignancy. Smith and colleagues[23] evaluated 19 cases of IM and found no evidence carcinoma at follow-up (mean 4.4 years[23]). Additionally, although 37% of the cases with IM had co-existing carcinoma, the investigators believed that the association between the 2 processes did not imply that IM was the precursor lesion. One study has suggested that pure adenocarcinomas of the urinary bladder (as opposed to urothelial carcinoma with glandular differentiation) are derived from IM, but attempts to definitively associate IM as premalignant have yet to be proven.[25] Extensive IM has been suggested to predispose patients to a greater risk for developing adenocarcinoma, but this frequently cited association is based on a single study[26] and no additional evidence has been identified in the current literature.

Glandular Metaplasia with Dysplasia

Glandular metaplasia (sometimes used interchangeably with IM[24]) has been associated with cytologic atypia in rare cases and can be further divided into glandular metaplasia with low-grade/high-grade dysplasia.[27] Low-grade dysplasia shares morphologic features with tubular adenomas of the colon, including columnar nuclei that maintain polarity and uniformity. In contrast, adenocarcinoma in situ (glandular metaplasia with high-grade dysplasia) demonstrates overt atypia, including nuclear stratification, atypical mitoses, and nuclear pleomorphism (**Fig. 13**).[28]

Villous adenomas of the urinary tract (also referred to as glandular metaplasia with an exophytic growth pattern[8]) histologically appear identical to colonic villous adenomas and consist of pseudostratified columnar mucosa with mucin-secreting cells and epithelial projections of variable size. Villous adenomas in the bladder have been associated with invasive adenocarcinoma, squamous cell carcinoma, and urothelial CIS.[29] These lesions are exceedingly rare but, when identified without concurrent carcinoma, seem to have

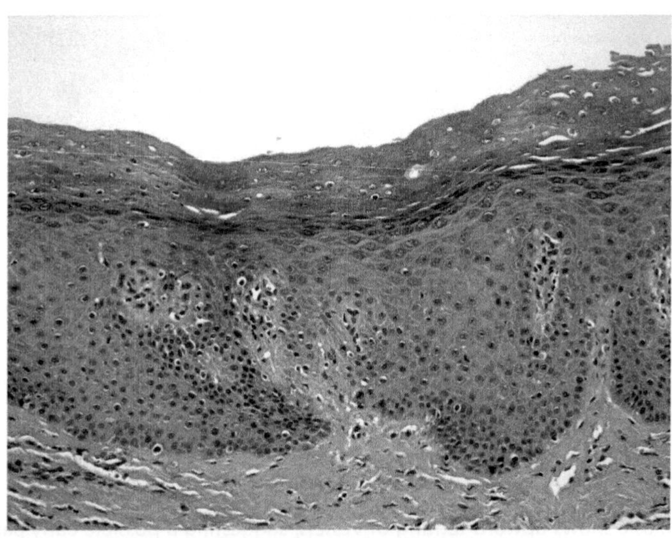

Fig. 10. Keratinizing squamous metaplasia (hematoxylin-eosin, original magnification ×20).

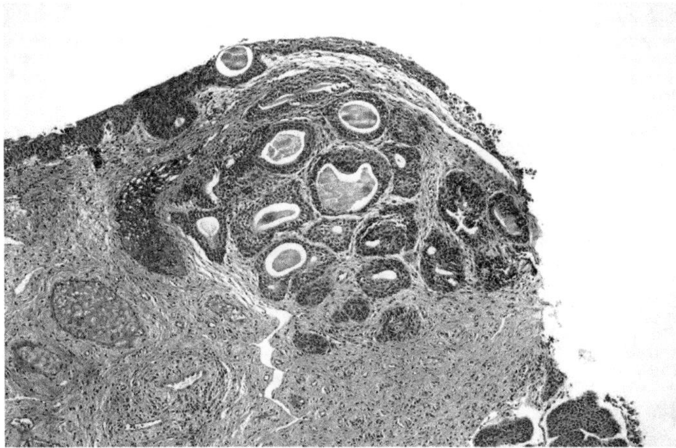

Fig. 11. CCEG (hematoxylin-eosin, original magnification ×10).

an excellent prognosis for patients.[30] As with villous adenomas of the colon, extensive sampling is imperative to definitively rule out stromal invasion or focal adenocarcinoma in situ.[8]

TREATMENT EFFECT AS A CAUSE OF ATYPIA AND DYSPLASIA

Nonsurgical intervention for bladder and/or prostate neoplasia involves a variety of treatments, including systemic chemotherapy, intravesicular therapy, and radiotherapy. Each treatment modality poses its own challenge to pathologists secondary to the inflammation and atypia associated with each intervention. Accurate determination of the cytologic and morphologic changes secondary to treatment effect requires a detailed understanding of what effects should be expected with individual therapies. Although several therapies may induce many reactive changes that may be interpreted as atypia, some—like radiation cystitis—may be a risk factor for the development of bladder neoplasia as well.

Radiation Therapy

Approximately one-fourth of all patients with muscle invasive bladder carcinoma undergo some form of radiotherapy.[31] In addition, many patients diagnosed with prostate cancer also undergo various forms of radiation therapy that can ultimately affect the bladder lining based on its proximity. On cystoscopy, edema, ulceration, and erythema are common findings in addition to areas of mucosal hemorrhage. Histologically, the urothelium shows radiation atypia, which includes cellular enlargement, multinucleation, vacuolization, and chromatin clearing (**Fig. 14**).[31] In addition to

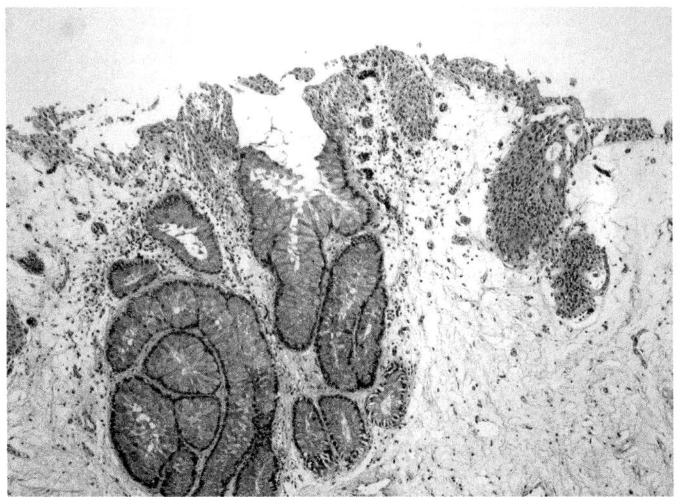

Fig. 12. IM showing mucin-containing goblet cells (hematoxylin-eosin, original magnification ×10).

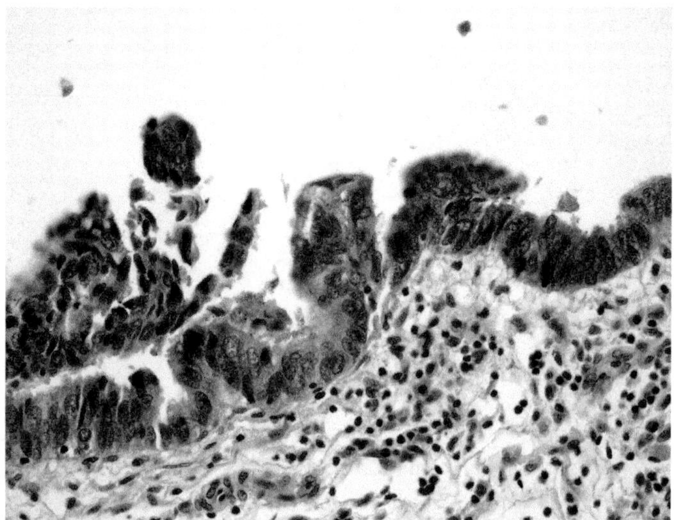

Fig. 13. Adenocarcinoma in situ (glandular metaplasia with high-grade dysplasia) shows overt neoplastic alterations (hematoxylin-eosin, original magnification ×40).

inflammation and cytologic atypia identified in the epithelium, vascular changes secondary to the radiation include edema, vascular proliferation, vessel wall hyalinization, and thrombosis. Ischemic changes caused by exposure to radiation can lead to long-term sequelae, such as mucosal denudation, contractures, and fistula formation.[32]

Chemotherapy

Chemotherapeutic regimens in the treatment of bladder cancer consist of intravesical and/or systemic agents, many of which can incite atypia of the urothelium. Two of the most common intravesical agents are triethylenethiophosphoramide (thiotepa) and mitomycin C. Thiotepa (an alkalating agent) and mitomycin C (an antibiotic with antitumor properties) both produce similar cytologic and architectural changes to the urothelium, including denudation and atypia of the umbrella cells with features of increased size, multinucleation, and vacuolization.[31] Additional forms of cellular atypia that occur following treatment with these 2 agents include degenerative changes and membrane alterations that may incite a diagnosis of atypia. Other intravesicular topical agents, such as doxorubicin and epirubicin, have been implicated in causing cystitis and similar cytologic changes, but details of these changes have not been studied thoroughly.[31]

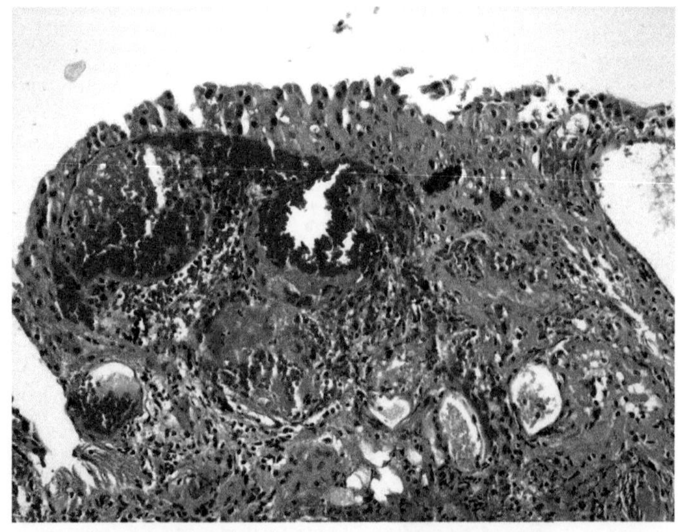

Fig. 14. Radiation atypia with a background of inflammation, nuclear atypia and edema (hematoxylin-eosin, original magnification ×20).

In addition to intravesicular chemotherapy with the oxazaphoshporine class of alkylating agents, systemic chemotherapy with cyclophosphamide has been identified as a cause of bladder urothelial atypia.[33,34] Often used in the therapy of autoimmune conditions, such as systemic lupus erythematous and rheumatoid arthritis, and lymphoproliferative disorders, this alkylating agent undergoes metabolism to produce acrolein and phosphoramide mustard, which are excreted in the urine and are exposed to the superficial bladder mucosa.[35] Clinically, patients can present with urinary symptoms and hematuria, which may prompt clinicians for cystoscopic evaluation and biopsy. Grossly, the mucosal surface can appear erythematous, edematous, and possibly hemorrhagic. Microscopically, large multinucleated cells are seen, caused by the arrest of cell division secondary to exposure to the active metabolites of cyclophosphamide. Nuclei are variably enlarged with irregular membranes, coarse chromatin, and irregularly sized and shaped nucleoli.[31] These effects are similar to changes induced by radiation therapy. Cyclophosphamide has also been associated with hemorrhagic cystitis.[36]

From a pathologist's perspective, one of the greatest difficulties in the setting of chemotherapeutic treatment is determining whether atypia is the result of therapy or whether the atypia represents early neoplastic changes secondary to new or recurrent disease. Several studies have determined that cyclophosphamide therapy is associated with an up to 9-fold increase in the development of bladder carcinoma.[37] Furthermore, chemotherapeutic agents have been associated with benign epithelial proliferations, which can mimic invasive carcinoma due to an infiltrative growth pattern into the lamina propria of the bladder mucosa.[38] These pseudocarcinomatous proliferations cause several challenges for pathologists due to the elevated risk for developing cancer in patients treated with chemotherapy and the limited sampling on biopsy.[38]

Bacillus Calmette-Guérin Therapy

Bacillus Calmette-Guérin (BCG) therapy is the most common intravesicular immunotherapy agent used worldwide for the treatment of superficial and noninvasive high-grade bladder neoplasia.[39] BCG is a pleiotropic immune stimulator that can limit tumor progression by recruitment of an antitumoral immune response.[28] Microscopically, BCG therapy most notably causes acute and chronic inflammation associated with noncaseating granulomas but may also induce mucosal ulceration, denudation, and reactive urothelial atypia.[40]

Photodynamic Therapy

Photodynamic therapy is a newer, less common modality used in treatment of bladder neoplasia.[41] Photodynamic treatment is administered either systemically or intravesicularly, subsequently inducing necrosis of tumor cells when exposed to a light source.[42] In addition to inducing coagulative necrosis and hemorrhage, adjacent benign mucosa may be affected by the treatment. Cytologic atypia is not traditionally associated with this therapy and should raise suspicion if identified on microscopy examination.[28]

Ketamine Cystitis

An exceedingly rare, but notable, mimicker of CIS is ketamine cystitis, which can occur in the setting of chronic exposure to this drug. These patients typically report clinical symptoms of dysuria, urgency, hematuria, and incontinence. On cystoscopy, a small capacity, erythematous bladder is seen. Microscopically, ulceration and acute inflammation are the most common findings. A 2009 study from Oxley and colleagues[43] looked at 17 patients with reported ketamine cystitis, 10 of which were described as having significant urothelial atypia on histologic examination concerning for CIS. The investigators reported that despite nuclear enlargement and disorganization of cells seen on biopsy, the changes identified were likely reactive and did not represent a preneoplastic process.

IMMUNOHISTOCHEMISTRY AS AN ANCILLARY TOOL

Although extensively studied, the use of IHC in the diagnosis of urothelial neoplasia has remained somewhat challenging. As discussed previously, discerning reactive atypia from dysplasia and CIS remains one of the greatest topics of contention in urologic pathology. Several studies have examined the utility of IHC in noninvasive lesions of urothelium, in particular atypia and CIS, to determine what role, if any, they may serve in reaching the appropriate diagnosis.

Several studies have been done to determine which IHC markers could be useful to pathologists to differentiate reactive atypia from dysplasia. In 2001, 1 study evaluated 25 cases of non-neoplastic urothelium (15 cases of reactive atypia and 10 cases of normal urothelium) using 3 common IHC stains: cytokeratin 20, CD44, and p53.[44] Cytokeratin 20 stains cytoskeletal intermediate filaments found in gastrointestinal mucosa, urothelium, and Merkel cells and is generally restricted to the umbrella cell layer in normal urothelium. p53 is a tumor suppressor gene implicated in many malignancies, including bladder carcinoma[45]; under normal conditions, p53 demonstrates a weak cytoplasmic signal in the urothelium. Finally, CD44 is an immunomarker previously studied as a possible prognostic factor in papillary urothelial neoplasms and has been found under normal conditions to reside in the basal layers of the urothelium.[45] A combinatorial approach has been used with these 3 IHC markers to aid in the distinction between normal urothelium with atypia and CIS. Specifically, intense nuclear p53 expression (that correlates with p53 mutation) coupled with full-thickness CK20 expression and loss of CD44 favors CIS.[44,46] Although this overall finding in larger studies seems promising, use of these markers routinely on individual cases can often be problematic, with variability in intensity and distribution of markers common.

SUMMARY

Evaluation of the bladder urothelium is a diagnostically challenging process that involves not only subtleties in morphologic evaluation but also an awareness of patient history to elucidate sources of atypia unrelated to neoplastic transformation. Common challenges in distinguishing the categories of reactive atypia from atypia of uncertain significance and dysplasia include the presence of inflammation, therapy, and prior instrumentation. Despite improved investigation into the utility of IHC markers, microscopic assessment remains the definitive approach to achieving the most accurate urothelial diagnosis possible.

REFERENCES

1. Epstein JI, Amin MB, Reuter VR, et al. The World Health Organization/International Society of Urological Pathology consensus classification of urothelial (transitional cell) neoplasms of the urinary bladder. Bladder Consensus Conference Committee. Am J Surg Pathol 1998;22(12):1435–48.
2. Epstein JI, Amin MB, Reuter VE. Normal bladder anatomy and variants of normal histology. In: Epstein JI, Amin MB, Reuter VE, editors. Biopsy interpretation of the bladder. Philadelphia: Lippincott Williams & Wilkins; 2010. p. 1–13.
3. Reuter VE. Urinary bladder, ureter, and renal pelvis. In: Mills S, editor. Histology for pathologists. 3rd edition. Philadelphia: Lippincott Williams & Wilkins; 2010. p. 910–22.
4. Banerjee SK, Lopez-Beltran A. Urothelial dysplasia and its mimics. Pathol Case Rev 2008;13(4):149–53.
5. Amin MB, McKenney JK, Paner GP, et al. ICUD-EAU International consultation on bladder cancer 2012: pathology. Eur Urol 2013;63:16–35.
6. Koss LG. Tumors of the urinary bladder, Fasicle 11. Washington, DC: Armed Forces Institute of Pathology; 1975.
7. Gorin MA, Ayyathurai R, Soloway MS. Diagnosis and treatment of bladder cancer: how can we improve? Postgrad Med 2012;124(3):28–36.
8. Sesterhenn I, van det Kwast KT, Mazerolles C. Preneoplastic non-papillary lesions and conditions of the urinary bladder: an update based on the Ancona International Consultation. Virchows Arch 2002; 440(1):3–11.
9. Sauter G, Algaba F, Amin MB, et al. Tumours of the urinary system. In: Epstein JI, Eble JN, Sesterhenn I, et al, editors. World Health Organization Classification of Tumours Pathology and Genetics: Tumours of the Urinary System and Male Genital Organs. Lyon (France): IARC Press; 2004. p. 89–157.
10. Cheng L, Cheville JC, Neumann RM, et al. Natural history of urothelial dysplasia of the bladder. Am J Surg Pathol 1999;23(4):443–7.
11. Filiatrault L, McKay RM, Patrick DM, et al. Antibiotic resistance in isolates recovered from women with community-acquired urinary tract infections presenting to a tertiary care emergency department. CJEM 2012;14(5):295–305.
12. Epstein JI, Amin MB, Reuter VE. Cystitis. In: Epstein JI, Amin MB, Reuter VE, editors. Biopsy interpretation of the bladder. Philadelphia: Lippincott Williams & Wilkins; 2010. p. 226–59.
13. Lane Z, Epstein JI. Polypoid/papillary cystitis: a series of 41 cases misdiagnosed as papillary urothelial neoplasia. Am J Surg Pathol 2008;32(5):758–64.
14. Young RH. Papillary and polypoid cystitis. A report of eight cases. Am J Surg Pathol 1988;12(7):542–6.
15. Herawi M, Parwani AV, Chan T, et al. Polyoma virus-associated cellular changes in the urine and bladder biopsy samples: a cytohistologic correlation. Am J Surg Pathol 2006;30(3):345–50.
16. Wojcik EM, Miller MC, Wright BC, et al. Comparative analysis of DNA content in polyomavirus-infected urothelial cells, urothelial dysplasia and high grade transitional cell carcinoma. Anal Quant Cytol Histol 1997;19(5):430–6.
17. Koss LG, Sherman AB, Eppich E. Image analysis and DNA content of urothelial cells infected with human polyomavirus. Anal Quant Cytol 1984;6(2): 89–94.
18. Taylor DC, Bhagavan BS, Larsen MP, et al. Papillary urothelial hyperplasia. A precursor to papillary neoplasms. Am J Surg Pathol 1996;20(12):1481–8.
19. Swierczynski SL, Epstein JI. Prognostic significance of atypical papillary urothelial hyperplasia. Hum Pathol 2002;33(5):512–7.

20. Abbas AK, Aster JC, Fausto N, et al. Cellular responses to stress and toxic insults: adaptation, injury, and death. In: Robbins SL, Kumar V, Cotran RS, editors. Robbins and Cotran pathologic basis of disease, professional edition. 8th edition. Philadelphia: Saunders; 2009. p. 3–42.
21. Epstein JI, Amin MB, Reuter VE. Flat urothelial lesions. In: Epstein JI, Amin MB, Reuter VE, editors. Biopsy interpretation of the bladder. Philadelphia: Lippincott Williams & Wilkins; 2010. p. 14–42.
22. Lagwinski N, Thomas A, Stephenson AJ, et al. Squamous cell carcinoma of the bladder: a clinicopathologic analysis of 45 cases. Am J Surg Pathol 2007; 31(12):1777–87.
23. Smith AK, Hansel DE, Jones JS. Role of cystitis cystica et glandularis and intestinal metaplasia in development of bladder carcinoma. Urology 2008;71(5): 915–8.
24. Corica FA, Husmann DA, Churchill BM, et al. Intestinal metaplasia is not a strong risk factor for bladder cancer: study of 53 cases with long-term follow-up. Urology 1997;50(3):427–31.
25. Behzatoğlu K. Malignant glandular lesions and glandular differentiation in invasive/noninvasive urothelial carcinoma of the urinary bladder. Ann Diagn Pathol 2011;15(6):422–6.
26. Elem B, Alam SZ. Total intestinal metaplasia with focal adenocarcinoma in a Schistosoma-infested defunctioned urinary bladder. Br J Urol 1984;56(3): 331–3.
27. Chan TY, Epstein JI. In situ adenocarcinoma of the bladder. Am J Surg Pathol 2001;25(7):892–9.
28. Montironi R, Lopez-Beltran A, Scarpelli M, et al. Morphological classification and definition of benign, preneoplastic and non-invasive neoplastic lesions of the urinary bladder. Histopathology 2008; 53(6):621–33.
29. Seibel JL, Prasad S, Weiss RE, et al. Villous adenoma of the urinary tract: a lesion frequently associated with malignancy. Hum Pathol 2002; 33(2):236–41.
30. Cheng L, Montironi R, Bostwick DG. Villous adenoma of the urinary tract: a report of 23 cases, including 8 with coexistent adenocarcinoma. Am J Surg Pathol 1999;23(7):764–71.
31. Lopez-Beltran A, Luque RJ, Mazzucchelli R, et al. Changes produced in the urothelium by traditional and newer therapeutic procedures for bladder cancer. J Clin Pathol 2002;55(9):641–7.
32. Pavlidakey PG, MacLennan GT. Radiation cystitis. J Urol 2009;182(3):1172–3.
33. Siddiqui A, Melamed MR, Abbi R, et al. Mucinous (colloid) carcinoma of urinary bladder following long-term cyclophosphamide for Waldenstrom macroglobulinemia. Am J Surg Pathol 1996;20:500–4.
34. Wall RL, Clausen KP. Carcinoma of the urinary bladder in patients receiving cyclophosphamide. N Engl J Med 1975;293:271–3.
35. Plotz PH, Klippel JH, Decker JL, et al. Bladder complications in patients receiving cyclophosphamide for systemic lupus erythematosus or rheumatoid arthritis. Ann Intern Med 1979;91(2):221–3.
36. Lawrence HJ, Simone J, Aur RJ. Cyclophosphamide-induced hemorrhagic cystitis in children with leukemia. Cancer 1975;36:1572–6.
37. Fairchild WV, Spence CR, Solomon HD, et al. The incidence of bladder cancer after cyclophosphamide therapy. J Urol 1979;122(2):163–4.
38. Lane Z, Epstein JI. Pseudocarcinomatous epithelial hyperplasia in the bladder unassociated with prior irradiation or chemotherapy. Am J Surg Pathol 2008;32(1):92–7.
39. Pinke LA, Lamm DL. "Intravesical immunotherapy: BCG." In: Lerner S, Schoenberg M, Sternberg C, editors. Textbook of bladder cancer. 1st edition. Oxon (UK): Taylor & Francis; 2006. p. 353–8.
40. Bassi P, Milani C, Meneghini A, et al. Clincial value of pathologic changes after intravesical BCG therapy of superificial bladder cancer. Urology 1992;40: 175–9.
41. Pinthus JH, Bogaards A, Weersink R, et al. Photodynamic therapy for urological malignancies: past to current approaches. J Urol 2006;175(4):1201–7.
42. Jichlinski P, Leisinger HJ. Photodynamic therapy in superficial bladder cancer: past, present, and future. Urol Res 2001;29:396–405.
43. Oxley JD, Cottrell AM, Adams S, et al. Ketamine cystitis as a mimic of carcinoma in situ. Histopathology 2009;55(6):705–8.
44. McKenney JK, Desai S, Cohen C, et al. Discriminatory immunohistochemical staining of urothelial carcinoma in situ and non-neoplastic urothelium: an analysis of cytokeratin 20, p53, and CD44 antigens. Am J Surg Pathol 2001;25(8):1074–8.
45. Netto GJ, Epstein JI. Immunohistology of the Prostate, Bladder, Kidney, and Testis. In: Dabbs D, editor. Diagnostic immunohistochemistry. 3rd edition. Philadelphia: Saunders; 2010. p. 593–661.
46. Hodges KB, Lopez-Beltran A, Emerson RE, et al. Clinical utility of immunohistochemistry in the diagnoses of urinary bladder neoplasia. Appl Immunohistochem Mol Morphol 2010;18(5):401–10.

Restaging Transurethral Resection for Non-Muscle Invasive Bladder Cancer

Who, Why, When, and How?

Chad R. Ritch, MD[a], Peter E. Clark, MD[a], Todd M. Morgan, MD[b,*]

KEYWORDS

• Non-muscle invasive bladder cancer • Transurethral resection • Repeat resection • Second-look cystoscopy • Restaging • Upstaging • Understaging

KEY POINTS

- Understaging rates of up to 40% for non-muscle invasive bladder cancer have been reported based on radical cystectomy data.
- Absence of muscularis propria MP in the specimen leads to a significantly higher rate of understaging (60%–78%).
- Patients with high-grade (HG) Ta and HG T1 tumors, regardless of presence of muscle, are strongly encouraged to undergo a restaging transurethral resection (TUR).
- Repeat resection should be performed 2 to 6 weeks following initial TUR.
- Deep biopsies in the base and periphery of the old resection site should be performed.

Non-muscle invasive bladder cancer (NMIBC) comprised the vast majority of the estimated 73,510 new cases of bladder cancer diagnosed in the United States in 2012.[1] Approximately 70% to 75% of patients with bladder cancer initially present at a low stage (stage 1), a category that includes carcinoma in situ (Tis – 1–10% alone as primary), tumors confined to the urothelial mucosa (Ta – 70%–80%), and those that invade only the underlying lamina propria (T1 – 20%).[2–4] The prognosis for patients with NMIBC is generally good, with approximately 80% to 90% of patients alive at 5 years.[2] In contrast, muscle-invasive bladder cancer, which represents about 25% of cases, has a significantly lower relative 5-year survival rate of 17% to 66% depending on tumor stage.[2,5] Epidemiologic evidence demonstrates that these trends in incidence and survival for noninvasive and invasive bladder cancer have remained relatively stable since 1993.[2] The most significant risk factor for bladder cancer is cigarette smoking.[6] While the risk may decrease with smoking cessation, former smokers still have a higher risk of bladder cancer than never smokers.[6] Additionally, in patients with NMIBC, current tobacco use and cumulative lifetime exposure are closely associated with recurrence and progression.[7,8] There is no currently accepted genetic or inheritable cause of urothelial carcinoma of the bladder, but studies suggest that polymorphisms in 2 carcinogen-detoxifying genes, GSTM-1 and NAT-2, may be responsible for increased susceptibility to developing bladder cancer in certain patients.[9]

Disclosures: None.

[a] Department of Urologic Surgery, Vanderbilt University Medical Center, A-1302 Medical Center North, Nashville, TN 37232, USA; [b] Department of Urology, University of Michigan, 1500 East Medical Center Drive, Ann Arbor, MI 48109, USA

* Corresponding author.

E-mail address: tomorgan@med.umich.edu

Urol Clin N Am 40 (2013) 295–304

http://dx.doi.org/10.1016/j.ucl.2013.01.009

0094-0143/13/$ – see front matter

WHO TO RESTAGE

Understanding the Predictors of Understaging, Recurrence, and Progression

Patients with NMIBC represent a heterogeneous group and demonstrate a broad range of outcomes with respect to recurrence, progression, and survival. Accurate staging and a fundamental understanding of the pathologic findings that predict outcome are therefore of utmost importance in clinical management. Thus, when considering the value of restaging transurethral resection (TUR), the first question that must be addressed is "who?" That is, which patients may benefit from additional resection rather than proceeding to intravesical chemotherapy/surveillance cystoscopy? Importantly, restaging TUR, which assumes a complete initial TUR, is distinguished here from a repeat resection performed when a complete initial TUR cannot be accomplished.[10]

Most (55%–75%) of Ta tumors are low grade (LG), and patients with high-grade (HG) tumors are at much greater risk of recurrence, progression, and death from bladder cancer compared with those with LG disease.[2,11,12] Long term follow-up of Ta LG tumors demonstrates that the overall recurrence rate is 55%, with 6% and 20% experiencing progression of stage and/or grade, respectively.[13] In contrast, 30% to 35% of Ta HG tumors will progress to at least T1 disease.[11,12] Ta HG urothelial cancer is associated with a significant risk of progression and death as manifested by progression-free survival and disease-specific survival rates of 61% and 74%, respectively, according to 1 study.[14] This has important implications when considering the merits of restaging TUR, since adequate tumor stage and grade information clearly guides future management decisions, including administration of intravesical therapy or a recommendation for early cystectomy in patients found to be understaged at initial TUR.

Along with Ta HG bladder cancer, carcinoma in situ (CIS) and T1 cancers are all considered high-risk NMIBC. Clinical stage T1 tumors, those invading beyond the mucosa but confined to the lamina propria at the time of TUR or biopsy, represent approximately 20% of NMIBC and behave more aggressively than Ta tumors. They may also be classified as HG or LG, but in contrast to stage Ta, most T1 tumors are HG and therefore have a high risk of progression.[12,15] Within stage T1 urothelial cancer, studies have shown that deeper invasion into the lamina propria leads to higher progression rates (58%) compared with superficial invasion (36%), and depth of invasion (as measured by muscularis mucosae involvement) is a significant independent predictor of progression.[15–17] While this is likely related in part to increased aggressiveness of more deeply invading tumors, this may also be indicative of the increased likelihood of an incomplete endoscopic resection in patients with tumors invading into the muscularis mucosae. Thus, adequate TUR is critical not only to ensure accurate staging and guide future management options, but also to remove all tumor from the bladder.

It should be emphasized that invasion of the muscularis mucosae is still considered non-muscle invasive disease in contrast to muscularis propria (MP) invasion, which is the hallmark of true muscle invasion (stage T2). Therefore, a TUR specimen with only muscularis mucosae and no MP is still considered inadequate for determination of muscle invasion. **Fig. 1** demonstrates a cT1 tumor with MP present in the specimen and not involved by cancer. **Fig. 2** demonstrates a cT1 tumor with only muscularis mucosae present in the specimen; it is therefore inadequate for the determination of muscle invasion due to lack of MP. The ability to distinguish between the MP and muscularis mucosae is challenging, however, as these images show. MP is a distinct layer of muscle fibers, whereas muscularis mucosae is typically a few smooth muscle cells arranged in fibers dispersed throughout the lamina propria.[18]

Sylvester and colleagues[19] reviewed 7 European Organisation for the Research and Treatment of Cancer (EORTC) trials in NMIBC and found that the probability of progression for T1HG disease ranged from 20% to 48% at 5 years, and the

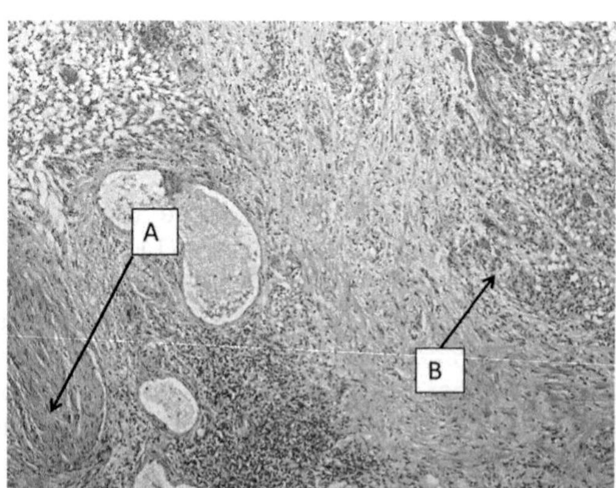

Fig. 1. TUR specimen demonstrating muscularis propria present in the specimen but not involved by urothelial carcinoma. Image shows a thick bundle of muscle fibers (*A*) that are seen in the resected specimen and are separate from the area of tumor (*B*). The tumor is high grade, demonstrating significant cytologic atypia with a desomplastic reaction and lamina propria invasion (stage T1). (*Courtesy of* Lan Gellert MD, PhD, Department of Pathology, Vanderbilt University.)

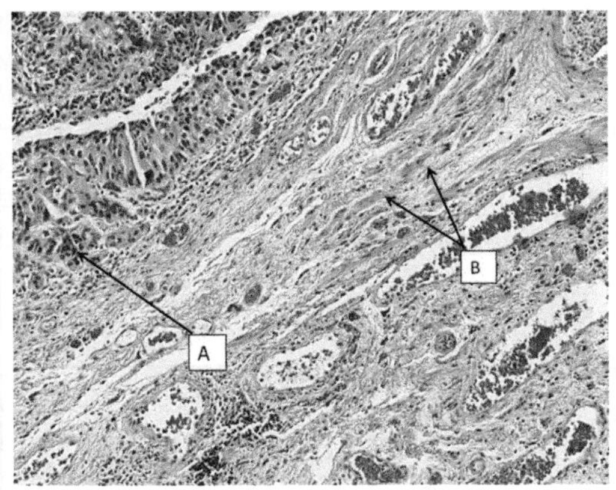

Fig. 2. TUR specimen demonstrating muscularis mucosae present in the specimen but no evidence of muscularis propria. Image shows an HG urothelial carcinoma with invasion of the lamina propria (*A*). There are scant fibers of smooth muscle cells that represent the muscularis mucosae (*B*) present in the lamina propria, but there is no evidence of distinct thick muscle bundles as would be seen if muscularis propria were present in the specimen. (*Courtesy of* Lan Gellert MD, PhD, Department of Pathology, Vanderbilt University.)

most important predictive factor was the presence of concomitant CIS. Patients who had T1 HG urothelial cancer without CIS had a 29% probability of progression at 5 years, whereas those with concomitant CIS had a 74% probability of progression at 5 years.[19] Similarly, in a multivariate analysis of predictors of recurrence, progression, and survival in primary Ta and T1 urothelial cancer, Millan-Rodriguez and colleagues[20] demonstrated that patients with CIS had almost twice the risk of recurrence and progression and 3 times the risk of mortality than those without CIS. CIS as a stand-alone entity is rare and represents only 1% to 10% of NMIBC. Additionally, although it is a noninvasive lesion, its presence is considered a strong indicator of risk for progression and HG disease.[3,4,21] Patients with CIS in the primary TUR specimen in combination with Ta or T1 tumors should therefore be strongly considered to undergo restaging TUR for accurate staging and prognosis as they can potentially harbor more aggressive disease.

To better understand which patients require restaging TUR, factors besides grade, stage, and CIS need to be considered. Several studies have found that the number of prior recurrences, multiple tumors, large tumor size (>3 cm), and the presence of hydronephrosis are all predictors of recurrence and progression and are additional indicators of high-risk disease.[19,20,22] In particular, tumor size and hydronephrosis are associated with muscle invasion and therefore often indicate tumor understaging in patients thought to have non-muscle invasive disease.[22] Additional pathologic findings that are concerning for progression and highrisk of disease-specific mortality are micropapillary variants of urothelial carcinoma and lymphovascular invasion (LVI).[23,24] The group at MD Anderson Cancer Center reviewed its experience with the micropapillary variant of urothelial carcinoma and found that in those who underwent intravesical bacillus calmette-guerin (BCG) therapy (all T1), only 19% (5/27) of patients were disease-free at a median follow-up of 30 months.[23] Early cystectomy is typically strongly considered in these patients, and restaging TUR is imperative if a bladder preservation strategy is employed, in light of the high risk of progression. With respect to LVI, Cho and colleagues[24] demonstrated that it was an independent predictor of recurrence and progression in 118 patients with NMIBC. Similarly, Resnick and colleagues demonstrated that patients with LVI at TUR were more likely to experience upstaging at the time of radical cystectomy.[25] Finally, there may eventually be a role for molecular profiling to better define the need for restaging TUR. Known markers of disease progression include p53, p16, fibroblast growth factor 3 (FGFR3), E-cadherin, and urokinase-plasminogen activator.[26–28] Future research may help to determine whether these markers can predict which patients may have occult invasive disease and more accurately stratify for risk patients with NMIBC after initial TUR.

In summary, given the data on upstaging, recurrence, and progression in patients with high-risk NMIBC, restaging TUR is indicated in any patient found to have high-grade and/or T1 disease but no MP in the specimen, unless radical cystectomy is planned. Both the 2007 American Urological Association (AUA) guidelines and the 2011 European Association of Urology (EAU) guidelines for the management of NMIBC unequivocally recommend restaging TUR in this setting.[29,30] The clinical relevance of this is apparent in light of contemporary reports revealing only 47% of patients with muscle present in the specimen on initial TUR.[31] Whether restaging TUR is necessary in high-risk patients despite the presence of MP in the initial TUR specimen has historically been an area of debate. However, as will be discussed further, there is a substantial risk of upstaging even when MP is present in the initial TUR specimen, and therefore restaging TUR is increasingly considered standard of care in any patient with HG and/or T1 disease planning on proceeding with a bladder-sparing approach. According to the EAU guidelines, a second restaging TUR is recommended in any patient with HG and/or T1 bladder cancer on initial TUR, regardless of the presence of MP in the specimen (level of evidence 2a).[30,32] The AUA guidelines also suggest that it is appropriate to consider restaging TUR in patients with HG T1 with MP and also HG Ta patients in an effort to improve the accuracy of clinical staging, although there is no explicit recommendation in favor of restaging TUR in these patients.[29]

WHY TO RESTAGE

Evidence for Understaging at Initial TUR

A central rationale for restaging TUR in high-risk NMIBC is the concern over clinical understaging given the specter of missing occult muscle-invasive disease. Available data from patients undergoing radical cystectomy for NMIBC suggests that there is a significant rate of clinical understaging. In an analysis of 78 patients who had radical cystectomy for non-muscle invasive disease Dutta and colleagues[33] demonstrated that 31 cases (40%) were clinically understaged, and most of these (80%) were cT1 based on their initial TUR. Of the 63 overall cT1 patients in the cohort, 26 (41%) had no MP in the specimen, and 16 (62%) of those without muscle were understaged compared with only 11 of 37 (30%) cT1 patients understaged with MP present and uninvolved.[33] These findings illustrate 2 salient points in TUR for NMIBC. First, the absence of MP at the time of pathologic analysis leads to a significant rate of understaging, and second, the rate of clinical understaging is as high as 30%, even with muscle in the specimen. Other contemporary studies have demonstrated similar rates of understaging.[34–36] In a series of 95 patients from the University of Michigan undergoing radical cystectomy for cT1 bladder cancer, 26 (27%) patients were understaged by TUR.[34] Bianco and colleagues reported an identical rate of 27% understaging for 66 cT1 patients following radical cystectomy.[35] **Table 1** illustrates the findings of several series comparing rates of clinical understaging based on review of radical cystectomy specimen. Thus, restaging TUR was first advocated in the setting of T1 disease without MP in the resection specimen in an effort to avoid the high rates of understaging found across these studies.

Risk factors for understaging relate primarily to the thoroughness of the TUR, with the main goal of any resection being to completely excise all tumor tissue with negative margins and obtain MP in the specimen for pathologic analysis. Absence of MP is an important indicator of a potentially incomplete resection.[37] A contemporary analysis by Badalato and colleagues[38] found that up to 78% of cT1 patients without MP in the specimen were upstaged at the time of cystectomy. However, as mentioned, understaging may occur even in the presence of muscle up to 30% of the time.[33] Muscularis mucosae involvement, mixed histology, and urethral involvement (in particular tumor in the prostatic urethra) are all additional predictors of understaging at initial TUR.[34,39] Demographic features that may independently predict understaging include female gender and age; however these may simply represent surrogate markers of a less aggressive TUR.[38,40]

Table 1
Rates of understaging in NMIBC based on radical cystectomy specimen

Study, Year	Number of Patients	Understaging (%)
Dutta et al,[33] 2001	78	30% (MP) 62% (no MP)
Badalato et al,[38] 2011	114	50% (MP) 78% (no MP)
Weizer et al,[63] 2009	95	27%
Gupta et al,[36] 2008	167	50%
Bianco et al,[35] 2004	66	27%
Fritsche et al,[40] 2010	1136	51%
Ficcara et al,[64] 2005	70	43%

Impact of Restaging TUR on Risk of Understaging

Several series have demonstrated significant improvement in the diagnostic accuracy of clinical staging following a restaging TUR. In a study of 150 patients undergoing a second TUR, Herr demonstrated that 24% of Ta cases (n = 38) were upstaged to T1 and 8% to T2. Similarly, 28% of all T1 tumors (n = 58) were upstaged to T2, and in T1 patients with no MP (n = 23) on primary TUR, 49% were upstaged to T2.[41] For all NMIBC patients (n = 96), the cT0 rate on restaging TUR was only 25%, and upstaging was present in 29% of cases.[41] Schwaibold and colleagues[42] reported similar findings following their experience in 136 patients who underwent restaging TUR, with 21% demonstrating an increase in T stage and 52% with residual tumor. Of those with residual tumor, 86% of disease was located in the prior resection site. However, other series, such as that reported by Schips and colleagues,[43] have reported lower rates of upstaging and residual disease. In this cohort of 110 patients, 40 (36%)

had residual disease. Of these, 22 (55%) patients were correctly staged; 9 (8%) patients were down-staged, and another 9 (8%) patients were up-staged following restaging TUR.[43] When broken down by stage, both cTa and cT1 tumors had similar rates of upstaging at 6.4% and 7.9%, respectively.[43] In another group of NMIBC patients (n = 710), Herr and colleagues found that 61% had residual disease on restaging TUR.[44] Importantly, restaging TUR pathology (T0 vs Tany) was a significant independent predictor of any tumor recurrence (HR 1.3) and stage progression (hazard ratio [HR] 6.9, *P*<.001 for both). They also found that none of the patients with LG NMIBC were upstaged on restaging TUR, supporting the general consensus that Ta LG tumors do not require restaging transurethral resection of bladder tumor (TURBT).[44]

The reported variation in these rates of upstaging is likely due to a combination of factors, including both TUR technique and pathologic interpretation.[18,45] Several studies have demonstrated that more experienced surgeons are more likely to obtain MP at TUR, and surgeon experience may impact the likelihood of recurrence following TUR.[37,46] However, in 1 cohort focusing on 523 patients with cT1 NMIBC seen at Memorial Sloan-Kettering Cancer Center (MSKCC) and undergoing restaging TUR either at MSKCC or elsewhere, a similar proportion of patients (21% MSKCC, 18% outside) were upstaged to T2 regardless of the institution where restaging TUR was performed.[31] This observation suggests that even in experienced hands, repeat TUR is necessary in patients with high-risk NMIBC. Additionally, 84 patients with NMIBC at restaging TUR went on to receive immediate cystectomy following repeated resection, and 19 (23%) were upstaged to pT2 or higher, demonstrating that even though a restaging TUR may improve the diagnostic accuracy, there is still a substantial risk of understaging.[31] **Table 2** summarizes and compares the rates of upstaging and residual disease reported in several contemporary series of NMIBC patients following restaging TUR. Data from these centers of excellence cumulatively support the fact that even in the best of hands, regardless of how thorough a resection for high-grade T1 disease, a repeat TUR should be performed to ensure accurate staging and for removal of any remaining residual noninvasive disease.

Table 2
Rates of upstaging and residual disease after repeat TUR

Study, Year	Number of Patients	Upstaging	Residual Tumor
Herr,[41] 1999	96	29%	75%
Schwaibold et al,[42] 2006	136	21%	52%
Schips et al,[43] 2002	110	8%	18%
Dalbagni et al,[31] 2009	523	20%	–
Divrik et al,[10] 2010	105	7%	33%

Impact of Restaging TUR on Response to Intravesical Therapy

Favorable response rates following intravesical therapy after a second TUR have been demonstrated in multiple studies when compared with a treatment following a single TUR. In a study from MSKCC comparing 215 patients who underwent restaging TUR followed by 6-week induction intravesical BCG with 132 who underwent a single TUR then received BCG therapy, the recurrence rate at 1 year and progression rate at 3 years were 17% and 7%, respectively for those who had a second TUR compared with 61% and 34% for those who had no restaging.[47] The rate of tumor presence at first cystoscopy after intravesical therapy was almost twice as high in those who were not restaged (57%) compared with those who had a second TUR (29%). On multivariate analysis, restaging TUR before intravesical BCG was a significant independent predictor of lower rates of recurrence and progression.[47] In a contemporary analysis of patients undergoing a repeat TUR followed by induction and maintenance BCG, those who were confirmed to have no residual tumor had improved response rates, with only 11% experiencing recurrence during follow-up (2.7 years) compared with 28% of those who had tumor present at second TUR.[48] Data from a prospective, randomized clinical trial of mitomycin C (MMC) following TUR also support the findings of improved response rates for those undergoing repeat resection. One hundred forty-two patients were randomized to either single versus restaging TUR (at 2–6 weeks) followed by a perioperative (within 24 hours – mean 2 hours) dose of intravesical MMC and then weekly instillations for 7 more weeks.[49] Recurrence-free survival (RFS) was significantly better for patients undergoing restaging TUR (74%) compared with a single TUR (37%). The median RFS was 27 months for the restaging TUR group versus 12 months for the single TUR group. However, there was no significant difference in progression during the follow-up period (mean follow-up 31.5 months).[49] While a single perioperative dose of MMC has been well established for its role in decreasing recurrence following TUR, there is not strong evidence of an impact on disease progression, potentially explaining the similar progression rates in this study.[50] These studies support the hypothesis that restaging TUR improves the accuracy of staging, thereby appropriately allocating patients to the correct treatment groups, and for those with residual tumor, restaging TUR decreases tumor burden and appears to improve the likelihood of a complete response to subsequent therapy.[47,51]

Impact of Restaging TUR on Cancer-Related Outcomes

As with other treatment decisions in NMIBC, the efficacy of restaging TURBT must be evaluated in terms of its effect on recurrence, progression, and survival. Evidence supporting a difference in recurrence for those undergoing restaging TUR versus single TUR has been shown by the analysis of Grimm and colleagues,[52] who reported a 63% versus 40% 5-year RFS for repeat compared with single TUR. Similarly, other studies have reported a significant difference in 5-year RFS of 59% for patients undergoing second resection versus 32% for a single TUR.[10] With respect to progression, the same group also demonstrated a significant improvement in 5-year progression free survival (PFS), with a rate of 93% for restaging TUR versus 79% for single resection.[10] In addition, despite a small number of patients dying of disease (16/65, 25%), they were able to show a significantly better cancer-specific mortality for restaging TUR (5/30, 16.7%) compared with single TUR (11/35, 31.4%). On multivariate analysis, a second TUR was an independent predictor of both recurrence (HR 2.482, P = .001) and progression (HR 3.487, P = .007).[10] These studies suggest that restaging TUR, in addition to providing accurate diagnostic information for better treatment allocation, may directly impact cancer-related outcomes by decreasing intravesical tumor burden.

WHEN AND HOW TO PERFORM RESTAGING TRANSURETHRAL RESECTION

Timing

Most studies suggest that restaging TUR should be performed within 2 to 6 weeks of the initial resection,[41,53] and, in light of these data, the EAU guidelines recommend performing restaging TUR within this time window.[30] However, studies have reported waiting as long as 7 weeks for restaging TUR, and others have defined restaging TUR as any resection performed less than 3 months following initial resection.[31,52] There is limited evidence to definitively support a single optimal time for repeat resection, and further investigations may help clarify this issue. Waiting for 2 weeks is likely sufficient to promote healing of the urothelium and thereby minimize the risk of perforation following sampling of previously resected areas. Delaying restaging TUR beyond 6 weeks, without a strong clinical indication, could potentially have adverse effects, including persistent hematuria from residual disease and, most importantly, disease progression due to delay of definitive treatment with intravesical therapy or radical cystectomy. It has been well demonstrated that prolonging the wait time from TUR to cystectomy increases the risk of overall mortality.[54] Particularly in light of the high rates of upstaging to muscle-invasive disease at restaging TUR, these data lend support to minimizing the lag time before second TUR to less than 6 weeks.

Technique

A restaging TUR is typically performed in the standard fashion of the initial TUR; however, particular attention is paid to deep sampling of the old resection bed.[45] The erythema and edema that occur around the time of the initial resection will have resolved, thus affording the opportunity to reassess whether a complete resection was performed at the time of the initial TUR.[55] Any evidence of residual tumor should be completely resected. A TUR loop resection should be performed of the old scar followed by a cold-cup biopsy of the base and resection edges of the old scar. It is imperative to resect detrusor muscle from the tumor bed, even if at the risk of bladder microperforation. Small asymptomatic bladder perforations are common, and do not appear to pose significant risk to the patient.[56] Each biopsy is sent in a separate container, which may potentially improve pathologic staging accuracy.[45] In addition, care should be taken to limit excess cautery, as this may lead to pathologic artifact and difficult interpretation of the specimen (**Fig. 3**). The larger sampling obtained with the TUR loop helps with a more definitive pathologic analysis, and the TUR loop can be used simultaneously to remove any residual non-muscle invasive disease. In addition to residual tumor at the site of the original resection, Brausi and colleagues demonstrated that 53% (166 of 316 patients) of patients with recurrence at the time of second TUR had tumor found at other sites. These tumors should be managed in the standard fashion and sampled separately using either cold-cup biopsy or TUR depending on size and suspicion for higher-grade disease.[45,57]

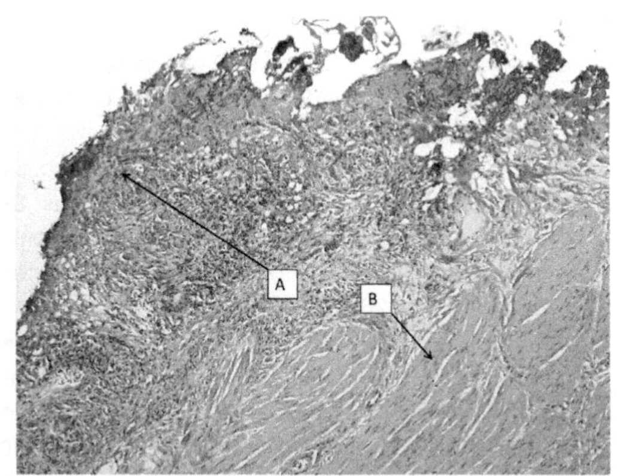

Fig. 3. TUR specimen demonstrating cautery artifact. Image shows resected tissue that is difficult to interpret due to poor cytologic detail with debris and distortion as a result of excessive cauterization (*A*). There are also thick muscle bundles present in the specimen (*B*), consistent with the presence of muscularis propria. (*Courtesy of* Lan Gellert MD, PhD, Department of Pathology, Vanderbilt University.)

Finally, there is increasing interest in photodynamic diagnosis (PDD) using a photosensitizer (5 aminolevulinate [5-ALA] or hexylaminolevulinate [HAL]). The dye is instilled and absorbed most rapidly by hypermatabolic or dysplastic tissue, emitting an intense red color that facilitates detection.[58] While the authors are not aware of any studies specifically addressing the use of PDD at restaging TURBT, there is strong evidence that these dyes aid in detection of tumors that would be otherwise missed by white light cystoscopy.[59–61] Furthermore, Karaolides and colleagues recently randomized 102 patients with NMIBC to TURBT with either white light alone or with the aid of PDD.[62] Their results suggest more successful complete tumor resection in the setting of HAL, with significant improvements in recurrence-free rates in the HAL cohort relative to the white light cohort. Whether similar results will be observed when PDD is used for restaging TUR remains to be seen, but it seems highly likely based on these data that PDD could offer both improved staging accuracy and tumor clearance in this high-risk population.

SUMMARY

The goal of restaging TUR is threefold: to improve staging accuracy, resect any residual tumor, and potentially to improve the response to intravesical treatment.[32,49] While patients with LG Ta cancer do not require restaging TUR, a second TUR is indicated in those patients with a high risk of being understaged or harboring residual disease. This most directly applies to patients with HG T1 disease, particularly with no MP present in the initial TUR specimen. However, patients with HG Ta are also at a significant risk of understaging and tumor recurrence, and restaging TURBT is appropriate in this population also. Other features that have been shown to increase the risk of recurrence and progression in NMIBC such as large tumors, presence of CIS, and multiple tumors may prompt restaging TUR in an effort to ensure accurate staging and improve the response rates to intravesical therapy compared with a single TUR. The second TUR should be done within 2 to 6 weeks of the initial TUR, and the base and margins of the old scar should be sampled separately for pathologic analysis. Lastly, proper patient counseling regarding prognosis is highly reliant on accurate diagnostic information and cannot be achieved without restaging TUR when clinically indicated.

REFERENCES

1. Siegel R, Naishadham D, Jemal A. Cancer statistics, 2012. CA Cancer J Clin 2012;62:10–29.
2. David KA, Mallin K, Milowsky MI, et al. Surveillance of urothelial carcinoma: stage and grade migration, 1993-2005 and survival trends, 1993-2000. Cancer 2009;115:1435–47.
3. Lopez-Beltran A, Montironi R. Noninvasive urothelial neoplasms: according to the most recent WHO classification. Eur Urol 2004;46:170–6.
4. Donat SM. Evaluation and follow-up strategies for superficial bladder cancer. Urol Clin North Am 2003;30:765–76.
5. Stein JP, Lieskovsky G, Cote R, et al. Radical cystectomy in the treatment of invasive bladder cancer: long-term results in 1054 patients. J Clin Oncol 2001;19:666–75.
6. Freedman ND, Silverman DT, Hollenbeck AR, et al. Association between smoking and risk of bladder cancer among men and women. JAMA 2011;306:737–45.
7. Rink M, Xylinas E, Babjuk M, et al. Impact of smoking on outcomes of patients with a history of recurrent nonmuscle invasive bladder cancer. J Urol 2012;188:2120–8.
8. Lammers RJ, Witjes WP, Hendricksen K, et al. Smoking status is a risk factor for recurrence after transurethral resection of nonmuscle-invasive bladder cancer. Eur Urol 2011;60:713–20.
9. Garcia-Closas M, Malats N, Silverman D, et al. NAT2 slow acetylation, GSTM1 null genotype, and risk of bladder cancer: results from the Spanish Bladder Cancer Study and meta-analyses. Lancet 2005;366:649–59.
10. Divrik RT, Sahin AF, Yildirim U, et al. Impact of routine second transurethral resection on the

long-term outcome of patients with newly diagnosed pT1 urothelial carcinoma with respect to recurrence, progression rate, and disease-specific survival: a prospective randomised clinical trial. Eur Urol 2010;58:185–90.

11. Samaratunga H, Makarov DV, Epstein JI. Comparison of WHO/ISUP and WHO classification of noninvasive papillary urothelial neoplasms for risk of progression. Urology 2002;60:315–9.
12. Pan CC, Chang YH, Chen KK, et al. Prognostic significance of the 2004 WHO/ISUP classification for prediction of recurrence, progression, and cancer-specific mortality of nonmuscle-invasive urothelial tumors of the urinary bladder: a clinicopathologic study of 1,515 cases. Am J Clin Pathol 2010; 133:788–95.
13. Leblanc B, Duclos AJ, Benard F, et al. Long-term follow-up of initial Ta grade 1 transitional cell carcinoma of the bladder. J Urol 1999;162:1946–50.
14. Herr HW. Tumor progression and survival of patients with high grade, noninvasive papillary (TaG3) bladder tumors: 15-year outcome. J Urol 2000;163: 60–1 [discussion: 61–2].
15. Cheng L, Neumann RM, Weaver AL, et al. Predicting cancer progression in patients with stage T1 bladder carcinoma. J Clin Oncol 1999;17:3182–7.
16. Holmang S, Hedelin H, Anderstrom C, et al. The importance of the depth of invasion in stage T1 bladder carcinoma: a prospective cohort study. J Urol 1997;157:800–3 [discussion: 4].
17. Bernardini S, Billerey C, Martin M, et al. The predictive value of muscularis mucosae invasion and p53 over expression on progression of stage T1 bladder carcinoma. J Urol 2001;165:42–6 [discussion: 6].
18. Miyamoto H, Epstein JI. Transurethral resection specimens of the bladder: outcome of invasive urothelial cancer involving muscle bundles indeterminate between muscularis mucosae and muscularis propria. Urology 2010;76:600–2.
19. Sylvester RJ, van der Meijden AP, Oosterlinck W, et al. Predicting recurrence and progression in individual patients with stage Ta T1 bladder cancer using EORTC risk tables: a combined analysis of 2596 patients from seven EORTC trials. Eur Urol 2006;49:466–77 [discussion: 75–7].
20. Millan-Rodriguez F, Chechile-Toniolo G, Salvador-Bayarri J, et al. Multivariate analysis of the prognostic factors of primary superficial bladder cancer. J Urol 2000;163:73–8.
21. Lamm DL. Carcinoma in situ. Urol Clin North Am 1992;19:499–508.
22. Divrik RT, Sahin A, Altok M, et al. The frequency of hydronephrosis at initial diagnosis and its effect on recurrence and progression in patients with superficial bladder cancer. J Urol 2007;178:802–6 [discussion: 6].
23. Kamat AM, Gee JR, Dinney CP, et al. The case for early cystectomy in the treatment of nonmuscle invasive micropapillary bladder carcinoma. J Urol 2006; 175:881–5.
24. Cho KS, Seo HK, Joung JY, et al. Lymphovascular invasion in transurethral resection specimens as predictor of progression and metastasis in patients with newly diagnosed T1 bladder urothelial cancer. J Urol 2009;182:2625–30.
25. Resnick MJ, Bergey M, Magerfleisch L, et al. Longitudinal evaluation of the concordance and prognostic value of lymphovascular invasion in transurethral resection and radical cystectomy specimens. BJU Int 2011;107:46–52.
26. Cordon-Cardo C, Zhang ZF, Dalbagni G, et al. Cooperative effects of p53 and pRB alterations in primary superficial bladder tumors. Cancer Res 1997;57:1217–21.
27. Hitchings AW, Kumar M, Jordan S, et al. Prediction of progression in pTa and pT1 bladder carcinomas with p53, p16 and pRb. Br J Cancer 2004; 91:552–7.
28. Sanchez-Carbayo M, Cordon-Cardo C. Molecular alterations associated with bladder cancer progression. Semin Oncol 2007;34:75–84.
29. Hall MC, Chang SM, Dalbagni G, et al. Guideline for the management of nonmuscle invasive bladder cancer: (stages Ta, T1 and Tis): 2007 update. J Urol 2007;178(6):2314–30.
30. Babjuk M, Oosterlinck W, Sylvester R, et al. EAU guidelines on nonmuscle-invasive urothelial carcinoma of the bladder, the 2011 update. Eur Urol 2011;59:997–1008.
31. Dalbagni G, Vora K, Kaag M, et al. Clinical outcome in a contemporary series of restaged patients with clinical T1 bladder cancer. Eur Urol 2009;56:903–10.
32. Kulkarni GS, Hakenberg OW, Gschwend JE, et al. An updated critical analysis of the treatment strategy for newly diagnosed high-grade T1 (previously T1G3) bladder cancer. Eur Urol 2010;57:60–70.
33. Dutta SC, Smith JA Jr, Shappell SB, et al. Clinical under staging of high-risk nonmuscle invasive urothelial carcinoma treated with radical cystectomy. J Urol 2001;166:490–3.
34. Weizer AZ, Wasco MJ, Wang R, et al. Multiple adverse histological features increase the odds of under staging T1 bladder cancer. J Urol 2009;182: 59–65 [discussion: 65].
35. Bianco FJ Jr, Justa D, Grignon DJ, et al. Management of clinical T1 bladder transitional cell carcinoma by radical cystectomy. Urol Oncol 2004;22: 290–4.
36. Gupta A, Lotan Y, Bastian PJ, et al. Outcomes of patients with clinical T1 grade 3 urothelial cell bladder carcinoma treated with radical cystectomy. Urology 2008;71:302–7.

37. Mariappan P, Zachou A, Grigor KM, et al. Detrusor muscle in the first, apparently complete transurethral resection of bladder tumour specimen is a surrogate marker of resection quality, predicts risk of early recurrence, and is dependent on operator experience. Eur Urol 2010;57:843–9.
38. Badalato G, Patel T, Hruby G, et al. Does the presence of muscularis propria on transurethral resection of bladder tumour specimens affect the rate of upstaging in cT1 bladder cancer? BJU Int 2011; 108:1292–6.
39. Huguet J, Crego M, Sabate S, et al. Cystectomy in patients with high risk superficial bladder tumors who fail intravesical BCG therapy: pre-cystectomy prostate involvement as a prognostic factor. Eur Urol 2005;48:53–9 [discussion: 9].
40. Fritsche HM, Burger M, Svatek RS, et al. Characteristics and outcomes of patients with clinical T1 grade 3 urothelial carcinoma treated with radical cystectomy: results from an international cohort. Eur Urol 2010;57:300–9.
41. Herr HW. The value of a second transurethral resection in evaluating patients with bladder tumors. J Urol 1999;162:74–6.
42. Schwaibold HE, Sivalingam S, May F, et al. The value of a second transurethral resection for T1 bladder cancer. BJU Int 2006;97:1199–201.
43. Schips L, Augustin H, Zigeuner RE, et al. Is repeated transurethral resection justified in patients with newly diagnosed superficial bladder cancer? Urology 2002;59:220–3.
44. Herr HW, Donat SM. A re-staging transurethral resection predicts early progression of superficial bladder cancer. BJU Int 2006;97:1194–8.
45. Nieder AM, Manoharan M. The role of the surgeon and transurethral resection in the treatment of superficial bladder cancer. ScientificWorldJournal 2006;6: 2626–31.
46. Han KS, Joung JY, Cho KS, et al. Results of repeated transurethral resection for a second opinion in patients referred for nonmuscle invasive bladder cancer: the referral cancer center experience and review of the literature. J Endourol 2008; 22:2699–704.
47. Herr HW. Restaging transurethral resection of high-risk superficial bladder cancer improves the initial response to bacillus Calmette-Guerin therapy. J Urol 2005;174:2134–7.
48. Guevara A, Salomon L, Allory Y, et al. The role of tumor-free status in repeat resection before intravesical bacillus Calmette-Guerin for high grade Ta, T1 and CIS bladder cancer. J Urol 2010;183: 2161–4.
49. Divrik RT, Yildirim U, Zorlu F, et al. The effect of repeat transurethral resection on recurrence and progression rates in patients with T1 tumors of the bladder who received intravesical mitomycin: a prospective, randomized clinical trial. J Urol 2006;175:1641–4.
50. Sylvester RJ, Oosterlinck W, van der Meijden AP. A single immediate postoperative instillation of chemotherapy decreases the risk of recurrence in patients with stage Ta T1 bladder cancer: a meta-analysis of published results of randomized clinical trials. J Urol 2004;171:2186–90 [quiz: 435].
51. Herr HW. Is repeat transurethral resection needed for minimally invasive T1 urothelial cancer? Pro. J Urol 2011;186:787–8.
52. Grimm MO, Steinhoff C, Simon X, et al. Effect of routine repeat transurethral resection for superficial bladder cancer: a long-term observational study. J Urol 2003;170:433–7.
53. Dalbagni G, Herr HW, Reuter VE. Impact of a second transurethral resection on the staging of T1 bladder cancer. Urology 2002;60:822–4 [discussion: 824–5].
54. Kulkarni GS, Urbach DR, Austin PC, et al. Longer wait times increase overall mortality in patients with bladder cancer. J Urol 2009;182:1318–24.
55. Herr HW, Donat SM. Quality control in transurethral resection of bladder tumours. BJU Int 2008;102: 1242–6.
56. Balbay MD, Cimentepe E, Unsal A, et al. The actual incidence of bladder perforation following transurethral bladder surgery. J Urol 2005;174:2260–2 [discussion: 2262–3].
57. Brausi M, Collette L, Kurth K, et al. Variability in the recurrence rate at first follow-up cystoscopy after TUR in stage Ta T1 transitional cell carcinoma of the bladder: a combined analysis of seven EORTC studies. Eur Urol 2002;41:523–31.
58. Kriegmair M, Baumgartner R, Knuechel R, et al. Fluorescence photodetection of neoplastic urothelial lesions following intravesical instillation of 5-aminolevulinic acid. Urology 1994;44:836–41.
59. Grossman HB, Stenzl A, Fradet Y, et al. Long-term decrease in bladder cancer recurrence with hexaminolevulinate enabled fluorescence cystoscopy. J Urol 2012;188:58–62.
60. Inoue K, Fukuhara H, Shimamoto T, et al. Comparison between intravesical and oral administration of 5-aminolevulinic acid in the clinical benefit of photodynamic diagnosis for nonmuscle invasive bladder cancer. Cancer 2012;118:1062–74.
61. Kausch I, Sommerauer M, Montorsi F, et al. Photodynamic diagnosis in non-muscle-invasive bladder cancer: a systematic review and cumulative analysis of prospective studies. Eur Urol 2010;57: 595–606.
62. Karaolides T, Skolarikos A, Bourdoumis A, et al. Hexaminolevulinate-induced fluorescence versus white light during transurethral resection of noninvasive bladder tumor: does it reduce recurrences? Urology 2012;80:354–9.

63. Weizer AZ, Wasco MJ, Wang R, et al. Multiple adverse histological features increase the odds of under staging T1 bladder cancer. J Urol 2009; 182(1):59–65.

64. Ficarra V, Dalpiaz O, Alrabi N, et al. Correlation between clinical and pathological staging in a series of radical cystectomies for bladder carcinoma. BJU Int 2005;95(6):786–90.

Optimal Risk-Adapted Surveillance Strategies for NMIBC, Including Upper Tract Imaging

Michael C. Large, MD, Joshua A. Cohn, MD*,
Gary D. Steinberg, MD

KEYWORDS

• Non-muscle invasive • Bladder cancer • Guidelines • Surveillance • Treatment • Imaging

KEY POINTS

- The financial burden of non-muscle invasive bladder cancer (NMIBC) continues to increase, underscoring the importance of efficient, evidence-based management of this disease. Management varies by risk (low, intermediate, or high).
- One of the treatment challenges rests in the heterogeneity within the umbrella diagnosis of NMIBC: mortality rates from low-risk disease are nonexistent, whereas those from high-risk disease approach 30% at 10 years. As such, there is concern for overtreatment of low-risk disease and undertreatment of high-risk disease.
- Following transurethral resection of bladder tumor (TURBT), consideration may be given to a single perioperative dose of intravesical chemotherapy. A European Organization for Research and Treatment of Cancer meta-analysis concluded that this practice was associated with a 12% reduction in tumor recurrence and a 39% reduction in the odds of recurrence. This finding was reportedly independent of the agent selected. An American Urological Association meta-analysis concluded there was a 17% absolute reduction in recurrence relative to TURBT alone across all risk groups. Evidence suggests, however, that the benefit of single-dose perioperative intravesical chemotherapy is limited for multiple or recurrent tumors or in cases of high-grade disease when bacillus Calmette-Guérin (BCG) therapy is planned.
- For those pursuing a bladder-sparing approach in pathologic Ta high-grade, Tis, and/or T1 disease, an induction course of intravesical BCG followed by maintenance BCG is a recommendation, with a meta-analysis suggesting a 5-year recurrence rate of 34% for those receiving TURBT and BCG maintenance.
- One of the foremost challenges to the urologist treating NMIBC is deciding when to abandon bladder-sparing therapies in favor of cystectomy. The morbidity of cystectomy is considerable, with short-term complication rates greater than 60%. However, it is also known that 40% to 50% of patients with Tis will fail BCG and nearly 25% will be pT2 or greater and 5.8% pN+ at cystectomy.

Funding sources: None.
Conflict of interest: Dr Cohn and Dr Large: None; Dr Steinberg: Consultant for Photocure, Abbott Molecular, Endo Pharmaceuticals, Predictive Biosciences, and Archimedes.
Section of Urology, The University of Chicago Medical Center, 5841 South Maryland Avenue, MC 6038, Chicago, IL 60637, USA
* Corresponding author.
E-mail address: joshua.cohn@uchospitals.edu

Urol Clin N Am 40 (2013) 305–315
http://dx.doi.org/10.1016/j.ucl.2013.01.013
0094-0143/13/$ – see front matter

INTRODUCTION

In 2012, there were an estimated 73 510 new cases of bladder cancer diagnosed in the United States.[1] Approximately 90% of bladder cancers are urothelial cell carcinoma (UC), with subtypes of squamous cell carcinoma and adenocarcinoma or other variants composing 5% and 2% or less of cases, respectively.[2] Seventy percent of newly diagnosed bladder cancer is non-muscle invasive bladder cancer (NMIBC). Although historically known as *superficial bladder cancer*, this term has been replaced by the stratification of NMIBC into 3 risk categories: low, intermediate, and high.[3] Although all major guidelines agree that risk stratification of NMIBC is appropriate, there is not consensus on the definitions of each risk category (**Table 1**).[4–6]

One of the treatment challenges rests in the heterogeneity within the umbrella diagnosis of NMIBC: mortality rates from low-risk disease are nonexistent, whereas those from high-risk disease approach 30% at 10 years.[7] As such, there is concern for overtreatment of low-risk disease[8] and under treatment of high-risk disease.[9] Improper management of NMIBC can be costly for patients and the health care system. Bladder cancer is estimated to be the ninth most expensive cancer in the United States, with total costs of approximately $3.98 billion in 2010, a number expected to increase to $4.9 billion by 2020.[10] It is estimated that $39 293 of the $65 158 average lifetime cost of treatment is associated with surveillance and management of recurrence, underscoring the importance of efficiency and quality in delivery of care for NMIBC.[11]

Evidence-based guidelines from the American Urological Association (AUA), the European Association of Urology (EAU), and the National Comprehensive Cancer Network (NCCN) have been established to simplify the diagnosis and treatment of this heterogeneous disease. This article reviews the consensus diagnostic and treatment algorithms for NMIBC, divided into 3 risk categories, and highlights the similarities and differences in recommendations across the AUA, EAU, and NCCN guidelines. The treatments discussed include (1) transurethral resection of bladder tumor (TURBT); (2) perioperative, postoperative, and maintenance intravesical therapy; and (3) cystectomy. When appropriate, rates of recurrence, progression, and mortality are addressed.

DIAGNOSIS, DETECTION, AND SURVEILLANCE TOOLS

This section describes the presentation of bladder cancer as well as the tools available to the urologist in its diagnosis and surveillance. Its purpose is to outline both routine and investigational tools intended to improve the management of NMIBC. Any specific recommendations regarding the use of these agents are described in subsequent sections.

The diagnosis of bladder cancer is usually preceded by hematuria. Patients with macroscopic hematuria have reported rates of bladder cancer between 13.0% and 34.5%, with microscopic hematuria associated with bladder cancer at a rate of 0.5% to 10.5%.[12–16] New-onset irritative voiding symptoms may also indicate underlying malignancy, with or without hematuria.[17,18]

Although cystoscopy is the mainstay of bladder cancer diagnosis and surveillance, cytology and urinary markers are often used in an adjunctive role. Urinary cytology, which involves microscopic examination of voided or barbotaged urine, has a sensitivity of between 4% and 31% for the diagnosis of low-grade disease, with an overall sensitivity and specificity of 34% and 99%.[19] Its sensitivity improves for high-grade disease, particularly carcinoma in situ (CIS); however, cytology may miss up to 60% of high-grade tumors.[20]

Tumor marker assays have been developed in an effort to improve on cytology for the detection of bladder cancer with variable success. Commercially available tumor marker assays include bladder tumor antigen (BTA), ImmunoCyt, nuclear matrix protein 22 (NMP22), and UroVysion. BTA assays detect human complement factor H–related protein. Results can be impacted by hematuria from other causes. The overall sensitivity and

Table 1
Risk groups by guideline panel

	Low Risk	Intermediate Risk	High Risk
AUA 2007	Small-volume Ta, low grade	Multifocal and/or large-volume Ta low grade	Ta high grade, T1, Tis
ICUD-EAU 2012	Ta low grade	—	Ta high grade, T1, Tis
NCCN	Ta low grade	Ta high grade	T1 high grade, Tis

Abbreviations: AUA, American Urological Association; ICUD-EAU, International Consultation on Bladder Cancer–European Association of Urology; NCCN, National Comprehensive Cancer Network.

specificity of the BTA stat test have been estimated at 57% to 83% and 60% to 92%, respectively.[20] ImmunoCyt combines cytology and immunofluorescence from monoclonal antibodies against carcinoembryonic antigen and 2 bladder cancer–associated mucins. It has a reported sensitivity of 50% to 100% and a specificity of 69% to 79%. False positives are associated with benign prostatic hyperplasia and cystitis, and it is generally only recommended for monitoring rather than diagnosis. NMP22 detects nuclear matrix protein and is approved for use in bladder cancer surveillance as well as detection of cancer in at-risk patients. Sensitivity and specificity have been reported at 47% to 100% and 60% to 90%, respectively. Specificity is markedly decreased with coexistent inflammation or instrumentation, leading to a relatively high false-positive rate that has limited its utility in clinical practice.[21]

UroVysion is a fluorescent in situ hybridization (FISH) assay that detects loss of 9p21 and aneuploidy of chromosomes 3, 7, and 17 and is approved for use in bladder cancer surveillance and detection.[22] Sensitivity of FISH is reported at 74% overall and 100% for high-grade disease, outperforming cytology in a meta-analysis with an area under the receiver operating characteristic curve of 0.87 versus 0.63.[23] FISH has been associated with the additional benefit of anticipatory positives; multiple studies report the development of cancer within 12 months in a high percentage of cases that seemed to be false positives based on initial cystoscopy.[24,25] The weakness of FISH relative to cytology is its high rate of false positives, which can be improved by combining with cellular morphology. Nonetheless, the specificity when combined with morphology is only 65%.[26] Similar to FISH, several markers designed to detect specific gene mutations common that are common in bladder cancer have shown promise but at this time are still investigational.[20]

Photodynamic agents including 5-aminolevulinic (5-ALA) acid or hexaminolevulinate (HAL) are approved in 26 European countries for the detection of bladder cancer. Neoplastic cells preferentially uptake these agents and fluoresce in the red part of the spectrum under blue-violet light excitation. A meta-analysis by Kausch and colleagues[27] concluded that combined with white-light cystoscopy, the use 5-ALA or HAL resulted in the detection of 20% more tumor-positive patients with NMIBC and 39% more with CIS. The odds of residual tumor being found were significantly less with photodynamic agents than with white-light cystoscopy alone (odds ratio 0.28; 95% confidence interval 0.15–0.52), and recurrence-free survival was significantly higher at 12 and 24 months. Photodynamic agents are not yet part of routine practice in the United States; however, several ongoing clinical trials will help define its role in bladder cancer diagnosis and surveillance in future practice (www.clinicaltrials.gov).

Upper tract imaging is indicated in the context of gross or microscopic hematuria not explained by obvious underlying causes, such as active infection, menstruation, or recent instrumentation.[28] Historically, intravenous urography (IVU) was the imaging study of choice for its availability and cost. It is estimated to detect up to 60% of known bladder tumors and approximately two-thirds of upper tract lesions.[29–31] IVU has, however, been almost entirely replaced by other imaging modalities for the evaluation of the upper tracts.[32] Ultrasound avoids ionizing radiation, although its sensitivity is poor for the detection of renal pelvis tumors, and it does not evaluate the ureters. Its sensitivity for the detection of bladder tumors is highly variable, having been reported at 26.0% to 91.4%.[32,33] Three-dimensional virtual and contrast-enhanced sonography may provide additional benefit for tumor detection within the bladder; however, the clinical utility of these modalities is unclear.[34,35]

Computed tomography (CT) and CT urography (CTU) have become the American College of Radiology's test of choice for the evaluation of the upper tracts in hematuria.[36] In a study by Turney and colleagues,[37] in 200 patients with hematuria with a cancer prevalence of 24% on cystoscopy, CTU had a sensitivity, specificity, and negative predictive value of 93%, 99%, and 98%, respectively. The sensitivity for the detection of bladder tumors seems to be best in patients with gross hematuria.[38] CTU can fail to pick up smaller tumors (<5–10 mm) and has limited ability to distinguish cancer from mucosal changes related to recent cystoscopic procedures.[39,40] Renal impairment can prevent the use of contrast in CTU, which limits its utility in this setting.

Gadolinium-enhanced magnetic resonance imaging (MRI) urography may be even better than CTU for tumor detection, with one head-to-head study reporting sensitivity of 93% versus 100% for CTU versus MRI urography and another suggesting superior ability to detect small (<10 mm) tumors.[41,42] Diffusion-weighted MRI seems to have further advantages over standard MRI in the detection of lesions and in distinguishing benign from malignant disease.[43,44] Although MRI does have the advantage of avoiding ionizing radiation, contrast administration is, as in CT, limited in those with poor renal function (estimated glomerular filtration rate <30 mL/min).[32] Its relatively higher cost and lack of availability have also limited its use in clinical practice relative to CTU; however, given its advantages relative to CT in local staging, the use of MRI is increasing in some centers. Virtual cystoscopy with either CT or MRI, although an interesting concept, is associated with a higher cost and increased radiation exposure relative to conventional CT and has no role in routine workup of hematuria.[45]

LOW-RISK DISEASE

Low-risk disease is defined by the AUA's guidelines as small, solitary, low-grade, primary disease.[4] Differing slightly from the AUA, as evident from **Table 2**, the International Consultation on Bladder Cancer–European Association of Urology's (ICUD-EAU) guidelines and the NCCN's Clinical Practice Guidelines in Oncology (NCCN's guidelines) define low-risk disease as Ta low grade.[5,6]

Approximately 20% of NMIBC presents as Ta low-grade disease, with an additional 20% presenting as papillary urothelial neoplasm of low malignant potential (PUNLMP) and 10% as papilloma.[46] Papillomas are urothelial outgrowths with otherwise completely normal urothelium and cellular architecture. A PUNLMP is defined by orderly but slightly altered cellular architecture with minimal nuclear atypia.[47] Papillomas and PUNLMPs are essentially benign lesions; however, distinguishing these entities from low-grade urothelial carcinoma can be challenging for pathologists less familiar with the changes made in the 2004 World Health Organization/International Society of Urological Pathology's consensus classification. Additionally, the potential for a small focus of cancer within or adjacent to one of these lesions means the rate of progression to invasive disease is close to but is not zero.

The consensus from the guidelines of the AUA, NCCN, and EAU for initial management involves complete transurethral resection (TURBT) of the lesion.[4–6] For lesions appearing superficial, small, and low-risk, a deep resection may not be necessary. Removal of the lesion with biopsy forceps or with a superficial swipe with the resectoscope loop provides an adequate specimen for pathologic review without exposing patients to the attendant risks of bladder perforation and bleeding.[48]

Following TURBT, consideration may be given to a single perioperative dose of intravesical chemotherapy. The EORTC's meta-analysis concluded that this practice was associated with a 12% reduction in tumor recurrence and a 39% reduction in the odds of recurrence.[49] This finding was reportedly independent of the agent selected. The AUA's meta-analysis concluded there was a 17% absolute reduction in recurrence relative to TURBT alone across all risk groups.[50] Evidence suggests, however, that the benefit of single-dose perioperative intravesical chemotherapy is limited for multiple or recurrent tumors[51] or in cases of high-grade disease when BCG therapy is planned.[52] The AUA's guidelines, therefore, recommend a single, immediate postoperative instillation of intravesical chemotherapy only for those with apparent low-risk NMIBC. If NMIBC is confirmed following TURBT, surveillance should consist of periodic cystoscopy with neither duration nor interval defined.

The ICUD-EAU's guidelines state that single intravesical administration of mitomycin C or epirubicin should be offered immediately after TURBT for apparent low-risk disease. Induction chemotherapy with or without maintenance may be offered to these patients for "unclear but potential" benefit.[5] Routine upper tract images are not recommended for isolated Ta low-grade disease, and surveillance is limited to periodic cystoscopy.

The NCCN's guidelines recommend consideration of single-dose postoperative intravesical chemotherapy in the setting of low-grade Ta disease.[6] Upper tract imaging is recommended for staging, and surveillance cystoscopy should be done at 3 months and then increasing intervals as deemed appropriate.

Adverse events following single-dose postoperative chemotherapy instillation have been reported in up to 22% of cases. Although most of these are mild, serious side effects and rarely death have been reported in cases of unrecognized bladder perforation.[52] Because 50% to 70% of low-grade Ta lesions recur but only 5% progress, expectant management of low-grade recurrence is advocated by some investigators.[8,53]

At the authors' institution, they do not routinely use single-dose postoperative chemotherapy based on the risks relative to the modest benefits. If following the initial TURBT there is no tumor at the 3-month in-office surveillance cystoscopy and cytology is negative, the authors perform repeat office cystoscopy 9 months later. Provided there is no recurrence, patients will undergo cystoscopy every 6 to 9 months for 5 years. Upper tract imaging is only performed if patients have symptoms or hematuria.

INTERMEDIATE-RISK DISEASE

AUA index patients with intermediate-risk disease have multifocal, recurrent, and/or large-volume Ta low-grade UC.[4] The NCCN guidelines consider Ta high grade as intermediate-risk, whereas the

Table 2
Individual panel recommendations, stratified by risk group

	Low-Risk	Intermediate-Risk	High-Risk
AUA 2007	• TURBT or biopsy with complete eradication of all visible tumors • Single instillation of intravesical chemotherapy immediately postoperatively (recommendation)	• Induction course of intra vesical BCG or mitomycin C • Maintenance BCG or mito mycin C (option)	• Repeat TURBT if T1 and muscularis propria not sampled • Induction course of intravesical BCG followed by maintenance (recommendation) • Cystectomy (option)
ICUD-EAU 2012	• TURBT with complete resection of all tumors; repeat TURBT if unsure of completeness of resection • Immediate post-TUR intravesical chemotherapy by instillation of mitomycin C or epirubicin	—	• TURBT with complete resection of all tumors; repeat TURBT if unsure of completeness of resection • BCG instillation in patients with pTa high grade urothelial carcinoma • For T1 disease ○ BCG following repeat TUR with initial diagnosis ○ Cystectomy for high-risk T1 and BCG failures
NCCN	• TURBT Adjuvant treatment • BCG (option) • Mitomycin C (option) • Observation (option) • Repeat TURBT if incomplete[a]	• TURBT • Repeat TURBT if incomplete, no muscle in specimen, large or multifocal[a] Adjuvant treatment • BCG • Mitomycin C (option) • Observation (option)	Tis • TURBT + multiple selective and/or random biopsies • Prostate urethral biopsy (option) Adjuvant treatment • BCG T1 • TURBT • Cystectomy (consideration) • Repeat TURBT (if no cystectomy)[a] Adjuvant treatment • No residual ○ BCG (preferred) or mitomycin C • Residual disease ○ BCG or cystectomy T1 with particularly high-risk: multifocal, LVI, BCG refractory • Cystectomy (recommendation)

Abbreviations: BCG, bacillus Calmette-Guérin; ICUD-EAU, International Consultation on Bladder Cancer–European Association of Urology; LVI, lymphovascular invasion.
[a] Within 6 weeks.

ICUD-EAU's guidelines do not explicitly define an intermediate-risk category.[5,6]

The AUA recommends complete TURBT followed by an induction course of bacillus Calmette-Guérin (BCG) or mitomycin C, with a meta-analysis suggesting a decrease in recurrence risk of 24% and 3%, respectively, versus TURBT alone.[4] Maintenance BCG or mitomycin C is an option, with meta-analysis demonstrating reduction in recurrence by 31% and 18%, respectively, versus induction therapies alone. The investigators note, however, that the surgeon must balance this benefit with the cost and side effects of therapy. The AUA's guidelines emphasize that it is unclear if any intravesical therapy decreases the rate of progression.

The NCCN guidelines advocate complete TURBT for Ta high-grade disease (NCCN intermediate-risk), with repeat TURBT within 6 weeks if the tumor is large, multifocal, or incompletely resected or if muscularis propria is absent from the specimen.[6] BCG induction is the preferred adjuvant treatment, with mitomycin C or observation provided as options. BCG induction therapy should be initiated within 4 weeks of TURBT, with a maximum of 2 induction courses. The investigators note that some data suggest maintenance therapy is beneficial. In cases of bacteriuria, gross hematuria, and traumatic catheterization, BCG should be withheld; for severe local symptoms, dose reduction is encouraged. Surveillance cystoscopy and cytology are indicated every 3 to 6 months for 2 years, then increasing as appropriate with consideration of upper tract imaging every 1 to 2 years. Urinary marker studies are optional.

The authors' institutional preference for surveillance in intermediate-risk disease is cystoscopy, cytology, and reflex FISH (ie, if cytology is atypical) every 3 months for 2 years, every 6 months for 2 years, and then annually thereafter. Routine surveillance is stopped if patients have been completely recurrence-free for 5 years. The authors obtain upper tract imaging only if warranted by symptoms and/or hematuria. Intravesical BCG or chemotherapy with maintenance is selectively given to those patients with multiple, multifocal recurrences requiring TURBT.

HIGH-RISK DISEASE

The AUA's and the ICUD-EAU's guidelines include Ta high-grade (approximately 20% of pTa disease is high grade[5]), T1, and Tis cancers as high-risk disease, whereas the NCCN's guidelines include only T1 high grade and Tis.[4–6]

According to the AUA's algorithm, a repeat TURBT should be performed in patients considering a bladder-sparing option with T1 disease but no muscularis propria on initial TURBT.[4] This algorithm is consistent with the findings of Herr[54] who showed that patients with T1 or Ta high-grade tumors, with or without concomitant CIS, who underwent restaging TURBT had an improved response to BCG and decreased recurrence rates. For those pursuing a bladder-sparing approach and pathologic Ta high-grade, Tis, and/or T1 disease, an induction course of intravesical BCG followed by maintenance BCG is a recommendation, with a meta-analysis suggesting a 5-year recurrence rate of 34% for those receiving TURBT and BCG maintenance versus 62% for those with TURBT and mitomycin C maintenance. Up-front radical cystectomy with pelvic lymph node dissection is provided as an option. Patients with recurrent disease after prior intravesical therapy but without sampling of muscularis propria should undergo repeat resection (standard) before further intravesical therapy. The panel recommends cystectomy as the preferred treatment of patients with recurrence of Ta high grade, Tis, and/or T1 after previous intravesical therapy for high-risk disease. Intravesical therapy is an option that may be appropriate for those with late recurrences, but it also may put those at high risk for progression at risk for metastatic or muscle-invasive disease.

The 2012 ICUD-EAU's guidelines state that TURBT with complete resection of all tumors should be performed; repeat TURBT should be done if uncertainty of complete resection exists; upper tract imaging should be obtained; and in the case of CIS, narrow-band cystoscopy should be performed if available.[5] Going forward, there may be a role for the routine use of photodynamic agent-assisted cystoscopy in this setting. For patients with Ta high-grade disease, BCG instillation should be initiated. BCG is recommended for patients with Tis, with at least 1 year of maintenance recommended. For those with T1 disease desiring a bladder-sparing approach, BCG following repeat TURBT should be administered. Cystectomy should be offered for those with high-risk T1, with the risk of progression based on tumor grade, size, and number, timing of recurrence, concomitant CIS, involvement of the prostate, depth of lamina propria invasion, and micropapillary or nested variants. Patients with persistent or recurrent high-risk disease after BCG should also be offered cystectomy.

The response to BCG should be assessed at 3 months, per the ICUD-EAU; those with no response may be offered cystectomy, a second 6-week induction course of BCG, or 3 weekly boosters.[5] For those with BCG failure (defined as disease after induction at 6 months and maintenance 3 months later), cystectomy is deemed the gold standard. The best option for both BCG-resistant disease (defined as persistent disease 3 months after the induction cycle) and BCG-relapsing disease recurring after a disease-free period of 6 months is repeat TURBT followed by BCG.

The NCCN's guidelines are concordant with the other two guidelines, recommending BCG for Tis disease, noting that some data suggest maintenance therapy provides a benefit.[6] The NCCN recommends TURBT with multiple selective and/or random biopsies and mentions prostatic urethral biopsy as a diagnostic option. For T1 high-grade disease, repeat TURBT within 6 weeks is recommended in patients pursuing bladder-sparing treatments while cystectomy is a consideration. Patients with no residual disease at repeat TURBT should preferentially be offered BCG, with mitomycin C listed as an option; those with residual disease may be offered either BCG or cystectomy. Surveillance cystoscopy and cytology should be offered every 3 to 6 months for 2 years, then at greater intervals as appropriate with upper tract imaging considered every 1 to 2 years. Urinary marker studies are optional. Lastly, for patients with T1 disease at particularly high risk of progression (multifocal, BCG refractory, and/or with lymphovascular invasion), cystectomy is recommended.

At the authors' institution, high-risk disease NMIBC is managed with repeat TURBT followed by 6 weeks of induction BCG if a bladder-sparing approach remains appropriate. One-third dose maintenance BCG is given for 3 doses at 3, 6, and 12 months following repeat TURBT. Cystoscopy, cytology, and reflex FISH (for atypical cytology) are performed every 3 months for 2 years, every 6 months for 2 years, and every 9 to 12 months annually thereafter. Upper tract imaging (preferably CTU) is performed on patients with symptoms and/or hematuria, recurrence in the bladder, or every 2 to 3 years.

FUTURE DIRECTIONS

In addition to some of the limitations outlined earlier, additional areas for future investigation remain. One of foremost challenges to the urologist treating NMIBC is deciding when to abandon bladder-sparing therapies in favor of cystectomy. The morbidity of cystectomy is considerable, with short-term complication rates greater than 60%.[55] However, it is also known that 40% to 50% of patients with Tis will fail BCG,[5] and nearly 25% will be pT2 or greater and 5.8% pN+ at cystectomy.[56] For patients with T1 disease, long-term follow-up suggests that roughly one-third will be alive with their native bladder, one-third will be alive having undergone cystectomy, and one-third will be dead of their disease.[7] When reviewing their experience with cystectomy in patients with Tis, Ta high-grade, and/or T1 disease, Herr and Sogani[57] found that disease-free survival (DFS) at 15 years was 69% for patients undergoing cystectomy within 2 years of initial BCG therapy versus 26% for those deferring cystectomy more than 2 years. Likewise, Denzinger and colleagues[58] reported a 78% 10-year cancer-specific survival for patients with T1 disease treated with early cystectomy versus 51% with deferred cystectomy. Although upstaging was found in 30% of cases, no risk factor was found to be predictive.

For patients treated with BCG, Fernandez-Gomez and colleagues[59] have developed a scoring system to predict recurrence and progression. Their Spanish Urological Club for Oncological Treatment (CUETO) model incorporates age, gender, CIS, and tumor grade, number, T stage, and recurrence to arrive at a risk profile. Similarly, Sylvester and colleagues[60] used the EORTC's risk tables to formulate a scoring system for the prediction of recurrence and progression in Ta high-grade and T1 disease. The calculator, found at https://www.eortc.be/tools/bladdercalculator, factors tumor number, size, recurrence rate, T stage, grade, and presence/absence of CIS. Although these nomograms are helpful in counseling patients, the best time for the abandonment of bladder-sparing protocols remains largely unknown. The study of molecular markers may provide further elucidation of predictive genetic factors for progression and recurrence that has the potential to greatly improve future guidelines.

The duration of maintenance BCG therapy also remains unclear. The Southwest Oncology Group (SWOG) study, the largest to demonstrate the benefit of maintenance BCG therapy, enrolled patients with an increased risk of recurrence, defined as those having 2 or more tumors within 1 year, 3 or more within the last 6 months, and/or CIS.[61] Maintenance BCG, per protocol given at 3, 6, 12, 18, 24, 30, and 36 months, was associated with increased recurrence-free survival. Of note, only 16% of patients received all 7 planned BCG treatment cycles. Because the study constitutes the best available evidence for maintenance usage, by default its regimen is frequently cited. The AUA acknowledges, however, that "the optimal maintenance schedule and duration has yet to be determined."[50]

The role of maintenance BCG therapy is also debated. This point is reflected in the difference between the AUA's and the ICUD-EAU's guidelines, both of which recommend maintenance BCG for high-risk patients, and the NCCN's guidelines, which merely mention that some data suggest a benefit from maintenance therapy.[4–6] In contrast to the aforementioned SWOG study and others, Herr's experience has suggested that DFS for patients with high-risk NMIBC treated with TURBT and induction BCG did not improve with the addition of maintenance therapy.[62]

Lastly, details of timing and duration of surveillance for upper tract recurrence remain ill defined.

Disease has been reported 15 years following diagnosis of lower tract disease.[63] In their study of Surveillance Epidemiology and End Results Registry data, Wright and colleagues[64] found high tumor grade, low tumor stage, and location (orifice, trigone, and bladder neck) to be predictive of upper tract recurrence. At present, the AUA's guidelines simply suggest that periodic upper tract monitoring "is of value,"[4,50] whereas the ICUD-EAU's guidelines state that periodic surveillance upper tract imaging for patients with Tis is indicated.[5]

COMPLIANCE

Any discussion of guidelines must address the topic of compliance. First, for guidelines to decrease health care costs and improve efficiency, they should be accessible, cost conscious, and evidence based. Udell[65] showed that a lower-intensity surveillance strategy for patients with low-risk disease can result in savings of nearly $8000 over 5 years. Such analysis may become more prominent in the construction of future guidelines. Addressing the concern of whether sound, evidence-based medicine is used in guideline construction, Poonacha and Go[66] evaluated the NCCN's guidelines for the 10 most common malignancies and reported wide variation in the quality of evidence cited. The ICUD-EAU and NCCN currently list the level of evidence and/or consensus beside guidelines, whereas the AUA stratifies its guideline statements by "standard" versus "recommendation" versus "option," thus lending some transparency to their selection criteria.[4–6,50]

If the implementation of guidelines is lacking, barriers toward adherence must be addressed. Currently, a minority of patients with NMIBC receives guidelines-based care both in the United States and abroad.[67,68] To improve the implementation of guidelines, Miller and colleagues[69] have demonstrated the importance of physician awareness of their baseline practice patterns. By first characterizing urologists' preexisting use of radiographic tests for prostate cancer staging before providing education and feedback, the investigators were able to significantly improve the adherence to guidelines.

Lastly, although guidelines serve an important role in patient care, the physician must not forget to address aspects of the patients' care beyond the primary diagnosis and guideline-based algorithm; although smoking cessation may decrease recurrence rates of NMIBC, it will likely harbor an even greater long-term health benefit that should be appropriately emphasized.[70]

REFERENCES

1. Siegel R, DeSantis C, Virgo K, et al. Cancer treatment and survivorship statistics, 2012. CA Cancer J Clin 2012;62(4):220–41.
2. Lopez-Beltran A. Bladder cancer: clinical and pathological profile. Scand J Urol Nephrol Suppl 2008; 218:95–109.
3. Soloway MS. It is time to abandon the "superficial" in bladder cancer. Eur Urol 2007;52(6):1564–5.
4. Brausi M, Witjes JA, Lamm D, et al. A review of current guidelines and best practice recommendations for the management of nonmuscle invasive bladder cancer by the international bladder cancer group. J Urol 2011;186(6):2158–67.
5. Burger M, Oosterlinck W, Konety B, et al. ICUD-EAU international consultation on bladder cancer 2012: non-muscle-invasive urothelial carcinoma of the bladder. Eur Urol 2013;63(1):36–44.
6. National Comprehensive Cancer Network guidelines in clinical oncology (r). Referenced with permission from The NCCN Clinical Practice Guidelines in Oncology (NCCN guidelines(r)) for guideline bladder cancer V.2.2012. (c) National Comprehensive Cancer Network, Inc 2012. All rights reserved. To view the most recent and complete version of the guideline, Available at: www.nccn.org. Accessed November 10, 2012. National Comprehensive Cancer Network®, NCCN®, NCCN Guidelines®, and all other NCCN content are trademarks owned by the National Comprehensive Cancer Network, Inc.
7. Shahin O, Thalmann GN, Rentsch C, et al. A retrospective analysis of 153 patients treated with or without intravesical bacillus Calmette-Guerin for primary stage T1 grade 3 bladder cancer: recurrence, progression and survival. J Urol 2003; 169(1):96–100 [discussion: 100].
8. Soloway MS. Expectant treatment of small, recurrent, low-grade, noninvasive tumors of the urinary bladder. Urol Oncol 2006;24(1):58–61.
9. Nieder AM, Simon MA, Kim SS, et al. Radical cystectomy after bacillus Calmette-Guérin for high-risk Ta, T1, and carcinoma in situ: defining the risk of initial bladder preservation. Urology 2006;67(4): 737–41.
10. Mariotto AB, Yabroff KR, Shao Y, et al. Projections of the cost of cancer care in the United States: 2010-2020. J Natl Cancer Inst 2011;103(2):117–28.
11. Avritscher EB, Cooksley CD, Grossman HB, et al. Clinical model of lifetime cost of treating bladder cancer and associated complications. Urology 2006;68(3):549–53.
12. Varkarakis MJ, Gaeta J, Moore RH, et al. Superficial bladder tumor. Aspects of clinical progression. Urology 1974;4(4):414–20.
13. Golin AL, Howard RS. Asymptomatic microscopic hematuria. J Urol 1980;124(3):389–91.

14. Mohr DN, Offord KP, Owen RA, et al. Asymptomatic microhematuria and urologic disease. A population-based study. JAMA 1986;256(2):224–9.
15. Sultana SR, Goodman CM, Byrne DJ, et al. Microscopic haematuria: urological investigation using a standard protocol. Br J Urol 1996;78(5):691–6 [discussion: 697–8].
16. Khadra MH, Pickard RS, Charlton M, et al. A prospective analysis of 1,930 patients with hematuria to evaluate current diagnostic practice. J Urol 2000;163(2):524–7.
17. Tissot WD, Diokno AC, Peters KM. A referral center's experience with transitional cell carcinoma misdiagnosed as interstitial cystitis. J Urol 2004; 172(2):478–80.
18. Zincke H, Utz DC, Farrow GM. Review of Mayo Clinic experience with carcinoma in situ. Urology 1985;26(Suppl 4):39–46.
19. Lotan Y, Roehrborn CG. Sensitivity and specificity of commonly available bladder tumor markers versus cytology: results of a comprehensive literature review and meta-analyses. Urology 2003;61(1):109–18 [discussion: 118].
20. Tilki D, Burger M, Dalbagni G, et al. Urine markers for detection and surveillance of non–muscle-invasive bladder cancer. Eur Urol 2011; 60(3):484–92.
21. Sharma S, Zippe CD, Pandrangi L, et al. Exclusion criteria enhance the specificity and positive predictive value of NMP22 and BTA stat. J Urol 1999; 162(1):53–7.
22. Junker K, Boerner D, Schulze W, et al. Analysis of genetic alterations in normal bladder urothelium. Urology 2003;62(6):1134–8.
23. Hajdinjak T. UroVysion FISH test for detecting urothelial cancers: meta-analysis of diagnostic accuracy and comparison with urinary cytology testing. Urol Oncol 2008;26(6):646–51.
24. Skacel M, Fahmy M, Brainard JA, et al. Multitarget fluorescence in situ hybridization assay detects transitional cell carcinoma in the majority of patients with bladder cancer and atypical or negative urine cytology. J Urol 2003;169(6):2101–5.
25. Gofrit ON, Zorn KC, Silvestre J, et al. The predictive value of multi-targeted fluorescent in-situ hybridization in patients with history of bladder cancer. Urol Oncol 2008;26(3):246–9.
26. Daniely M, Rona R, Kaplan T, et al. Combined morphologic and fluorescence in situ hybridization analysis of voided urine samples for the detection and follow-up of bladder cancer in patients with benign urine cytology. Cancer 2007;111(6):517–24.
27. Kausch I, Sommerauer M, Montorsi F, et al. Photodynamic diagnosis in non–muscle-invasive bladder cancer: a systematic review and cumulative analysis of prospective studies. Eur Urol 2010;57(4): 595–606.
28. Davis R, Jones JS, Barocas DA, et al. Diagnosis, evaluation and follow-up of asymptomatic microhematuria (AMH) in adults: AUA guideline. J Urol 2012;188(Suppl 6):2473–81. http://dx.doi.org/10.1016/j.juro.2012.09.078.
29. ACR appropriateness criteria. Pretreatment staging of invasive bladder cancer. American College of Radiology. 2009. Available at: www.acr.org. Accessed November 15, 2012.
30. O'Malley ME, Hahn PF, Yoder IC, et al. Comparison of excretory phase, helical computed tomography with intravenous urography in patients with painless haematuria. Clin Radiol 2003;58(4):294–300.
31. Herranz-Amo F, Diez-Cordero JM, Verdú-Tartajo F, et al. Need for intravenous urography in patients with primary transitional carcinoma of the bladder? Eur Urol 1999;36(3):221–4.
32. Purysko AS, Leão Filho HM, Herts BR. Radiologic imaging of patients with bladder cancer. Semin Oncol 2012;39(5):543–58.
33. Datta SN, Allen GM, Evans R, et al. Urinary tract ultrasonography in the evaluation of haematuria–a report of over 1,000 cases. Ann R Coll Surg Engl 2002;84(3):203–5.
34. Nicolau C, Bunesch L, Sebastia C, et al. Diagnosis of bladder cancer: contrast-enhanced ultrasound. Abdom Imaging 2010;35(4):494–503.
35. Kocakoc E, Kiris A, Orhan I, et al. Detection of bladder tumors with 3-dimensional sonography and virtual sonographic cystoscopy. J Ultrasound Med 2008;27(1):45–53.
36. ACR appropriateness criteria. Hematuria. American College of Radiology. 2008. Available at: www.acr.org. Accessed November 15, 2012.
37. Turney BW, Willatt JM, Nixon D, et al. Computed tomography urography for diagnosing bladder cancer. BJU Int 2006;98(2):345–8.
38. Sadow CA, Silverman SG, O'Leary MP, et al. Bladder cancer detection with CT urography in an academic medical center. Radiology 2008;249(1): 195–202.
39. Jinzaki M, Tanimoto A, Shinmoto H, et al. Detection of bladder tumors with dynamic contrast-enhanced MDCT. AJR Am J Roentgenol 2007;188(4):913–8.
40. Kim JK, Park SY, Ahn HJ, et al. Bladder cancer: analysis of multi-detector row helical CT enhancement pattern and accuracy in tumor detection and perivesical staging. Radiology 2004;231(3):725–31.
41. Kim B, Semelka RC, Ascher SM, et al. Bladder tumor staging: comparison of contrast-enhanced CT, T1- and T2-weighted MR imaging, dynamic gadolinium-enhanced imaging, and late gadolinium-enhanced imaging. Radiology 1994;193(1):239–45.
42. Tanimoto A, Yuasa Y, Imai Y, et al. Bladder tumor staging: comparison of conventional and gadolinium-enhanced dynamic MR imaging and CT. Radiology 1992;185(3):741–7.

43. El-Assmy A, Abou-El-Ghar ME, Mosbah A, et al. Bladder tumour staging: comparison of diffusion- and T2-weighted MR imaging. Eur Radiol 2009; 19(7):1575–81.
44. Avcu S, Koseoglu MN, Ceylan K, et al. The value of diffusion-weighted MRI in the diagnosis of malignant and benign urinary bladder lesions. Br J Radiol 2011;84(1006):875–82.
45. Kim JK, Ahn JH, Park T, et al. Virtual cystoscopy of the contrast material-filled bladder in patients with gross hematuria. Am J Roentgenol 2002;179(3): 763–8.
46. Donat SM. Evaluation and follow-up strategies for superficial bladder cancer. Urol Clin North Am 2003;30(4):765–76.
47. Miyamoto H, Miller JS, Fajardo DA, et al. Non-invasive papillary urothelial neoplasms: the 2004 WHO/ISUP classification system. Pathol Int 2010;60(1): 1–8.
48. Pan D, Soloway MS. The importance of transurethral resection in managing patients with urothelial cancer in the bladder: proposal for a transurethral resection of bladder tumor checklist. Eur Urol 2012;61(6): 1199–203.
49. Sylvester RJ, Oosterlinck W, Van der Meijden AP. A single immediate instillation of chemotherapy decreases the risk of recurrence in patients with stage Ta, T1 bladder cancer: a meta-analysis of published results of randomized clinical trials. J Urol 2004;171(6 Pt 1):2186–90.
50. Hall MC, Chang SS, Dalbagni G, et al. Guideline for the management of nonmuscle invasive bladder cancer (stages Ta, T1, and Tis): 2007 update. J Urol 2007;178(6):2314–30.
51. Gudjónsson S, Adell L, Merdasa F, et al. Should all patients with non-muscle-invasive bladder cancer receive early intravesical chemotherapy after transurethral resection? The results of a prospective randomised multicentre study. Eur Urol 2009;55(4): 773–80.
52. Dobruch J, Herr H. Should all patients receive single chemotherapeutic agent instillation after bladder tumour resection? BJU Int 2009;104(2):170–4.
53. Jones JS, Larchian W. Non-muscle-invasive bladder cancer (Ta, T1, and CIS). In: Campbell-Walsh urology, vol. 3, 10th edition. Philadelphia: Saunders; 2011. p. 2335–6.
54. Herr HW. Restaging transurethral resection of high risk superficial bladder cancer improves the initial response to bacillus Calmette-Guerin therapy. J Urol 2005;174(6):2134–7.
55. Shabsigh A, Korets R, Vora KC, et al. Defining early morbidity of radical cystectomy for patients with bladder cancer using a standardized reporting methodology. Eur Urol 2009;55(1):164–74.
56. Tilki D, Reich O, Svatek RS, et al. Characteristics and outcomes of patients with clinical carcinoma in situ only treated with radical cystectomy: an international study of 243 patients. J Urol 2010;183(5): 1757–63.
57. Herr HW, Sogani PC. Does early cystectomy improve the survival of patients with high risk superficial bladder tumors? J Urol 2001;166(4): 1296–9.
58. Denzinger S, Fritsche HM, Otto W, et al. Early versus deferred cystectomy for initial high-risk pT1G3 urothelial carcinoma of the bladder: do risk factors define feasibility of bladder-sparing approach? Eur Urol 2008;53(1):146–52.
59. Fernandez-Gomez J, Madero R, Solsona E, et al. Predicting nonmuscle invasive bladder cancer recurrence and progression in patients treated with bacillus Calmette-Guerin: the CUETO scoring model. J Urol 2009;182(5):2195–203.
60. Sylvester RJ, Van der Meijden AP, Oosterlinck W, et al. Predicting recurrence and progression in individual patients with stage Ta-T1 bladder cancer using EORTC risk tables: a combined analysis of 2596 patients from seven EORTC trials. Eur Urol 2006;49(3):466–75 [discussion: 475–7].
61. Lamm DL, Blumenstein BA, Crissman JD, et al. Maintenance bacillus Calmette-Guerin immunotherapy for recurrent TA, T1 and carcinoma in situ transitional cell carcinoma of the bladder: a randomized Southwest Oncology Group Study. J Urol 2000; 163(4):1124–9.
62. Herr HW, Dalbagni G. Defining bacillus Calmette-Guerin refractory superficial bladder tumors. J Urol 2003;169(5):1706–8.
63. Herr HW, Cookson MS, Soloway SM. Upper tract tumors in patients with primary bladder cancer followed for 15 years. J Urol 1996;156(4):1286–7.
64. Wright JL, Hotaling J, Porter MP. Predictors of upper tract urothelial cell carcinoma after primary bladder cancer: a population based analysis. J Urol 2009; 181(3):1035–9 [discussion: 1039].
65. Udell I. Surveillance guidelines for low grade non-invasive bladder cancer: a cost comparison. In: Programs and abstracts of the 2012 American Urologic Association Annual Meeting. Atlanta, May 19–23, 2012.
66. Poonacha TK, Go RS. Level of scientific evidence underlying recommendations arising from the National Comprehensive Cancer Network clinical practice guidelines. J Clin Oncol 2011;29(2): 186–91.
67. Chamie K, Saigal CS, Lai J, et al. Compliance with guidelines for patients with bladder cancer: variation in the delivery of care. Cancer 2011;117(23): 5392–401.
68. Bolenz C, Ho R, Nuss GR, et al. Management of elderly patients with urothelial carcinoma of the bladder: guideline concordance and predictors of overall survival. BJU Int 2010;106(9):1324–9.

69. Miller DC, Murtagh DS, Suh RS, et al. Regional collaboration to improve radiographic staging practices among men with early stage prostate cancer. J Urol 2011;186(3):844–9.

70. Lammers RJ, Witjes WP, Hendricksen K, et al. Smoking status is a risk factor for recurrence after transurethral resection of non–muscle-invasive bladder cancer. Eur Urol 2011;60(4):713–20.

Index

Note: Page numbers of article titles are in **boldface** type.

Urol Clin N Am 40 (2013) 317–321
http://dx.doi.org/10.1016/S0094-0143(13)00026-8
0094-0143/13/$ – see front matter

Moving?

Make sure your subscription moves with you!

To notify us of your new address, find your Clinics Account Number (located on your mailing label above your name) and contact customer service at:

Email: journalscustomerservice-usa@elsevier.com

800-654-2452 (subscribers in the U.S. & Canada)
314-447-8871 (subscribers outside of the U.S. & Canada)

Fax number: 314-447-8029

Elsevier Health Sciences Division
Subscription Customer Service
3251 Riverport Lane
Maryland Heights, MO 63043

*To ensure uninterrupted delivery of your subscription, please notify us at least 4 weeks in advance of move.

Printed and bound by CPI Group (UK) Ltd, Croydon, CR0 4YY
03/10/2024
01040347-0012